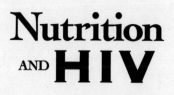

Nutrition
AND **HIV**

Nutrition
AND HIV

•

A New Model for Treatment

MARY ROMEYN, M.D.

Jossey-Bass Publishers • San Francisco

Substantial discounts on bulk quantities of Jossey-Bass books are available to corporations, professional associations, and other organizations. For details and discount information, contact the special sales department at Jossey-Bass Inc., Publishers (415) 433–1740; Fax (800) 605–2665.

For sales outside the United States, please contact your local Simon & Schuster International Office.

 Manufactured in the United States of America on Lyons Falls Turin Book. This paper is acid-free and 100 percent totally chlorine-free.

Library of Congress Cataloging-in-Publication Data

Romeyn, Mary, date.
    Nutrition and HIV : a new model for treatment / Mary Romeyn. — Rev. and updated ed.
        p.   cm.
    Includes bibliographical references and index.
    ISBN 0-7879-3964-1 (paperback)
    1. AIDS (Disease) — Nutritional aspects. 2. AIDS (Disease) — Diet therapy. I. Title.
    [DNLM: 1. Acquired Immunodeficiency Syndrome — diet therapy — popular works. 2. Self Care — popular works. WC 503.2 R764n 1998]
RC607.A26R634   1998
616-97'920654 — dc21
DNLM/DLC
for Library of Congress   97-41330

SECOND EDITION
PB Printing   10 9 8 7 6 5 4 3 2 1

CONTENTS

•

PART I

•

Nutrition and HIV

PART II

•

What You Can Do for Yourself

PART III
•
What You Can Do with Your Doctor

PART IV
•
Taking Charge: How to Direct Your Own Healing

APPENDIXES
•

For Paul, and Anthony,
and John and Eddie Lee

and Pat and Doug
and Mary Anne and Keith

and Ben and all the others

and Andrew, always Andrew

who come and wrap their hands
around my heart

PREFACE TO
THE SECOND EDITION

•

Much has happened since this book was first published in October 1995. HIV has found its way into mainstream culture, and into the heartland of America. Many more people are infected. A new bunch of kids has gotten older and feels as immortal and invincible as its elders did at the same age. Rates of infection continue to rise in injection drug users. And what's going on in the United States is mirrored and amplified in other countries. We're only beginning to grasp the economic and social implications of HIV's unchecked spread through Asia, Africa, and other parts of the Third World.

In the same short time, we've made great strides. Our understanding of how the virus works has risen exponentially. Our expertise as warriors has advanced. Our weaponry is far superior to anything we had to work with when this book was first released. We can monitor our successes, and our failures, much sooner.

Rapid and universal access to new information has made it possible to oppose those parts of the pressure for cost control that were purchased at the cost of people's lives. There is no longer any question about the value of aggressive, comprehensive, and early treatment. Insurance companies can no longer refuse those interventions that are proven to extend, perhaps give us back, our lives. Outcome studies even show that keeping people well is cheaper, in the long run, than taking care of people who are sick.

It's great that a book about HIV needs updating so quickly. It's a tribute to the researchers who do the basic science and design clinical trials. It's as great a tribute to the activists, who make bureaucrats move faster and hold profiteers to account. But it's most of all a tribute to the people who fight the virus every day in their own lives. Because so many people with HIV refuse to die politely, because they educate themselves as well as—and sometimes better than—their caregivers, because they thus can call those caregivers to a standard of excellence that they have themselves achieved, the tide is beginning to turn.

You can be a part of that revolution. If you are HIV-negative, this book will help you understand the challenges—and victories— the ones you love will face as they deal with their infection. If you are positive, understanding the enemy has never been more important.

We stand at the threshold of a whole new era in the fight against HIV. There is so much we can do now, not only to improve life but to dramatically lengthen it. For the first time since the start of the epidemic, people with HIV have a chance to live out a normal life span. But that chance doesn't come for free. It takes discipline and commitment, and an openness to change. Most of all it takes knowledge, and the choice to be a participant—the primary participant—in decisions that affect you so powerfully.

If you stand up to the challenge HIV infection poses, your journey will be exciting and rewarding. It will shape your life and the person you become. It may in fact give you your whole life back. And you will truly be the one in charge.

It can be done. You are the one to do it. And now is the time to start.

Acknowledgments
•

I am grateful for the growing sense of community in HIV advocacy and activism. As we learn to depend on each other, we become more and more effective. And I have to think of this book, also, as a community effort.

Many friends and activists again reviewed the new material. I'm grateful for their counsel. My research assistant, Brad Shapiro, became an authority on Internet access and drinking water safety—critical new issues for people with HIV. He's done a great job; next book, I'm working for him.

Since the first edition, the Andrew Ziegler Foundation has been born, has grown, and now promotes access to cutting-edge HIV education and treatment. So special thanks to Bruce McMurray, Tom

LeNoble, Mark Bowers, Paula Fener, and Diane Cenko. I couldn't care for patients, offer research, tilt at windmills, and still write books without their love and support.

Thanks also to my patients, still my greatest teachers; the women of my office, who will put up with anything; and the doctors and nurses and social workers and therapists and revolutionaries who still believe that we can and should take *excellent* care of each other, *always*, and who help me remember I'm not crazy.

November 1997   Mary Romeyn, M.D.
                                                         San Francisco, California

PREFACE TO
THE FIRST EDITION

•

I moved to San Francisco in 1988, to begin my internship in internal medicine. My sons were grown; I had a grandchild, and another was on the way. I knew that I wanted not only to practice healing, but to be involved as fully as possible in the fight against HIV. I was excited by the opportunity, and felt prepared for anything.

What I was not prepared for was the streets of San Francisco. Many people, everywhere I went, were wasting away, sometimes to skeletal form. As my eyes became more attuned, the subtler manifestations—a translucence to the skin, a sharpening of feature—showed me there were many who would follow. I saw starvation in face after face.

There was little known about wasting then, and even less being done.

Things are different now. All over the world, researchers are investigating—successfully—this aspect of HIV. We have learned its importance and many of its mechanisms. And we are learning how to fight it. But much of the work is still at the research stage. What has been published has not yet been publicized; patients lack access to the medical literature; doctors, trained to treat illness, are less concerned with wellness and prevention and are overburdened. So mostly, the word isn't out yet.

Many of the men and women with HIV in this country have taken matters into their own hands, using the resources available to them to address and defend against wasting. It is to those people I dedicate this book: to the ones who don't wait for instructions to take care of their bodies; who seek their own ways, when the ways of medicine are too slow; who, given an opportunity to learn what is known about wasting, will take it; and who, if we will listen, will teach us. For their courage, their research, and their willingness to share it, I am grateful.

This book is written for people living with HIV and for those who provide their care. It offers a conceptual approach to understanding the nature and progression of HIV infection, particularly from the standpoint of nutrition. It describes how HIV attacks the body's ability to maintain its core, and it outlines the effects of that attack. It reports on new research into how to defend and fight back. Finally, it offers some practical approaches to recognizing, diagnosing, treating, and preventing the causes of wasting in HIV and AIDS. I have also tried to share some of the wisdom offered by my own patients, whose courage is matched only by their generosity.

No part of HIV management is more critical to survival than the maintenance of nutritional status. And nutritional status can only be maintained if all parts of HIV management are addressed with equal effort. People with HIV must play a strong part in that effort.

This is a time of expansive progress in our understanding of HIV, and in the tools we have to fight it. Paradoxically, it is also a time of shrinking resources. Doctors are pressured to see more and more patients and to spend less and less on their care. The more we are able to do as scientists, the less we are expected to do as clinicians. If patients are to survive and do well in such an era, they must be their own advocates. They will need to ask for the level of care they deserve. And to do that effectively, they must understand not only what they need, but why they need it.

For those doctors, nurses, dieticians, and other caregivers whose work is dedicated to fighting HIV, I have included references from the medical literature that support or explain more fully what is dealt with in the text. We are more powerful advocates for our patients when we are armed with facts.

One final note: although my own status is negative, I frequently use the word "we" in addressing issues or feelings of people with HIV. When the battle is so important, and your life is built around it, it's hard to separate yourself. I think that's appropriate, and I left it as I wrote it. This is indeed a battle for all of us.

Acknowledgments
•

I met Marc Hellerstein in 1991, when he spoke to residents in my program about HIV and the wasting syndrome. At my request he designed and supervised a program of study that introduced me to concepts and research already in place and prepared me to go forward independently. I am grateful for the time and intellect he offered so generously, and for the doors to understanding he helped open. He has been a true teacher, and his teaching has shaped my practice.

Yvette Garcia-Shelton, of San Francisco General Hospital, helped me work out my assessment forms and shared her own hands-on tricks. Kristen Weaver, of HIV Care at Saint Francis Memorial Hospital, reviewed the book and tested formulas for accuracy. Much of what I know about HIV nutrition has come from listening to her speak over the years.

Ronald Baker, editor of *BETA*, offered his time to review the manuscript. So did Martin Delaney of Project Inform. Mark Bowers, medical writer and HIV activist with Project Inform, has freely shared his knowledge and advocacy with me and with my patients. Leonard Robinson has introduced me to the practice of alternative medicine. These are true warriors against HIV, and I thank them for their help.

Special thanks also to my research assistant, Corey Wallach, for hours spent on the drudgery of research, and for his input and support. I couldn't have done it without him.

Jeremy Hollinger, HIV Bereavement Coordinator for Visiting Nurses and Hospice, helped keep me honest. Alan Rinzler, my editor, taught me how to write a book. My children shook their heads and grinned at one another, and did without a mother for another two years. Mark, Jeannette, Ian, and Corey, I'm grateful and I love you.

The patients who have taught me are too numerous to name. You know who you are, and I thank you.

July 1995   Mary Romeyn, M.D.
                                                              San Francisco, California

Nutrition
AND HIV

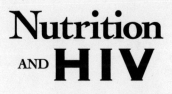

PART I

Nutrition
and HIV

CHAPTER 1

•

A New Model for Treatment

In order to understand the importance of nutrition in HIV-infected people, let's begin with some basic definitions. HIV, or human immunodeficiency virus, is an organism acquired by contact with blood or body fluids from an infected person. The virus enters the cells of the body, taking control of cellular mechanisms and using them to reproduce itself. As more and more virus is made, HIV infection spreads throughout the body.

Current methods used to screen routinely for HIV are based on finding antibodies to the virus in your blood. These antibodies are your first line of defense against the virus. It takes your body time to develop these antibodies. Normally we can expect to find them, and diagnose infection, from one to six months after infection has occurred. If we have reason to suspect infection at a more recent time, we can look for the presence of the virus, or parts of the virus, in the blood before antibodies have developed. For this we have a test for HIV viral load, or for a part of the virus that stimulates the later antibody response. Using these methods, we may in fact detect HIV as early as three or four days following infection.

People are called HIV-positive at the point when any of these tests show the presence of HIV in the body.

AIDS, or acquired immunodeficiency syndrome, is a precise and formal term. It is used to define a specific stage of HIV infection, involving a progression to symptoms or a decrease in the number of certain immune-system cells, called T-helper cells, in the blood, which indicates progression to a more critical stage. The exact criteria for a diagnosis of AIDS, as defined by the Centers for Disease Control (CDC), can be found in Appendix I. There are also formal definitions for stages of AIDS, once diagnosed.

You can have HIV disease without having AIDS. You can't have AIDS without having HIV disease.

HIV disease actually begins at the moment of infection: before there are any symptoms or observable changes in your body; before there is evidence of the virus, by standard testing methods, in your blood; often many years before a diagnosis of AIDS can be made. A small group of people who have been shown to be HIV-positive have not had progression of disease, although they remain infected, and some partners of people with HIV have evidence in their blood of exposure to, but not infection by, the virus. There are even a few babies who were HIV-infected at birth, and who seem to have cleared their infection.

Based on that information, researchers are now attempting to eradicate the virus from a small group of people who were diagnosed shortly after infection. But generally, those infected with HIV remain infected.

For practical purposes—you don't know it's there if you haven't been tested—people generally date the onset of HIV disease from the time of a positive test.

Much of the work on HIV management has focused on the care of AIDS and its problems. It is only recently that we have begun to see the importance of care and prevention—even suppression—in the earlier, less obvious stages of infection.

HIV Disease as a Continuum
•

I want to suggest that you consider the progression of HIV disease as a continuum—one whose stages, as the scientific community defines them, are artificial designations. They are particularly valuable for gathering information, and for finding out what treatments are most likely to work. The medical establishment does this by looking at large groups of people, generalizing about what has been learned, and using those generalizations to make statistically based recommendations for treatment of individuals. It's a good place to start and a way to discard approaches that do not show general value.

For you, however, as one person who carries the virus, these stages are less important. And, particularly for those who wish to involve themselves in their own healing, their own adaptations and response to HIV, it is important not to get caught up in them.

You are not home free if you don't have AIDS. And you are not appreciably sicker on the day you are diagnosed with AIDS than you were the day before.

In this book we will use the term *HIV disease,* or *HIV,* to refer to the whole spectrum of infection. We will use the term *AIDS* only as it is used in the medical literature, and as it has been defined above.

There are many ways to look at the overall picture of HIV disease. We know that it begins with infection. The HIV virus enters your body and establishes itself in your cells. From that point on, we do not yet understand how to end its continuing presence.

We know that the virus enters the cells of your immune system and duplicates itself there, eventually weakening your capacity to fight and contain it. Thus it is possible to look at HIV and AIDS as stages in a disease of the immune system, using this model to seek ways to strengthen and defend that system.

We also know that HIV infection can be followed by an increased susceptibility to other infections as well. Much of the attention in HIV research has been devoted—productively—to helping your body overcome, or contain, these secondary infections. So, many doctors caring for people with HIV work from a concept or model of AIDS as a disease of progressive secondary infections and devote their energy to treating those infections, or to anticipating them and treating to avoid them.

A Nutritional Model of HIV
•

I want to propose another model—a nutritional model of HIV infection. Working from this model does not in any way detract from the ones mentioned above, but it does give us a different way to look at the illness, and a rationale for pursuing treatments that have not been widely known or recommended. And although it does not offer a cure, it does offer ways to extend life as well as vigor while waiting for a cure.

Almost from the very beginning, HIV infection causes changes in your nutritional status. You may have already seen this in its most obvious form, as weight loss. But this weight loss generally occurs farther along. Weight loss represents a visible step in what has already been a long progression of changes in the body—changes we can recognize, measure, and defend against, *before* they are apparent to the naked eye.

There are ways to get a head start on this process. You can monitor your own intake, for example, so you will notice if you begin to eat less, or less well—normally a silent process that goes on a long time before it's detected.

We can tell from blood tests that your body is beginning to use its nutrients differently, and perhaps less efficiently.

We have means of assessing how well you are holding on to the lean tissue in your body, which you need to maintain in order to survive, and of monitoring your body for change. Some of these means involve simple physical measurements, which dieticians are trained to do. With the advent of new, relatively cheap technology and equipment, even more precise measurements should soon be widely available.

If we know, early on, that there are changes in our body, we can adapt to them and resist them before they go too far. Obviously such early attention and response will result in people who are stronger and feel better. What we have also seen is that longer life can result as well. And while there has been a great deal of exciting research on this, it has not yet received the attention it deserves from the medical community. This means that the more you know, the more you can work to help yourself—and even to educate your doctor to share in that work.

Some of the research in this area is highly complex and may take some effort to understand. It's worth it, though. You will be able to use this information to promote and maintain your own health. In addition, you will have access to more care, earlier and more complete investigation, and more treatment from your doctors if you can argue for such care, investigation, and treatment from a scientific basis.

Thus the more you know, the more you are likely to get—both from yourself and from the system. That makes it important for you to know not only what you need, but why. And that's what this book is about.

Wasting
•

HIV disease is characterized by wasting—the loss of nutritional status. The process by which this occurs is different from simple starvation. While people with HIV do tend to eat less under certain circumstances, other factors cause their bodies to use what they eat less efficiently. They may absorb the food less well. In the presence of diarrhea, they may eliminate food more rapidly, before it can be absorbed. And certain of the body's responses to infections can cause what *is* absorbed to be used less efficiently.

We see these changes in other illness as well—particularly in the case of overwhelming bacterial infections. But these are brief events; with successful treatment, the body's nutritional efficiency returns. In HIV, however, there is always a smoldering response to infection, because the virus is always there. Thus any additional insult to the body can cause us to deplete our nutritional resources and make it hard to rebuild them when we've stabilized again.

Where we have seen the effects of wasting as weight loss, it can be more precisely defined as a loss of lean body mass: a progressive reduction of the part of your body that lies within cell membranes and does not include fat. Lean body mass is the part of your body that you need to keep.

This is an important distinction. Since the early changes that occur in HIV disease include an increase in the amount of water found outside your cells, measurement of weight alone is deceptive. Any loss of lean body mass can be masked by the extra water. You look the same. You weigh the same. But silently, invisibly, your lean body mass—the stores you need to live on—may be depleting. And it's hard to fix a problem that you don't know you have.

While lean body mass is harder to measure than total body weight, ways have been found to measure it, or to estimate it fairly reliably. In the research setting, we've been doing this for years. Thus we already know many of the factors that contribute to wasting, and many that oppose it.

Studies on AIDS patients in the 1980s showed that their degree of wasting was intimately connected to the timing of decline and death. One study showed that people seemed to die as they reached a particular point in the wasting process—regardless of which particular infection or illness they appeared to die from. This critical point was at about 66 percent of their ideal body weight, or 54 percent of their original lean body mass. Interestingly, this seems to match the point at which people die from simple starvation, though the pathways to that point are not the same. These results suggest that many of the people who have died from HIV died not from the causes listed on their death certificates, but in fact from wasting—starvation from within.

This is a revolutionary concept. If death in HIV disease is in fact death from wasting—from a special and complex type of starvation—it is critical to understand and counteract the forces and events that lead to that starvation. It gives us a whole new way to approach, study, and fight this process. It points us to ways to prolong life. It offers us a chance to buy time—which may be critically important, as better treatments are found, more is learned, and researchers race for a cure.

Early in the history of HIV, when we knew much less about how to treat it, patterns of wasting were much more extreme than they are now. You can still see similar patterns in underdeveloped countries, where hygiene is poor and medical care is primitive or unavailable. In Africa, for instance, AIDS was first known as "slim disease" and was characterized by rapid and steady weight decline, with death coming quickly. In populations where medical care is better and resources are greater, we now see a stepwise pattern—periods of relative stability in lean body mass, interspersed with periods of rapid decline during secondary infections. These periods of active decline can be shortened if we diagnose secondary infections early and treat them quickly. The time between these periods can be lengthened if we protect against the onset of those infections.

Recently a more encouraging pattern has been reported: some of what has traditionally been lost during periods of decline can be maintained with aggressive feeding regimens. Some, when we stabilize, can be restored. There are even ways, if we start early, to build up the stores we're conserving, through progressive resistance exercise.

Over the past two years, we have found ways to actually reverse wasting already in place, and to regain lean body mass already lost—even, in some cases, when wasting has been far advanced. This is why it's so important not to just give up. The course of wasting can, in fact, be altered at almost any point along the continuum. We now know that this translates into longer and healthier life.

So the bottom line is this: HIV is a disease of decreasing nutritional status; people die when their nutritional status can no longer support life; we already have ways to delay, limit, or reverse that decline; and more are on the way. In the race with time against HIV, we have new ways to buy more time. And for some of us, the goal to "Be Here for the Cure" may actually be within our grasp.

REFERENCES

Beach, R. S. "Nutrition and HIV/AIDS in developing countries." *Nutrition and HIV/AIDS*, 1992, *1*, 43–51.

Bower, R. "Nutrition and immune function." *Nutrition in Clinical Practice*, 1990, *5*, 189–195.

Brozek, S. S., and others. "Medical aspects of semistarvation in Leningrad (siege 1941–1942)." *American Review of Soviet Medicine*, 1946, *4*, 70–86.

Busch, M. P., and others. "Time course and dynamics of viremia during early stages of HIV seroconversion." *4th Conference on Retroviruses and Opportunistic Infections*, Washington, D.C., January 1997, *749*, 203.

Centers for Disease Control. "Revision of the CDC surveillance case definition for acquired immunodeficiency syndrome." *MMWR*, 1987, *36*(Supplement 1S), 3S–14S.

Centers for Disease Control and Prevention. "1993 revised classification system for HIV infection and expanded case surveillance definition for AIDS among adolescents and adults." *MMWR*, 1992, *41*, 1–19.

Chlebowski, R. T., and others. "Nutritional status, gastrointestinal dysfunction, and survival in patients with AIDS." *American Journal of Gastroenterology*, 1989, *4*(10), 1288–1292.

Dworkin, B. M., and others. "Dietary intake in patients with acquired immunodeficiency syndrome (AIDS), patients with AIDS-related complex, and serologically positive human immunodeficiency virus patients: Correlations with nutritional status." *Journal of Parenteral and Enteral Nutrition,* 1990, *14*(6), 605–609.

Grunfeld, C. M., and Feingold. "Metabolic disturbances and wasting in the acquired immunodeficiency syndrome." *New England Journal of Medicine,* 1993, *327*(5), 329–337.

Hecker, L. M., and Kotler. "Malnutrition in patients with AIDS." *Nutrition Reviews,* 1990, *48*(11), 393–401.

Ho, D. "Can HIV be eradicated from an infected person?" *4th Conference on Retroviruses and Opportunistic Infections,* Washington, D.C., January 1997, *S1,* 1.

Kotler, D. P., and others. "Body composition studies in patients with the acquired immunodeficiency syndrome." *American Journal of Clinical Nutrition,* 1985, *42,* 1255–1265.

Macallan, D. C., and others. "Prospective analysis of patterns of weight change in stage IV human immunodeficiency virus infection." *American Journal of Clinical Nutrition,* 1993, *58,* 417–424.

Schnittman, S. M., and Fauci. "Human immunodeficiency virus and acquired immunodeficiency syndrome: An update." *Advances in Internal Medicine,* 1994, *39,* 305–355.

Serwadda, D., and others. "Slim disease: A new disease in Uganda and its association with HTLV-III infection." *Lancet,* 1985, *2,* 849–852.

CHAPTER 2

•

Understanding the Process of Wasting

To understand the wasting process, we need to understand how people normally build and maintain their bodies. It's a fairly complex process. In its simplest form, it involves the following:

Intake: What foods we eat, and how much.

Absorption: How we break down foods into simpler elements and move them across the walls of our digestive tract, or gut, into our body. Problems with elimination can impact on this also.

Metabolic rate: The rate at which we break down nutrients and use or store them. Also, the speed or intensity of our body processes (heart rate, temperature, and so on).

Metabolism of nutrients: The way we break down nutritional elements and either use them for immediate energy or for building and maintaining body structures or store them as energy reserves.

HIV infection can attack—and be attacked at—every point in this cycle.

Intake
•

We know that symptomatic HIV-positive patients often have less appetite. This is actually part of a trend that begins much earlier. Even healthy, asymptomatic people who carry the virus have been shown to take in fewer calories than healthy HIV-negative people.

Studies have shown that HIV-positive people who have previously had a secondary infection, giving them a diagnosis of AIDS, but who currently have no such infection and no symptoms, take in fewer calories than healthy HIV-positive people. Thus food intake seems to decrease further with progression to AIDS, even when an active secondary infection is not present. But the most significant reduction in intake is seen in people who have AIDS *and* an active secondary infection. Some of this, as we'll see later, is due to metabolic changes caused by the response of our immune system to infection.

Medicines used to treat HIV and related infections can also lower appetite. Poor absorption can leave undigested food in our system; this can cause a feeling of fullness, or even nausea, until it is eliminated. Enlargement of the liver or the spleen can cause pressure on the gut, making us feel full. This is not commonly seen except in more advanced stages of illness, but any illness affecting the liver or the spleen can result in enlargement.

Even the act of eating can be unpleasant, if there are infections of the mouth or esophagus. Swallowing may be difficult or painful; such pain may override hunger. If people have diarrhea, they may fear they will set it off by eating.

Depression, fatigue, dementia, or poverty can also contribute to the problem. If you're too sad too eat, too tired to prepare food, too confused to remember to eat, or too poor to afford nourishing, appealing food, the problems can be overwhelming. And for those who are homeless, they are nearly insurmountable. This is where social supports are so important. Friends and family, community organizations, and organized feeding programs can make a big difference.

Absorption

Think of your body as a closed system, with your gut, or digestive tract, as part of the outside, serving as a carefully controlled means of entry. Food in the gut is broken down; substances the body can tolerate safely and use are transported across the gut wall by elegant, complicated systems, using specialized cells in the highly organized tissues that make up that wall. If those tissues are injured by HIV infection, or if the regulation of those transport systems is disturbed, absorption is affected. Nutrients you eat may not make it into your body. Also, if diarrhea results, from infection or another process, food moves through more quickly. Thus there is even less opportunity for the injured gut to extract what nutrients it can.

The gut wall also serves as a protective barrier, keeping out bacteria, the products of bacteria, and other toxic wastes. When the barrier breaks down, this protection is lost.

The HIV virus enters and lives in the cells of the gut wall, changing its architecture and disturbing its function. Other infections can cause inflammation and swelling, further reducing its efficiency. Some infections are irritants as well, reducing transit time by speeding up movement in the gut, so that the already injured system has less time to extract nutrients as the food moves by. In the worst case, the wall may become so damaged that proteins already in the body leak out, to be washed away and lost.

Another early effect of HIV on the gut wall is the loss of lactase, an enzyme that breaks down the sugars in milk for absorption. Left unabsorbed, these sugars ferment, causing lactose intolerance. This is the reason many HIV-positive people feel gassy and bloated after eating milk or milk products.

Ironically, antibiotics used to fight infection, in the gut and elsewhere, are indiscriminate: they kill not only the bad germs, but also the good ones that help to digest food and prepare it for absorption. Thus some of the solutions are also part of the problem. In other cases, in the absence of antibiotics, an impaired immune system may allow bacterial overgrowth. This can also alter the balance of friendly bacteria needed for good absorption.

Lastly, malnutrition itself damages the gut wall. Thus poor nutrition further weakens immunity, predisposing the body to further infection—which further disturbs absorption, increasing malnutrition. It's a vicious cycle.

Remember, these are *potential* effects. There is much we can do to intervene.

Metabolic Rate
•

Resting energy expenditure, the energy your body spends while doing nothing, is increased in people living with HIV. The patterns of increase are as we would expect: a slight increase in the asymptomatic, a greater one in people with AIDS, and the greatest in those with an active secondary infection. It's not a big part of the picture, actually; the body responds by reducing the energy spent on activity. That adaptation, though, is partly responsible for the fatigue and lethargy felt by people with HIV—so the price, in terms of quality of life, is high.

Ordinarily, an adaptation made in people whose rate of energy expense is increased—pregnant women, growing adolescents, athletes—is to adjust the way the body uses its resources, reducing by up to 50 percent its use of protein stores to provide the extra calories it needs. But people with HIV don't do this. Their protein—an essential part of lean body mass—isn't conserved preferentially when their energy needs go up.

Metabolism of Nutrients
•

Changes in metabolic pathways—the series of chemical reactions through which our cells use absorbed nutrients to form tissues and other structural elements, manufacture enzymes, and store fats— are among the most important factors contributing to wasting. They are also the most complex. The changes seen in people with HIV disease and AIDS, largely involving the making and spending of fats in the body, are triggered by immune-system changes in response to HIV.

There are cells in the immune system called monocytes that, when stimulated, produce factors with widespread effects on the body. These factors, called monokines or cytokines, can first of all reduce appetite, causing us to take in fewer calories. In addition, they affect what we do with the calories we do take in.

The healthy human body converts its nutrients to sugars (the body's immediate energy source), proteins (used for making muscle and other tissues, for carrying substances needed for reactions in the body, and for making the substances that cause those reactions to occur), and fats (for storing energy, to be available for breakdown when needed). To use an analogy, think of sugars as the body's cash flow, proteins as its working assets, and fats as its capital, invested and stored, to be ready to take over when the cash reserves get low.

Normally the body, when it has spent all its sugars as energy, converts its economy from one that runs on sugars to one that runs on fats, broken down and converted to energy sources. Thus, it spares the structures it needs in times of high demand, in order to continue to function. Only if the body has been starved, and has used up its available reserves of sugars *and* fats, will it begin breaking down its own structures for its energy requirements. And it will use the calories it takes in for energy, not for storage as fat, in order to protect those structures.

HIV, particularly in association with secondary infections, interferes with this natural process of protecting one's core. Nutrients are directed to the liver, where they are converted, inappropriately, into fats. What protein manufacturing the liver does accomplish is directed more toward acute phase reactants—proteins used to fight the virus—and less toward structural protein synthesis. Thus the structural proteins of your body are spent and not properly repleted.

Fats, which are normally converted into energy in the liver, are not broken down. This means that energy needs continue to be met by sugars—and when these sugars are gone, proteins must be converted to make more. These proteins come, in large part, from muscle, especially skeletal muscle. Thus lean body mass is lost, and wasting is accelerated. And, because the liver continues to make fats preferentially, new proteins are not assembled to replace those that are lost.

Some of this process is set in motion just by HIV infection alone. However, all else being equal, we seem to be able to compensate for this. But in the presence of additional infection, activating monocytes and releasing cytokines, the process is speeded up. We still cannot adapt enough to preserve our protein stores.

• • •

Thus, the study of nutrition in HIV infection takes us beyond the level of what to eat and how much. It goes to the very root of the way we use our food. While it is a complicated matter, it is crucial to our understanding. It offers many more opportunities to reduce, overcome, even reverse the process of wasting in HIV. There is a great deal of exciting research under way, looking for ways to manipulate the process. Some of it is already bearing fruit.

REFERENCES

Abrams, B., and others. "A prospective study of dietary intake and acquired immune deficiency syndrome in HIV-seropositive homosexual men." *Journal of Acquired Immune Deficiency Syndromes and Human Retrovirology*, 1993, *6*(8), 949–958.

Coodley, G. O., and others. "The HIV wasting syndrome: A review." *Journal of Acquired Immune Deficiency Syndromes and Human Retrovirology*, 1994, *7*, 681–694.

Feingold, K. R., and others. "Tumor necrosis factor stimulates hepatic lipid synthesis and secretion." *Endocrinology*, 1989, *124*, 2336–2342.

Folks, T. M., and others. "Tumor necrosis factor alpha induces expression of human immunodeficiency virus in a chronically infected T-cell clone." *Proceedings of the National Academy of Science USA*, 1989, *86*, 2365–2368.

Griffin, G. E. "Human immunodeficiency virus and the gastrointestinal tract." *Bailliere's Clinical Gastroenterology*, 1990, *4*(1), 110–134.

Griffin, G. E. "Malabsorption, malnutrition and HIV disease." *Bailliere's Clinical Gastroenterology*, 1990, *4*(2), 361–373.

Grunfeld, C., and others. "Hypertriglyceridemia in the acquired immunodeficiency syndrome." *American Journal of Medicine*, 1989, *86*, 27–31.

Grunfeld, C., and others. "Persistence of the hypertriglyceridemic effect of tumor necrosis factor despite development of tachyphylaxis to its anorectic/cachectic effects." *Cancer Research*, 1989, *49*, 2554–2660.

Grunfeld, C., and others. "Circulating interferon-alpha levels and hypertriglyceridemia in the acquired immunodeficiency syndrome." *American Journal of Medicine*, 1991, *90*, 154–162.

Grunfeld, C., and others. "Lipids, lipoproteins, triglyceride clearance, and cytokines in human immunodeficiency virus and the acquired immunodeficiency syndrome." *Journal of Clinical Endocrinology and Metabolism*, 1992, *74*, 1045–1052.

Grunfeld, C., and others. "Metabolic disturbances, anorexia and wasting in HIV/AIDS." *Nutrition and HIV/AIDS*, 1992, *1*, 9–15.

Harris, H. W., and others. "Chylomicrons alter the fate of endotoxin, decreasing tumor necrosis factor release and preventing death." *Journal of Clinical Investigation*, 1993, *91*(3), 1028–1034.

Hellerstein, M. K., and others. "Interleukin-1-induced anorexia in the rat: Influence of prostaglandins." *Journal of Clinical Investigation*, 1989, *84*, 228–235.

Hellerstein, M. K., and others. "Current approach to the treatment of HIV-associated weight loss: Pathophysiologic considerations and emerging management strategies." *Seminars in Oncology*, 1990, *17*(6), 17–33.

Hellerstein, M. K. "Pathophysiology of lean body wasting and nutrient unresponsiveness in HIV/AIDS." *Nutrition and HIV/AIDS*, 1992, *1*, 17–25.

Justice, A. C., and others. "A new prognostic staging system for the acquired immunodeficiency syndrome." *New England Journal of Medicine*, 1989, *320*, 1388–1393.

Kotler, D. P., and others. "Preservation of short-term energy balance in clinically stable patients with AIDS." *American Journal of Clinical Nutrition*, 1990, *51*, 7–13.

Kotler, D. P., and others. "Detection, localization, and quantitation of HIV-associated antigens in intestinal biopsies from patients with HIV." *American Journal of Pathology*, 1991, *139*(4), 823–830.

Kotler, D. P., and others. "Causes and consequences of malnutrition in HIV/AIDS." *Nutrition and HIV/AIDS*, 1992, *1*, 5–8.

Koyanagi, Y., and others. "Cytokines alter production of HIV-1 from primary mononuclear phagocytes." *Science*, 1988, *241*, 1673–1675.

Macallan, D. C., and others. "A longitudinal study of body composition during weight change in men with AIDS." *11th International Conference on AIDS*, Vancouver, July 1996, TuB *2379*, 331.

Molina, J. M., and others. "Production of cytokines by peripheral blood monocytes/macrophages infected with human immunodeficiency virus type 1 (HIV-1)." *Journal of Infectious Diseases*, 1990, *161*, 888–893.

Read, T. E., and others. "Chylomicrons enhance endotoxin excretion in bile." *Infection and Immunology*, 1993, *61*(8), 3496–3502.

Ullrich, R., and others. "Small intestinal structure and function in patients infected with human immunodeficiency virus (HIV): Evidence for HIV-induced enteropathy." *Annals of Internal Medicine*, 1989, *111*, 15–21.

PART II

•

What You Can Do for Yourself

•

CHAPTER 3

•

Starting Your
Own Assessment

Wherever you are in the course of HIV, now is the time to start with a nutritional assessment. At whatever level you do this—on your own or with a dietician's help—such an assessment will give you a baseline, a way to check your progress and react aggressively if you start to lose ground.

Looking at Yourself

•

You already have much of the information you will need, in an informal way, to see where you stand and what you need to do. Here are some important questions to ask yourself:

- How much do you weigh? How much did you weigh before HIV? Have you experienced periods of rapid weight loss? If so, were they during periods of illness?
- Do you try to stay thin or lose weight because of concerns about your appearance?

- How much do you eat? Do you tend to skip meals? If so, which ones, and why?
- Is your appetite better at some times of the day than at others? Does it seem to be affected by any of the medicines you take? By drugs you use for recreation? By any current illness or its symptoms?
- What are those symptoms? Do you sometimes feel bloated or nauseated? Is the act of eating painful? Or do you have pain after you eat? Does eating trigger diarrhea? If so, do you compensate by not eating?
- What kinds of food do you eat? Are there types of food you avoid, which might lead to nutritional deficiencies? Do you avoid some foods because they make you feel uncomfortable or ill?
- Do you do your own shopping? If so, do you try to buy nutritious food?
- Can you *afford* nutritious food? Do you have a place, and the will, to prepare it? If not, are there community organizations, family members, or friends available to help?
- Do you use fresh food quickly or discard it? Do you wash fresh fruits and vegetables before you eat them? Do you ever eat raw meat or fish, such as tartar steak or sushi?
- Are there foods that make you feel happy or safe or that evoke old memories that are precious to you? Do you comfort yourself with food when you are sad?

These are things to think about, for starters.

Your Diet Diary

Keep a record of what you eat for at least three days. Doing this will help you assess how much you're taking in, and what kind of nourishment you're feeding your body.

Appendix II gives you a diet diary to work from. You will want to record your intake at regular intervals, in a way that allows you to monitor for change. I suggest doing so every three months. Sometimes all it takes to eat more is to know you are eating less; you'll naturally start to make up for it.

Keeping track of calories every day is a lot of work, and there are simpler ways to monitor your intake. For the three days of your diet diary, though, it's worth the effort. You'll find a list of calorie equivalents for common foods in Appendix III.

Your Weight

Another way to assess whether you are eating enough is to monitor your weight. It's not as sensitive as lean body mass, which you won't be able to measure on your own; so if your weight is stable, you still have work to do. Your lean body mass may still be decreasing. But if your weight goes down, you know you must step up your efforts.

Day-to-day changes may be due to normal variation. I recommend weighing yourself at home once a week. Keeping a written record will help you to monitor for change.

Your Lean Body Mass

Monitoring lean body mass directly is an exciting new way to keep track of your progress in maintaining nutritional competence. This can be done by bioimpedance monitoring, or BIA, in some doctors' offices and clinics, particularly those that follow many people with HIV infection. Other methods used for research, which may be available by joining studies, are discussed in Chapter Twelve.

Your Nutritional Assessment
•

It helps to have defined goals to work toward. To begin with, it's important to know if you are getting enough protein, as well as enough calories. It's also important to get vitamins, minerals, and trace elements. The nutritional assessment form we use in my office is included in Appendix II. As you can see from this form, you already know much of the information you will need.

If you have completed your first three-day diet diary, you're ready to get down to business, keeping in mind the following points.

Section 1: Who You Are

Men and women have different body types, based largely on fat distribution and relative amount of lean body mass. Thus, their nutritional recommendations are different. Also, if you're a pregnant woman living with HIV, you and your baby will have even greater nutritional needs. The recommendations for food intake that follow will not take your pregnancy into account.

Section 2: Your HIV Status

This gives us an idea of what to stress: how much you can exercise, for instance, if you're recently infected or you have high T-cell counts; or the potential importance of malabsorption, even without diarrhea, if your counts are low. Knowing your stage of HIV progression helps us to focus our efforts. But remember, these stages are artificial. They are chosen to provide statistical information for large groups, and they don't tell us much about any individual. There's much we can do at *every* stage.

We all know of people who have gone for years with no T-helper CD4 cells, to speak of, with good quality of life. Many people using the new aggressive combination antiretroviral regimens that have become the standard of care for HIV management now have CD4 counts much higher than they once were. And we also now have access to viral load testing, with which we can directly measure the amount of virus now in your body, instead of simply measuring the damage done to your immune system after it has happened. These tests are widely available and should be used to monitor your health. For starters, though, we'll use the lowest CD4 count you've had on record (your CD4 nadir) to suggest which interventions may be the most important.

If you don't know your CD4 nadir, you can still target your interventions better by looking at the issues most relevant to your stage and the time since your infection.

Section 3: Your Weight Status

Keeping track of your weight helps you to see where you stand in relation to your status prior to infection. In addition, it can alert you to any increased immediate danger; a period of active wasting signals a pressing need for evaluation by your doctor.

The formulas used to determine ideal body weight represent only averages. In addition, these formulas were developed in an affluent society, with a population that tends toward obesity. Thus they have been used traditionally as weight *loss* goals, for people who are overweight. *This means that they may be biased in favor of leanness.* You may also be affected by that bias; our culture prizes slenderness, and many people living with HIV have been careful to keep their weight down, out of concern for their appearance. In your own case, you may find that your usual weight, before infection or diagnosis, was less than those figures recommend.

If your usual weight prior to HIV was lower than the ideal, ask yourself why. Were you dieting? Were you thinner than you should have been, due to drug use, prior illness, or some other reason? If that's the case, it's better to work with the recommended ideal weight as your goal. Were you working out, or were you highly athletic, so that fat was reduced without noticeable loss of muscle mass? Or have you always been on the thin side, without any effort on your part? If so, your usual pre-HIV weight is a good enough place to start from and to use as your goal.

In people with HIV whose current body weight is greater than their ideal body weight, the goal is maintenance of current weight, *not weight loss.* Remember, what you lose now is more likely to be protein, lean body mass, than fat.

Finding your estimated ideal weight requires some calculation. Table II.1 in Appendix II outlines the steps. Start by writing down your height. Then subtract five feet, and see how many inches remain.

For men: Multiply the result by 6 and add 106 pounds.
For women: Multiply the result by 5 and add 100 pounds.

The final sum will be the estimated ideal weight for a person of medium build.

Let's consider a couple of examples. Suppose you are a man and you're 6 feet 2 inches tall. Start by subtracting 5 feet from 6 feet 2 inches, which leaves 14 inches. Next, multiply 14 by 6, which gives you 84. Then add 106 to 84, which gives you 190. The ideal weight for a man who is 6 feet 2 inches tall and of medium build, then, is estimated to be 190 pounds.

Suppose you are a woman who is 5 feet 4 inches tall. Subtract 5 feet from this height, which gives you 4 inches. Multiply that result by 5, which gives you 20. Then add 100, to get 120. The ideal weight for a woman who is 5 feet 4 inches tall and of medium build, then, is about 120 pounds.

But what if you're not of medium build? Or what if you're not sure whether your frame—the skeletal structure your body is built around—is smaller or larger than the norm? There is actually a way to measure that, too. It's done by dividing your height by your wrist circumference; the result of this calculation is used to classify people as small-, medium-, or large-framed individuals. This calculation is also shown in Table II.1 in Appendix II.

Most of us can estimate our frame size. If you need to confirm it, you can use the calculations in Table II.1 and adjust accordingly.

Calculate your current weight as a percentage of your ideal body weight or usual weight, and record this value in Part I, Section 3, of your nutritional assessment. This will give you an idea of how well you are currently doing, and how close you are to maintaining nutritional competence. You will choose your goal weight, either ideal or usual, based on the considerations above. The percentage of your ideal or usual goal weight will tell you where you stand now and will help to give you a picture of the effects of HIV to date.

If you've had periods of wasting before, you probably noticed that they were associated with, or immediately preceded, the presence of a secondary infection. If you're losing weight rapidly now, this is probably also the case. It's urgent that you get to your doctor and look for a source of infection.

Section 4: What You're Eating

Much of the information for this section of your nutritional assessment can be taken from your diet diary summary sheet. Your average daily calorie count will help you gauge how much you're taking in. Use Table II.2 in Appendix II to help you assess how many calories you should have each day.

This section will also show you how much protein you are now getting. Common protein sources and amounts are listed in Table II.3 in Appendix II. At the bottom of Table II.2 is a formula to help you calculate how much protein you need.

To estimate your recommended protein intake, multiply your recommended calories by one of two numbers, as shown at the bottom of Table II.2. One is for maintenance; the other is for repleting lean body mass.

You'll also be able to see how your current diet supplies you with vitamins and other micronutrients—things we need in small amounts that are often found to be deficient in people with HIV.

It's important to note that while a well-balanced diet can supply a good portion of the vitamins, minerals, and trace elements your body needs for optimal performance, you should not rely on diet alone to give you all you need. Even in the presence of an excellent diet, rich in natural vitamin sources, deficiencies are common in the presence of HIV. In addition, there is good reason to suspect that increased supplementation of some vitamins may have special value in controlling the virus and minimizing its effects. This important part of your personal program will be discussed in Chapters Four and Five.

Section 5: How You Spend Your Energy

The number of calories you need is influenced by the amount of energy you spend during daily living. We'll use this information to help you set your calorie intake goals in your nutritional assessment.

• • •

Let's look at David, for example. David is fifty years old. He's six feet tall and hangs 180 pounds on a large frame. He has been athletically active most of his life.

David tested positive for HIV in 1990 and has a CD4 count of about 250. He has no current active infections. He works full time at a desk job, but he walks about a mile to and from work. He takes three flights of stairs to and from his office rather than using the elevator. He lives in a third-floor walkup. Thus, although he doesn't work out actively, he averages nine flights up, nine flights down, and two miles walked each day.

David's usual weight—his weight before he tested positive—was 204 pounds. He lost 19 pounds over four weeks fourteen months ago, during a bout with pneumocystis pneumonia. He regained 6 pounds but lost them again four months ago—this time during an episode of diarrhea, which resolved on antibiotics after two weeks. Since then, his weight has been stable. He is able to handle his job and a comfortable social life, but he does not feel up to an aggressive exercise program.

David's appetite is good, although he does tend to skip breakfast. The average daily calories from his diet diary are about 2,800.

David's ideal weight, according to Table II.1 of Appendix II, is 196 pounds (6 feet minus 5 feet equals 12 inches; 12 times 6 is 72; 72 plus 106 is 178; adding 10 percent for a large frame, or 18 more pounds, brings the total to 196). At his current weight of 180 pounds, David is at 92 percent of his ideal weight. He is at 88 percent of his usual weight. So he would like to gain.

Since his ideal body weight is *less* than his usual body weight, the ideal body weight is his goal. He'd like to increase lean body mass and gain 16 pounds. The calculations to determine David's daily calorie and protein needs follow (see Table II.2):

Add:

weight	180 pounds	×	6.2	=	1,116
height	6 feet				
number of inches over 5 feet					
	12 inches	×	12.5	=	150
plus					816
subtotal					2,082

Subtract:

age	50	×	6.8	=	(340)
subtotal					1,742

Multiply:

Activity level (choose one):

normal activity	× 1.3–1.5 =		2,267–2,613

Special factors (choose one):

attempting gain	×	1.2 =	2,720–3,136

Number of Calories Needed: 2,720–3,136

Amount of Protein Needed:

anabolism (repletion)	×	0.042 =	114–132 grams

The summary from Part I of David's assessment, then, will show that at most he must increase his intake by about 400 calories a day if he hopes to gain weight. He's doing pretty well, though.

Because he wants to maintain not only his weight but also his lean body mass, David must also be sure to get enough protein. He can do this by counting the average number of servings from each different food group and figuring each group's contribution to his protein intake, using Table II.3 in Appendix II. To estimate the amount of protein he eats each day, David simply needs to add up the appropriate per-serving amounts from this table.

In David's case, his current average protein intake is 104 grams. Because he is not wasting now, and he is trying to replete what he has previously lost, he will use the anabolism, or body mass repletion, formula. Thus his recommended intake of protein is 117 to 132 grams a day. This is a lot, but he can reach his goal by eating not only meat, fish, and dairy products, but carbohydrates and vegetables as well.

Monitoring Your Protein Intake
•

Keeping close track of your protein intake is important when you're first getting started. It's time-consuming, though, to do this on a daily basis. You may want to try this shortcut. It's less precise, but it's almost effortless. Just count your servings of meat, dairy, vegetables, and starches. Then assign them these average values:

Every egg and every ounce of meat, fish, or poultry is
  7 grams.
Every half-cup serving of cheese or glass of milk is 7 grams.
Every serving of vegetables (half cup cooked, full cup raw)
  is 2 grams.
Every half cup of complex carbohydrates or slice of bread
  is 3 grams.
Every cup of casserole or combination food is 13 to 20 grams.

Using this system David can plan his meals without difficulty, despite his high protein requirements. Two 4-ounce servings of meat and a glass of milk will total 70 grams. Two poached eggs in the morning add 14 grams. Adding a bagel or toast, and bread with lunch, contributes 12 more. Two servings of vegetables, a salad, and a potato add 12 more. Throw in a cup of casserole (13–20 grams), shake on a little grated cheese (7 grams), and he's home free. And there's still room for fruit, treats, and the other non-protein-rich foods he needs to balance his diet.

In fact, David's initial protein intake was well below the mark. Despite a good appetite and no digestive symptoms, he will need to work consciously to reach his goals.

Once you have arrived at your total calorie and protein intake goals, you too may find it hard to maintain them. Don't get discouraged. Habits change slowly. They change more easily as we begin to learn how to improve our health and increase our appetite and comfort. For starters, if you can meet even your maintenance goals, you're doing a good job. If not, just do the best you can. And be proud of it. Every step you take, however small, in increasing your calorie and protein intake is a step forward—and will help you come closer to meeting those goals.

REFERENCES

Friedman, B. "Acquired immunodeficiency syndrome." In G. Zaloga, *Nutrition in Critical Care* (pp. 783–800). St. Louis, Mo.: Mosby, 1994.

Hickey, M. S. *Handbook of Enteral, Parenteral and ARC/AIDS Nutritional Therapy.* St. Louis, Mo.: Mosby, 1992.

Lehmann, R. *Cooking for Life.* New York: Bantam Doubleday Dell, 1997.

Smith, L. C. "Nutritional assessment and indications for nutritional support." *Surgical Clinics of North America,* 1991, *71*(3), 449–457.

Zeman, F. J., and Ney. *Applications of Clinical Nutrition.* Upper Saddle River, N.J.: Prentice Hall, 1988.

CHAPTER 4

•

Vitamins, Minerals, and Trace Elements

To understand the role of vitamins and minerals, it helps to understand a little bit about the chemistry of your body. Living organisms rely on highly complex processes to perform and regulate those internal functions that are necessary to maintain life. Processes are in place to

- Build the cells that make up your body's structures
- Meet the separate needs of different types of cells
- Permit each of these different cell types to carry out its own specific functions
- Help maintain cellular structure and performance
- Alter the type and degree of cellular activity in the face of changing circumstances
- Communicate and coordinate each cell's activity with the activity of other cells and organs in the body
- Adjust cellular behavior, as needed, in ways that will permit a coordinated response of the whole organism to its environment

- Dispose of waste products
- Govern the disposal of cells when their job is done

The scientific term we use to describe all this is *homeostasis*.

Homeostasis can be defined, then, as the ability of a living organism to maintain its structure and function intact, separate from and invulnerable to the forces of its environment.

The maintenance of homeostasis is highly complex, requiring many series of chemical reactions, distinct and yet interrelated. Each step in each reaction requires the presence of specific substances, often in minute amounts. If these materials are not present, or are present in too small a quantity to perform their roles, the reactions that require them cannot proceed correctly.

Vitamins, minerals, and trace elements are among these necessary substances. With the exception of vitamin D, which can be made within the skin, they cannot be made in the body; they must be absorbed to be obtained. Some are produced for us within the gut, by bacteria that live there.

We don't need a lot of them. Given perfect health and a well-balanced diet, we can get what we need from the food we eat. Given states of altered metabolism, though, we may need more. And during or following an illness, the body's natural processes of healing and repair cannot go forward unless we have enough — sometimes more — of the vitamins required.

There is evidence that raises the possibility that higher amounts of some of these substances may actually improve our health even when we're not sick, by giving our bodies a richer source of materials to draw on in the face of normal stress. This view is controversial, but more and more research supports it.

HIV and Vitamin, Mineral, and Trace-Element Deficiencies
•

Some evidence suggests that in HIV, as in normal aging, we may benefit from more of some of these elements than we normally get from our diet or than was previously recommended. In addition, many people with HIV have been shown to have actual vitamin deficiencies — lower body stores of some vitamins than what is considered necessary even for a person in perfect health.

In some cases, the HIV virus itself can benefit directly from those deficiencies, increasing the rate of its production. This means that it's critical to avoid these deficiencies. It also offers hope for increasing our gains in the battle against HIV production in our own bodies.

As we have seen, HIV infection can cause you to eat less. Also, you may absorb nutrients less well. This is part of the reason for HIV-associated vitamin and mineral depletion.

Many vitamins, minerals, and trace elements are found to be deficient or in the low-normal range in people with HIV. This has been documented even early in the course of infection. Even people who eat an excellent, well-balanced diet are not immune to these deficiencies if they are HIV-positive. Therefore, even apart from the possible benefits of higher levels in some specific cases, it makes sense to supplement.

Supplementation
•

The best place to start—as simple as it seems—is to eat well. As Dr. Bruce Bistrian, of the Harvard nutrition team, puts it, "When we eat what God gave us, we're eating what's good for us. . . . You got to do it the hard way." We'll look at food sources that are naturally rich in each particular vitamin as we discuss it below.

But I don't believe you should stop there. You have too much at stake. Therefore, the recommendations in this chapter will be for supplementation—for taking vitamins daily—in addition to maintaining a healthy diet. And if for some reason you aren't sure your diet is healthy, supplementing it can help to protect you anyway.

Before we look at supplementation or institute a program, though, it's important to talk about the RDA. The RDA, or recommended dietary allowance, is a baseline figure. It is used to suggest the lowest amount of a given substance that we should take in, daily, from our diet. You'll see references to the RDA on labels for vitamins and for many prepared foods.

It's important to understand that this is not a recommended intake level. Rather, it represents the minimum amount required to prevent an overt, frank deficiency in healthy people with good absorption and the ability to maintain normal nutritional status. Thus the RDA holds very little meaning for you.

The RDA underestimates the requirements of an organism under stress. It is not a good guide for your nutritional or dietary intake. For vitamin C, for example, the RDA is 60 milligrams a day—just enough to prevent scurvy in a healthy sailor.

The RDA also does not take into account specific actions of a given vitamin that can be of special value in illness or that may promote your overall good health.

It's also important to define our goals for supplementation. First off, we don't want to compound the problems of HIV with the problems of vitamin deficiency—but we can do more than avoid that. We can improve our bodies' ability to fight the effects of injury, disease, and stress by knowing what can help, and taking it.

We already know which vitamins and trace elements tend to be reduced in HIV infection. We already have an idea of the benefits that higher levels of supplementation may offer. And we already know when it's too much of a good thing—when vitamin excess can work against your health. Popping a good multivitamin or two each day, along with a trace-element supplement, can be a good start. There is research in the literature that shows a real role for daily vitamin use. One study showed that people with HIV did better just by taking a multivitamin supplement every day.

If you want to consider more specific supplementation—and I believe you should—some suggestions follow. For certain vitamins in particular, high-dose supplementation is worth considering.

Vitamins That May Be Deficient in People with HIV
•

Note that in many cases the appropriate supplementation amount simply has not been determined. Where we don't know how much of a particular vitamin can help you, the RDA is given, just to give you a rock-bottom floor. Where we know that too much of a vitamin can hurt you, this is stated as well.

To understand the minute quantities that are needed, you have to know the relevant units of measure:

1,000 micrograms = 1 milligram
1,000 milligrams = 1 gram
28 grams = 1 ounce

Here are some of the vitamins you want to pay special attention to.

Vitamin B₁ (Thiamine)

Thiamine is needed for conversion of carbohydrates into energy, for transmission of signals from your nerves to your muscles, and for maintaining the structure of membranes in the nervous system.

It is absorbed high in the small intestine and stored mainly in muscle tissue. Raw fish, coffee, and tea can break it down. Deficiency can occur quickly, as the body can't store this vitamin for long. Malabsorption, malnutrition, alcohol, diarrhea, and low folate levels can all contribute to B₁ deficiency. Antacids and other medicines that reduce stomach acidity can destroy it.

Need is increased with fever, heavy exercise, or high caloric intake.

Deficiency can result in weight loss, irritability, poor appetite, and paresthesias—the burning or prickling sensations we associate with peripheral neuropathy—especially in the feet and lower legs. When deficiency is more severe, there can be weakness and changes in mental status. Supplementation at five times the recommended daily allowance has been shown to improve survival in HIV.

One to two milligrams a day is said to prevent frank deficiency. Excess thiamine goes out in the urine, so too much can't hurt you.

Most multivitamins contain 1½ to 3 milligrams of thiamine. High-potency pills and B-complex supplements contain 50 to 100 milligrams.

Dietary sources of thiamine include red meat, whole grains, potatoes, peas, beans, nuts, and yeast. As this nutrient is water-soluble, it can be lost when food is cooked in liquids.

Vitamin B₂ (Riboflavin)

Riboflavin is also absorbed in the small intestine. It is needed for many reactions in the body, and particularly for the metabolism—the energy economy—of amino acids, the basic units from which proteins are constructed. It is also needed to convert dietary vitamin B₆ to its active form in the body.

Riboflavin deficiency can develop within a week. Some drugs

can contribute to such deficiencies: Compazine, or prochlorperazine (used for nausea); major tranquilizers; and tricyclic antidepressants such as Elavil, or amitriptyline, often used for the treatment of foot pain in HIV, are among them.

Deficiency can result in burning and itching eyes, painful sensitivity to light, tongue and mouth pain, anemia, and personality changes. In addition, metabolism of drugs can be altered.

Three milligrams a day are recommended to prevent riboflavin deficiency. Five times that much has been shown to be associated with prolonged survival in HIV infection. Again, if you don't need it, you excrete it.

Supplementation in standard multivitamins is in the range of $1\frac{1}{2}$ to $3\frac{1}{2}$ milligrams. High-potency sources and B-complex preparations contain 75 to 100 milligrams.

People who supplement their B_2 notice that their urine shines a bright, fluorescent yellow. That's why you see this now, if you're taking a B-complex supplement.

Natural sources of riboflavin include dairy products, meat, fish, and green leafy vegetables. Whole-grain cereals are also good sources, as are egg whites. Riboflavin is broken down by light, so exposure while cooking (by broiling, for instance) can deplete it.

Vitamin B_6 (Pyridoxine)

Pyridoxine is also absorbed in the small intestine, and any excess is excreted in the urine. Deficiency can develop in two or three weeks. Like vitamin B_2, it is active in the metabolism of amino acids. It also plays a role in making neurotransmitters—the chemicals that brain cells use to communicate with one another. It is essential to many enzyme reactions.

Vitamin B_6 deficiency is relatively common in people with HIV. This has been reported in the early, asymptomatic phase of infection in particular. Isoniazid, or INH, commonly used to treat tuberculosis in people with HIV, further contributes to B_6 deficiency.

Symptoms include irritability, depression, and other changes in mental status, as well as skin rashes and tongue and mouth tenderness. Nausea and vomiting, as well as seizures, are late manifestations. B_6 deficiency can also cause anemia, and it has been shown to further impair immune function in people with HIV. People who are vitamin B_6–deficient also have impaired production of IL-2, a factor produced by immune cells and active in the immune response. The role of IL-2 and other cytokines is discussed in Chapter Twelve. Thus, adequate stores of B_6 may be needed in order to maximize our immune response against the virus.

One study reported that oral supplements of 20 milligrams or more a day successfully corrected deficiencies in people with HIV. Another has shown increased survival in HIV with increased intake. Twenty-five to 50 milligrams a day is better if you're taking INH. Standard multivitamin preparations contain 2 to 5 milligrams. B-complex pills can have 5 to 100 milligrams.

Foods rich in B_6 include meat, fish, egg yolks, beans, fruits, and vegetables. Liver is a good source, as are whole-grain cereals. Losses occur during cooking.

Vitamin B_{12} (Cobalamin)

Absorption of vitamin B_{12} is more difficult than that of the other B vitamins. Cells in the stomach produce a factor that binds to B_{12} and permits it to be absorbed in the small intestine. Thus there are two points in its journey at which oral absorption can be impaired. On the other hand, the body can recycle some of what gets in, shuttling it back and forth between the intestine and the liver, for reuptake and reuse. It is stored in the liver in ample quantities, so B_{12} deficiency takes longer to occur than other B-vitamin deficiencies.

Nonetheless, B_{12} deficiency is common; some studies have found vitamin B_{12} levels to be low in 20 to 36 percent of people with HIV. Many of these people showed no obvious symptoms of deficiency. Also, it's harder to detect clinically.

Most HIV-negative people with B_{12} deficiency have changes in their red blood cells—bigger cells, more hemoglobin per cell—that show up easily on a complete blood count, alerting their doctors to test B_{12} levels. HIV-positive people don't show this pattern. If their doctors are not looking specifically for B_{12} deficiency, they may never know it's there. Doctors may also not consider the enormous contribution of malabsorption to HIV nutritional status and disease progression, which might otherwise encourage them to check B_{12} levels automatically. Thus, when not checked routinely, B_{12} deficiency can often be missed.

A low level of vitamin B_{12} is especially important in the setting of HIV, because of its potential role in problems with nerve conduction or function (neuropathy) and spinal cord abnormalities (myelopathy). These conditions are seen with some frequency in the HIV-positive population, and they have substantial impact on quality of life. One study looked at people with relatively advanced HIV disease who were referred to a university neurology clinic. These people presented either with neuropathy or myelopathy. Of those who had both conditions, vitamin B_{12} was found to be low in more than half.

Vitamin B_{12} deficiency has also been associated with early, subtle changes in mental function in people with HIV. Those changes include the speed with which we process information and our performance on tasks requiring visual-spatial coordination. Because they are subtle, we may not pick these changes up.

Vitamin B_{12} is provided in the diet by meat, fish, and eggs, so vegetarians are particularly at risk. It can be obtained in lesser amounts from milk and milk products. Generally, it is not destroyed by cooking.

As with the above vitamins, there is no specific recommendation for supplementing in HIV-positive people; the studies just haven't been done. Your basic multivitamin has 6 to 18 micrograms of B_{12}. B-complex preparations include from 12 to 500 micrograms. Separate B_{12} oral supplements are also available, in doses from 25 to 1,000 micrograms. An excess of B_{12} won't hurt you, but it may not be necessary.

We'll talk more about vitamin B_{12} supplementation later. Because malabsorption is so frequently a factor in B_{12} deficiency, you may need some help from your doctor.

Folate

Folate changes into its active form after it has been absorbed by the body. It is excreted through the gastrointestinal tract. It is necessary for making red blood cells and for neurological function. Thus deficiencies in folate, as with vitamin B_{12} deficiencies, are associated with neurologic symptoms. This can be particularly important to people with HIV. More folate is needed in the presence of severe infection, cancer, and pregnancy.

One report measured folate in the cerebrospinal fluid—the fluid that bathes the brain and spinal cord—in children infected with HIV. Results showed a lower level of folate in that fluid than in the blood. Thus we may be folate-deficient where we need it most, even when we test in the normal range. And, as is found with vitamin B_{12} deficiencies, the red-blood-cell changes normally associated with folate deficiency are often not seen in the presence of HIV.

Zidovudine (AZT, ZVD) has been shown to contribute to folate deficiency. People taking zidovudine are therefore at greater risk. This is also true of other commonly used drugs. Trimethoprim, for example, part of the drug trimethoprim-sulfamethoxazole (Bactrim or Septra), which is widely used to protect against pneumocystis pneumonia, is a folate antagonist—it directly blocks folate. So do pyrimethamine, used for toxoplasmosis, and methotrexate, a common chemotherapy agent. Phenytoin, or Dilantin, a popular antiseizure medicine, blocks absorption of folate. So do barbiturates, used by some doctors for pain control or to help you sleep.

Alcohol is a special villain. It also blocks folate absorption, and people who regularly use substantial amounts of alcohol are often seriously deficient. Vitamin B_{12} deficiency can also lower available folate levels, as it is needed to change folate into its active form.

Loss of appetite, nausea, diarrhea, hair loss, and mouth and tongue pain can all be symptoms of folate deficiency. Fatigue is common too. As things get worse, changes in blood cells may be seen.

Folate deficiencies are treated with 1 to 2 milligrams a day. One milligram or less a day is given thereafter for maintenance. Oversupplementation is not thought to be dangerous.

Leafy vegetables, organ meats, and yeast are good dietary sources.

Multivitamin folate levels are usually set at 4 milligrams. Folate is not normally included in B-complex preparations.

Vitamins Not Frequently Requiring Supplementation in HIV
•

You'll see these vitamins listed on the labels of the multivitamin supplements you buy, as well as for sale separately. It's important that you know their role. Supplementing in large quantities is unnecessary and can in some cases be harmful. Supplementation in the small quantities used in standard multivitamin preparations won't hurt you, though.

Niacin

Niacin is needed for the metabolism of proteins, carbohydrates, and fats. It is absorbed throughout the intestine and excreted in the urine. In large doses, in HIV-negative people, it can have beneficial effects on cholesterol and triglyceride levels. But lowering these levels may not be essential if you are HIV-positive.

Without serious malnutrition, we rarely see nutritionally based niacin deficiency. Classically, deficiency has been found only in people who eat a corn-based and otherwise unbalanced diet. Still, one study has shown improved survival in HIV-positive people who took some form of niacin supplementation.

Five to 20 milligrams a day are enough to protect against niacin deficiency, and large amounts may not be good for you. What you get in your diet should go a long way toward meeting your needs. Beyond that, my patients stick to what they get in their multivitamin pills.

Symptoms of niacin deficiency include generalized weakness and indigestion. Headaches and insomnia can follow. Severe deficiency can cause characteristic skin rashes, massive and bloody diarrhea, and even dementia.

Symptoms of supplementation include flushing and temporary tingling and burning sensations. Oversupplementation can cause vomiting, diarrhea, and even fainting, due to a fast heart rate and low blood pressure. At very high doses ulcers, liver damage, and high blood sugar can also result. This is not a vitamin to play around with.

Standard preparations contain 20 to 30 milligrams, which is a minimal amount. B-complex supplements can contain up to 100 milligrams. Even at that dose you may get some flushing and a characteristic prickling feeling.

If you can tolerate this, it won't hurt you; doses totaling up to 300 milligrams or so a day are probably okay. But there's no reason to take it on its own. In particular, you should avoid the time-release preparations. They are more likely to damage your liver.

As an HIV doctor, I also prefer that most of my patients not take niacin in substantial quantities because it changes the lab values I use to monitor their health. Large amounts of niacin will lower cholesterol and triglyceride levels, so those levels no longer tell me what I need to know. It's important to remember, though, that many people with HIV are living out their full life span. Thus if there is heart disease, medicating to reduce cholesterol and tryclyceride levels may now be necessary.

Sound sources for obtaining sufficient niacin in the diet include meat, fish, eggs, and beans.

Biotin

Biotin is found in most foods and is absorbed throughout the gut. Bacteria in the colon make more. Therefore, less biotin will be available if gut bacteria are destroyed by powerful antibiotics. It is needed for metabolism of fats and carbohydrates. Raw egg whites contain a substance that inactivates biotin. Still, biotin deficiency has only been seen in severe malnutrition.

Rashes, muscle pain, and hair loss are symptoms of biotin deficiency, as are nausea and anemia. However, even in patients maintained entirely on total parenteral nutrition or TPN (food delivered through the veins for people who can't be fed otherwise), reports of deficiency are rare. For anybody who can eat, the amount in a normal multivitamin, about 30 to 300 micrograms, should suffice. B-complex vitamins contain 30 to 100 micrograms.

Pantothenic Acid

Easily absorbed and readily available in the diet, pantothenic acid contributes to the metabolism of carbohydrates and fats and to making steroids. Deficiencies are rare and have only been described in association with other vitamin deficiencies.

When deficiency has been caused experimentally, the result has been foot pain—the so-called "burning foot syndrome." For this reason, investigators have tried to treat those symptoms with 10 milligrams a day. Success has been limited, however.

No role has yet been found for individual supplementation with this vitamin. You'll get a little, about 10 milligrams, in most routine supplements. Vitamin B combinations can have 5 to 75 milligrams.

Vitamin D

Vitamin D is available in the diet, but the major portion is produced by skin synthesis. It is important for calcium and phosphate metabolism and may have a role in immune function. Vitamin D deficiencies are rare, occurring only with inadequate exposure to sunlight. There are no reported cases of vitamin D deficiency in people with HIV. Too much vitamin D can raise your calcium level, weaken your bones, and lead to kidney stones. If you want to ensure that you have enough vitamin D, don't look to your vitamins; just go to the park and lie in the sun. Because of the 1997 discovery that people with HIV lose bone mineral density, in my office we now test vitamin D levels.

Vitamin K

Vitamin K occurs in two forms. It can be obtained in the diet from green leafy vegetables and liver. Bacteria in the gut provide another form, which is less active. Vitamin K is stored in limited amounts in the liver, where it is used to make factors that promote blood clotting. Thus a vitamin K deficiency can result in anticoagulation. If the liver is damaged, it may not be able to use vitamin K, even when present or provided in adequate amounts.

Malabsorption or the long-term use of powerful antibiotics, which sterilize the gut, can lead to a vitamin K deficiency. So can long-term use of TPN. Such deficiencies respond to injections of vitamin K, if the liver is healthy. There is no report of vitamin K deficiency peculiar to HIV, and I know of no need to supplement it on your own. Multivitamins don't generally contain it.

When a deficiency is documented in people with long-term malabsorption and diarrhea, it sometimes will respond to oral treatment. You should discuss this with your doctor.

Antioxidant Vitamins
•

Antioxidant vitamins play a central role in regulating homeostasis. They are especially interesting because it is possible that increasing levels of supplementation may, in some cases, be of benefit.

To understand what an antioxidant is, we need to learn a little more about the way our bodies work. I'll try to keep this simple.

How Antioxidants Work

The body is made up of molecules, combinations of atoms constructed in a particular way to do a specific job.

The molecules that take part in or regulate processes in your body are held together by the forces between their electrons, which have a sort of magnetic attraction to one another and fit together based on that attraction.

Many molecules within your body exist periodically in what is called an oxidized state. This means that they have one or more unpaired electrons. They are looking for molecular partners, often at the expense of other important molecular relationships. When they are in this state, they are called free radicals.

These free radicals can react much more with their surroundings, often in ways that are damaging. They can interact with and disrupt many finely tuned processes that are needed to maintain the body.

In some cases, the presence of these active molecules, or free radicals, can be helpful. Cells of your immune system, for example, rely on the destructive power of free radicals and use them as ammunition, discharging them where infection is present in order to kill the invaders. But along with the destruction of unwelcome cells or organisms, there can be damage to nearby tissues and processes your body needs.

In other cases, however, free radicals are simply an unavoidable by-product of body processes—the leftovers, so to speak, of necessary reactions—and serve no useful purpose. In these cases they are like static on the radio: they mess things up a little, but the music keeps on playing.

All of this is true for every living body.

Our bodies contain natural substances, called antioxidants, that can gather up and neutralize free radicals, limiting their capacity for destruction. Often there are not enough to do the whole job.

At some stages or circumstances in our lives, free radicals and their damage are increased. Much of the deterioration we see in aging, for example, results from the presence of an increased amount of these reactive molecules. Our natural stores of antioxidants cannot successfully overcome the increase. In states of illness or infection, free radical presence is also increased and results in many of our symptoms. This is of special concern for people with HIV, in whom the normal antioxidant defense system is compromised.

Alcohol and other substances increase the number of free radicals, and hence the damage they do to the body. We'll talk more about that later, when we look at alcohol and HIV.

What makes all this very important is that, given the chance, the HIV virus uses free radicals to establish itself. Free radicals activate the critical step in the actual copying of genetic material needed to reproduce the virus. And the virus itself stimulates their increased presence. The more we can swamp them with extra antioxidants, the harder it is for HIV to grow.

This is currently the subject of substantial research around the world. We already know this:

- If you add antioxidants to a culture dish in which HIV is growing, activity of the virus is profoundly reduced, and HIV production is inhibited.
- If antioxidants are removed from a culture dish in which HIV is growing, production of the virus is increased.
- The amount of certain natural antioxidants is decreased in the blood of people with HIV, and antioxidant levels decrease progressively with increasing illness.
- The results of some studies suggest that *antioxidant supplementation may slow the progression of HIV.*

We can help our system to protect and repair itself by increasing its antioxidant supply. This chapter will look at some of the natural antioxidants our body uses, which we can easily increase with supplementation.

There are also some antioxidants not found naturally in the body that are being studied for their possible role in fighting HIV.

Vitamin C (Ascorbic Acid)

Vitamin C is the best-known, the most-studied, and the most frequently supplemented antioxidant. It is easily absorbed in the small intestine, as it is a simple carbohydrate, and it is excreted in the stool and urine. The kidney reabsorbs it from the urine when supplies are low. Absorption, both in the kidney and the small intestine, is reduced when intake is greater than 200 milligrams per day.

The bulk of its impact on wound healing is due to its role in making collagen, the building block of new tissue formation. Thus it helps maintain our very structure. It also may offer special protection to the lungs, by reducing damage to delicate lung tissues caused by activation of the cells of the immune system.

Vitamin C is involved in the manufacture of hormones, steroids, and neurotransmitters—the substances by which our nerve cells speak to one another. It is necessary for the conversion of folate into its active form. It also assists in iron absorption.

Our need for and utilization of vitamin C increases in the presence of infection or injury. We consume more with inflammation and fever. Major burns increase requirements by a hundredfold. And if we are malabsorbing, we must take in a lot to get in a little.

Frank vitamin C deficiencies are rare; they manifest as poor wound healing, easy bruising and bleeding, and anemia.

Vitamin C has been studied in the medical literature, and it is touted in the lay literature for its effects on the common cold—a viral infection—both for prevention and recovery. One study treated patients newly infected with colds, using either vitamin C (six grams a day for five days) or a placebo. (A placebo is an inactive substance made to look like the pill being studied, so that neither the doctor nor the patient can tell who gets the real thing.) Improvement was so striking in those receiving vitamin C that it was not possible to hide their identity from the doctors who observed them.

Other studies did not show a reduction in the number of colds contracted, but did show that colds were shorter and less severe with vitamin C supplementation. And fewer superimposed bacterial infections—which often follow colds when resistance is down— have been reported.

Let's look at the nature of vitamin C. We know that, except for guinea pigs, humans are the only mammals who can't make it. We know that, pound for pound, the average mammal makes the equivalent of up to ten grams a day for an organism our size. We know that this production is not static, but increases when an animal is stressed (for example, by infection). Rats, when stressed, have been shown to increase their production tenfold. We know that the amount of supplementation required to cause diarrhea, a side effect of high supplementation, increases when we have an infection, suggesting that we use more, if we have it, when we need it. Interestingly, levels of vitamin C have been found to be reduced in humans during infection with the common cold. We use more when we're sick, and we can't make more to replace it.

Part of the role of vitamin C in infection is to react with and neutralize free radicals. Cells of the immune system release toxic substances to kill an invading germ or virus; surrounding tissues are also damaged; and the free radicals that result can extend that damage further. This is particularly worrisome in people with HIV, because the virus needs just such an environment—one with excess free radicals, in an oxidized state—to reproduce itself. And vitamin C is a powerful antioxidant.

Vitamin C also helps increase the net antioxidant action of vitamin E. Some of vitamin E's actions can actually oppose its antioxidant effect, but in the presence of vitamin C this does not happen.

Perhaps because of its antioxidant properties, vitamin C use is associated with a reduced risk not only of infection but also of heart disease, cataracts, and some cancers. It helps protect against the ravages of cigarette smoke and city smog. Preliminary data suggest a role for vitamin C in treating or helping prevent heart attacks, adult-onset diabetes, some long-term side effects of psychiatric drugs, and other chronic disorders.

Some cells in the immune system contain up to fifty times as much vitamin C as is found in the blood. This may help protect these cells against the kind of damage they cause their surroundings, from the compounds they make to fight infection.

While there can be problems with oversupplementation of vitamin C, most of them occur only at very high doses. Diarrhea is the most common. It rarely occurs at doses of less than 4 grams, or 4,000 milligrams, a day, and it resolves when amounts are reduced. In fact, those who take high doses of this vitamin often choose their dose by increasing their intake daily until diarrhea appears. And, as we have said, that diarrhea is not present at the same dose during times when their system is stressed. It's a natural way to ask your body how much vitamin C it can handle.

There are people, some of them doctors, who advocate massive doses of vitamin C—up to 10 or more grams a day. But such doses are not without risk. Kidney stones can precipitate at very high intake levels.

At this point, until the results are in, I recommend an intermediate dose of 1 to 3 grams a day, as tolerated. During periods of active infection you can double or triple this dose; but I suggest no more, for now, than 6 grams a day. For those who are committed to higher doses, consider taking baking soda, to keep your urine alkaline and to reduce the risk of stones. Drinking large quantities of water can help prevent kidney stones, too.

Remember that we have no proof of what constitutes the perfect dose. But you and I just don't have time to wait. To quote a 1994 editorial in the *Journal of the American College of Nutrition:* "Antioxidant nutrients appear remarkably benign, even at high supplementary intakes. . . . [R]ecommendations to wait until every conceivable study has been designed and conducted to achieve a level of absolute certainty will result in the continuing cost of the disease to the individual and to society" (Hemila, 1992).

Basic multivitamin preparations contain 60 to 180 milligrams of vitamin C. You'll find some vitamin C in your B stress, or B-complex, vitamins. You need not count this in your total.

Vitamin E (Tocopherol)

Vitamin E is absorbed in and with fat; it requires pancreatic and biliary enzymes for absorption. Its antioxidant properties serve to protect and stabilize cell membranes. It is found in vegetable oils, and to a lesser degree in eggs, whole-grain cereals, and butter. You can get a little from vegetables. Frank deficiency is rare and takes a long time to occur, but can it be seen when there is lasting, severe fat malabsorption. It can also be seen after long-term TPN administration. Effects of vitamin E deficiency include peripheral neuropathy, poor position sense and balance, and a reduction in knee-jerk and other reflexes. Deficiency of this vitamin alone in those who are not HIV-positive can result in the same immune-system abnormalities found in people with HIV infection.

Cell membranes have a fat, or lipid, layer. Free radicals in these membranes react with oxygen and initiate a chain reaction, forming new free radicals at every step in the chain. Vitamin E counters this process by entering the lipid membrane and uniting with the free radical. The molecule that results has a different shape; it sticks its head out of the membrane, where it becomes visible to vitamin C. When attacked by vitamin C, it can be reduced back to a stable molecule, and the chain of damage is halted.

It's important to know what kind of vitamin E you're taking. If it's not naturally produced alpha tocopherol, vitamin C won't recognize it, and you won't get all of this effect. If it's gamma tocopherol, such as is found in soybean oil, it will be excreted quickly. So you should try to find supplements that contain natural alpha tocopherols. These have the most activity. Most vitamin E is sold in the alpha form.

Vitamin E is used in a variety of circumstances for its antioxidant effects. It is used with vitamin C and beta-carotene, for example, as supportive treatment for those with cholesterol disorders, along with appropriate cholesterol-lowering drugs. Its supplementation has been shown to increase cell-mediated immunity in healthy elderly people. This is exactly the type of immune response that is impaired, and eventually destroyed, by HIV disease. In each of these studies, the dosage used has been 800 units a day. Vitamin E is also one of the vitamins that can be taken in relatively large doses without toxicity.

Dietary supplementation of vitamin E is thought to increase zidovudine's effectiveness in fighting the virus. And, in the presence of HIV infection, vitamin E intake may decrease the speed of progression to AIDS.

We have already noted that, in laboratory cultures of HIV, addition of antioxidants slows the rate of growth of the virus. With high enough doses of vitamin E, growth may actually be halted; those doses, however, are so high that they kill the cells in which the virus has been cultured. Thus, the toxicity of vitamin E at super-high doses limits the extent of its effect. In moderately high doses, however, it may stimulate, and perhaps protect, some of the immune cells the virus is known to destroy.

Low levels of vitamin E have been found to correlate with the presence of HIV and other infections, particularly in immigrants from developing countries. The Italian studies that reported this finding did not investigate which abnormality—infection or vitamin E deficiency—might have come first. They did report, however, that vitamin E was found to be deficient in study subjects with AIDS, and in about a third of intravenous drug users who did not have evidence of HIV infection. This association of vitamin E deficiency with migrants from developing countries, and with intravenous drug users, was also reported in another Italian study, raising the possibility that low levels of vitamin E and other antioxidants might actually play a role in initial infection, as well as in progression to AIDS in those already infected.

In another study, blood levels of vitamin E were found to be low in 27 percent of HIV-positive men—four to five times as many as those who are deficient in vitamins A or C.

There are a few early reports of vitamin E toxicity in patients on aggressive protease inhibitor therapy.

Thus, we know that vitamin E helps slow the growth of the virus; we know that your vitamin E level may be deficient if you are infected; and we know that moderately high doses won't hurt you. Given these facts, it makes sense to supplement vitamin E.

Based on recommendations for other health conditions, I recommend 800 to 1,200 milligrams of vitamin E a day.

Your standard multivitamin has only about 30 milligrams of vitamin E. Centrum contains none.

Vitamin A

Like vitamin E, vitamin A is a fat-soluble vitamin. It occurs in its active form in milk products, meat, and saltwater fish. Green leafy vegetables, carrots and other yellow root vegetables, and yellow and orange fruits contain beta-carotene, which the body can convert to vitamin A. Depletion results from malabsorption of fats, or from the use of mineral oil as a laxative. Alcohol use can also contribute. Beta-carotene conversion to active vitamin A in the body can be defective in people with diabetes or hypothyroidism. Long-term TPN can promote deficiency, too.

Dry eyes, night blindness, and other eye conditions are symptoms of vitamin A deficiency. In extreme cases, blindness can result. Also, white cells can be reduced, as can red blood cells. Resistance to infection is impaired. Thus vitamin A deficiency can result in more, and more severe, diseases of many types. Even a mild deficiency has been shown to increase the risk of pneumonia, diarrhea, and even death in children. Vitamin A deficiency has been associated with an increased likelihood of transmission of HIV from mother to infant in India, Asia, and Africa. In a U.S. study published by Barbara Weiser in 1997, however, vitamin A supplementation did not affect rates of mother-infant transmission.

Supplementation with beta-carotene, the recommended form of vitamin A replacement, has been shown in one study to increase the number of T4 (CD4) lymphocytes in healthy, HIV-negative people. This kind of immune cell—the kind you want to hold on to—is entered, taken over, and eventually destroyed by HIV. One of the fourteen participants in this study reported diarrhea. No other side effects were seen.

And what about the particular need for supplementation in people with HIV? In a study of over one hundred HIV-positive patients with no symptoms other than enlarged lymph nodes, 18 percent were found to be deficient in vitamin A. Several studies have shown an association between vitamin A deficiency and reduced CD4 counts, as well as an association between moderate supplementation and increased survival. High levels of supplementation, however, appear to result in reduced survival, as does vitamin A deficiency. So we can get too much of a good thing.

So once again, we find that higher levels of a vitamin may help protect against HIV's effects on the immune system. We know that lower levels are likely to be found in the presence of HIV, just when its support is most needed. We know this can happen early. We also know, however, that an excess of vitamin A is toxic and must be avoided.

Too much vitamin A—called hypervitaminosis A—can result in high levels of blood calcium, as calcium is pulled from bone. Vomiting and headache can result. Bone and joint pain are features also. In extreme cases there can be liver damage. A recent study showed increased lung cancer in smokers who supplemented their vitamin A intake. This is of less concern for you, but it does point to the fact that inappropriate use of vitamin A, even as beta-carotene, can actually promote free radicals.

Hypervitaminosis A is one of the more common types of vitamin excess. You can monitor yourself for it by watching the color of your palms, and by looking for yellow coloration in the places where you sweat. But the best way is to monitor your intake.

Doctors have a shared joke: an alcoholic, they say, is a person who drinks more than her or his doctor. In my office we define a patient with hypervitaminosis A as someone whose palms are yellower than mine.

One of the ways we avoid vitamin A toxicity is to supplement in the form of beta-carotene. I do not recommend taking a direct vitamin A supplement. Nor do I recommend cod liver oil.

Even in the form of beta-carotene you shouldn't go overboard. I suggest 15 milligrams a day, which will give you the equivalent of 25,000 units of vitamin A. If you drink carrot juice most days, you can skip supplementation entirely. Hypervitaminosis A can even be seen in people who take no supplements, if they live their life on carrot juice.

You'll find about 3 milligrams, or 5,000 units, of vitamin A in most multivitamins. High-dose preparations can have up to three times this much.

Minerals
•

The regulation of mineral balance in the body is essential to survival. Like the body itself, each cell is a living organism and must maintain its internal environment. And it must interact with its surroundings in order to perform the functions assigned to it. The movement of minerals across cell membranes, between the extracellular and intracellular fluid, forms the basis for the body's most primary functions. Electrical activity is initiated; hearts beat, nerve cells signal. Muscles respond. Blood vessels tighten or relax. Water balance is maintained.

Here is a look at how some of these processes work, and a survey of the need to supplement in the setting of HIV.

Sodium and Potassium

These minerals, as they flow back and forth across cell membranes in controlled fashion, maintain homeostasis in the cell, and in the organ and the body that it is part of.

The body's ability to regulate and maintain its stores of sodium and potassium is impressive. Except in the case of severe illness, or the use of certain medications or intravenous fluids, there should be no special need to supplement. In those cases, your doctor will monitor your levels.

Calcium and Phosphorus

While there is a recommended dietary intake for calcium and phosphorus, deficiencies have not been studied in HIV. New data that suggest that bone, like muscle, can waste with advancing HIV are causing us to take a new look at calcium supplementation. Calcium will be found in your multivitamins in varying amounts; about 30 to 150 milligrams of phosphorus will be present in your daily vitamin, and it's commonly present in foods. If levels are low in the blood, it will be because you're sick, and your doctor will be watching them.

If you have lost a lot of weight, have recently been ill, or are now ill, you might want to monitor your phosphorus level. It's found on a routine chemistry panel.

Magnesium

Magnesium plays an active role in the metabolism of sodium, potassium, and calcium. It acts on your heart and blood vessels, your nerves and muscles, and your gut. Most of it is concentrated in tissue, so levels in the blood don't tell us much.

Kidneys spill magnesium. Losses also occur in the stool and through the skin. Malabsorption can reduce its availability from the diet. High alcohol use reduces it. Diuretics and some antibiotics deplete it.

Often, levels are low in states of severe infection and then rise in that setting, suggesting that tissue damage and cell death cause its release. Then it's carried out of the body and lost. Thus illness can deplete you rapidly, and your doctor may not know it, even if she or he tests you. Calcium deficiency can result from magnesium depletion and may not respond to treatment without magnesium supplementation.

Unlike calcium, there are no reserves in bone to draw on if

magnesium supplies get low. But you cannot get too much if your kidneys are healthy.

Recent studies show that magnesium supplementation can reduce lung injury from oxygen toxicity. It blocks blood vessel constriction, so it can augment blood flow. It has been shown to increase the speed of recovery from open-heart surgery, and to improve the likelihood of recovery from severe, life-threatening infection.

Since it can be hard to get magnesium in and easy to lose it, since it's so important, since you can't get too much, and since too much can't hurt you, it makes sense to supplement.

The only time you *shouldn't* supplement your magnesium is in the case of impaired kidney function. If you can't excrete it in the urine, magnesium can build up.

One hundred to 125 milligrams are found in most multivitamins. Theragram M has only 24 milligrams. Trace-element combinations generally contain 100 to 500 milligrams. The RDA for magnesium is 400 milligrams.

Given the exciting results of all the new research described above, you may want to beef up your program with a separate magnesium supplement. There's no way to know how much is enough. For now I suggest 500 extra milligrams a day, on top of whatever's in your combination pills. With frank magnesium deficiency, your doctor may prescribe more. If oral supplements don't work, magnesium can be given by vein.

Trace Elements
•

These are other elements whose quantities are small but whose contribution is enormous and essential. Seven essential trace elements are described in humans: chromium, copper, cobalt, iodine, iron, selenium, and zinc.

There is no known use for cobalt except as part of vitamin B_{12}. No deficiency of manganese has ever been reported. Iodine is important in thyroid metabolism, but it has no known potential role in HIV in the absence of thyroid disease. It's present in small amounts in combination pills. Supplementing this element aggressively may meddle with your thyroid levels, so I don't recommend it.

The remaining trace elements are discussed in the following pages.

Chromium

Chromium helps insulin perform, so it's needed by your cells to take up glucose. Thus when it is deficient, blood sugar levels can be elevated. Cholesterol and triglyceride levels rise too. Peripheral neuropathy has been reported, as has weight loss. Heavy exercise, infection, and injury increase its use, and hence its loss.

Chromium is found in good supply in brewer's yeast and in meats and cheeses.

The normal American diet is said to contain only about half of what we should have, but deficiencies have rarely been reported. And the above effects are the only ones we've seen.

The RDA, which is all we have to go by here, is 50 to 200 micrograms. There are no studies reported on its importance in HIV.

Multivitamins contain from 15 to 100 micrograms of chromium. Trace-element supplements can add another 100 micrograms or so.

Copper

Copper is a necessary part of some of the enzymes that help to in-activate free radicals. Thus it plays a part in antioxidant protection. It is also used for making blood cells. It is active in the metabolism of iron. Copper-containing enzymes are involved in immune function.

Absorption can be reduced by critical illness, by high-dose zinc supplementation, and by antacids. Deficiencies are rare except in severe wasting. Measurement is difficult. Excesses can be harmful and can lead to liver failure.

Specific copper supplementation is not normally recommended, except for those on TPN. However, copper deficiencies have been reported in people with HIV, and copper can be further reduced with zidovudine treatment. One study, though, showed higher levels of copper in people with HIV.

There is no RDA for copper. Two to 3 milligrams are generally found in daily multivitamins.

Iron

Iron is needed to make red blood cells. It can function as an antioxidant. Vitamin C promotes its absorption. When your body needs more iron, it absorbs more from your diet.

Deficiency leads to anemia. Malabsorption can result as well. When present in excess, though, iron can work against you. Iron is frequently sequestered in the body to prevent its use by bacteria as a source of fuel. Thus increasing iron inappropriately might lead to increased infection.

Iron attaches to proteins; it is first stored and then carried throughout the body by these proteins. But in states of chronic illness, the supply of these proteins is reduced. Storage capacity is thus limited. And when the body runs out of safe places to put its iron, what's left is deposited in tissues. The function of these tissues can be harmed by this process, particularly in the liver and the heart.

When present in excess, iron can actually *stimulate* free radical formation.

Unless you're menstruating, or otherwise losing blood regularly, there's no way to get rid of excess iron. And while insufficient iron can cause anemia, anemia may not mean that you need iron.

In one study, higher levels of iron were found in HIV-positive subjects than in HIV-negative subjects.

Low levels of iron should be interpreted by your doctor in the context of other tests, before you supplement your intake. These tests show not only what your level is but also whether you have a safe place to park it.

Supplementation *in documented deficiency states* is prescribed at 325 milligrams, one to three times a day.

You'll get about 18 milligrams in most vitamin supplements, and the same in trace and mineral combinations. If your multivitamin specifically advertises iron, in its name or loudly on its label, it may contain more. I suggest you stay with a regular multivitamin.

Iron is found in red meats, liver, beans, and peas. The RDA ranges from 7 milligrams a day to 14 for women who menstruate.

Because of its potential for harm when oversupplied, and until we can better interpret its role in people with HIV, I recommend not supplementing beyond what you get in combinations unless you are proven to be deficient and your total iron-binding capacity is in the normal range.

Selenium

Selenium is an especially important antioxidant for you. It has been found to be depleted in both the tissues and the blood of people with AIDS, suggesting a deficiency of long standing. Selenium deficiency has been found in patients with or without diarrhea and malabsorption. Eighteen percent of the men in one HIV study, all asymptomatic, were found to be selenium-deficient.

Levels go down if disease progresses. Selenium levels correlate with albumin levels, with lean body mass, and with total lymphocyte count—all markers of immune function. Supplementation has been shown to improve symptoms and blood levels, but not these other markers. Further studies of its use, in combination with other antioxidants, are under way.

Infection and increased metabolic rates compound the loss of selenium.

Selenium deficiency is associated with heart disease and with anemia. Thrush is more common, and CD4s drop. Some patients report that their thrush goes away when they start selenium supplementation.

Current trials will tell us more about the value of selenium supplementation. For now, I recommend it. The 10 to 100 micrograms you'll get in your daily vitamin and trace-element supplements are a start. I recommend an additional 50 micrograms from one to four times a day.

I don't advise huge amounts. Selenium functions with—and very much like—vitamin E. We know more about vitamin E, and we know it's safe to push the dose. We don't yet know that about selenium.

There is as yet no RDA for selenium.

Zinc

Zinc can be shuttled from blood to tissue in times of stress or illness. Thus plasma levels may not reflect its true concentration in the body. Zinc is absorbed in the small intestine. High-fiber diets and the presence of parasites can limit its absorption. Only 25 percent of what's ingested is absorbed, at best; with poor intestinal absorption, the amount can be even less.

Wound healing and the maintenance of membranes are among its tasks. It also plays a role in antibody production, and other aspects of immune response.

With zinc deficiency, immune response is impaired. Hair loss can result. Night vision is lost. We may think less clearly. Wound healing is slowed, and protein metabolism is impaired.

Diarrhea can be both a cause and a result of zinc deficiency, and thus can compound the problem. Zinc should always be supplemented in people with severe, chronic diarrhea.

A reduction or change in our sense of taste can also result from zinc deficiency. This can be especially disturbing, as it affects both appetite and absorption.

Levels of testosterone, a male hormone, drop in states of zinc deficiency. This is particularly interesting to men with HIV, up to 20 percent of whom are said to have low testosterone levels. In my own practice, I don't tend to see that so often—but I certainly see it in 10 percent of my male patients, and particularly in those with advanced illness. Loss of sexual desire and a decreased ability to build and maintain lean body mass are associated.

Some, but not all, studies have shown reduced zinc levels in people with HIV. Remember, though, that these are blood levels. They may not reflect tissue levels. Zidovudine lowers zinc levels.

Some investigators report improvement of symptoms with supplementation. When taken in excess, though, zinc can weaken immune-system function and lower calcium levels.

I'm particularly concerned about the results of a study set up in 1984 in which 288 HIV-positive men were asked what supplements they took, at the time they entered the study. They were then monitored for seven years for progression to AIDS. High daily intakes of vitamin C, biotin, and niacin were associated with slower progression to AIDS. High zinc intakes, however, were associated with *faster* progression, in a pattern consistent with the amount of intake. The authors concluded that high levels of zinc supplementation may have harmed immune status in these men.

In the past two years, multiple studies have reported a trend toward reduced survival with zinc supplementation. In fact, access to ample levels of zinc may support the assembly of new virus. I find that troubling, and I strongly recommend against aggressive zinc supplementation until we understand more about this.

The amount of zinc you get in a standard trace-element supplement, or a multivitamin with trace elements, is small. Beyond what you get in those pills, zinc normally should not be supplemented.

So we know we need some zinc, and we know we may have less in the setting of HIV infection. We also know that a little bit of it may help to reduce symptoms. And we know that too much may be bad for us.

Multivitamins usually contain about 15 milligrams of zinc. Trace-element supplements have 20 to 25 milligrams. Separate zinc supplements usually contain 50 to 60 milligrams. You'll get about 50 milligrams, then, if you take two multivitamins and a trace-element supplement each day. I think that should be enough.

The RDA for zinc is 15 milligrams.

What to Do
•

Now that you have all this information, you have to decide what to do with it—just how aggressive, how committed, you want to be.

To start with, you see how important it is to eat a healthy, varied diet, including the foods we've mentioned, to help supply these nutrients. Everyone should do that.

It is worth mentioning that even routine daily use of one multivitamin pill has been associated with a longer delay in progression from HIV to AIDS. We recommend this to all our patients.

The simplest schedule, then, is as follows:

- A multivitamin, without extra iron, twice a day
- A trace-element supplement once a day
- An antioxidant supplement once a day

While this may not offer you all of the possible benefits of the high-dose supplementation described below, it should help prevent frank deficiencies. And if it's hard for you to eat or to get pills down, or if money is a problem, this will give you a safe, supportive regimen that is easy and inexpensive.

If you want to do more, here's my recipe:

- A multivitamin, without extra iron, twice a day.
- A trace-element supplement once a day.
- A vitamin C supplement, 1,000 to 3,000 milligrams (as tolerated), once a day; or 3,000 to 6,000 milligrams (as tolerated), once a day during periods of active illness.
- A vitamin E supplement (alpha tocopherol preferred), 800 to 1,200 units, once a day.
- A beta-carotene supplement, 15 milligrams (with 25,000 units of vitamin A), once or twice a day.
- A vitamin B stress complex supplement twice a day. (These offer higher doses than an average B-complex supplement. They have a little added vitamin C, to promote their absorption. You needn't count this vitamin C toward your recommended vitamin C total.)
- A magnesium supplement, 250 milligrams, twice a day.
- A selenium supplement, 50 micrograms, one to four times a day.

This is imprecise, because these studies are in their infancy. But it's a good place to start. And it takes into account the dangers of over-supplementing.

If your own regimen currently calls for more than what I've outlined, or calls for different substances, be sure to consider the dangers we've looked at above. You don't want too much of a good thing.

It's a good idea to take your vitamins with food, if you can.

• • •

Here in the United States, vitamins are easy to buy. There are health food stores in every town; even supermarkets and drugstores routinely carry a supply of the basics. But in other countries, where attention to nutrition is less a part of the popular culture, they're harder to find.

I was surprised, in speaking with AIDS activists and with educators associated with the French HIV information service SIDA, to find that access to vitamins was so limited, and their cost so high, in Europe.

If you can't obtain vitamins where you live, a list of sources for reasonably priced, good vitamin supplements is included in Appendix IV.

REFERENCES

Abrams, B., and others. "A prospective study of dietary intake and acquired immune deficiency syndrome in HIV-positive homosexual men." *Journal of AIDS*, 1993, *6*(8), 949–957.

Adams, J. S., and others. "Vitamin D metabolite-mediated hypercalcemia and hypercalcuria in patients with AIDS- and non-AIDS-associated lymphoma." *Blood*, 1989, *73*(1), 235–239.

Alexander, M., and others. "Oral beta-carotene can increase the number of OKT4+ cells in human blood." *Immunology Letters*, 1985, *9*, 221–224.

Asfora, J. "Vitamin C in high doses in the treatment of the common cold." *International Journal for Vitamin and Nutrition Research*, 1987, *S16*, 219–234.

Baum, M. K., and others. "Association of vitamin B6 status with parameters of immune function in early HIV-1 infection." *Journal of Acquired Immune Deficiency Syndromes and Human Retrovirology*, 1991, *4*, 1122–1322.

Baum, M. K., and others. "Zidovudine-associated adverse reactions in a longitudinal study of asymptomatic HIV-1-infected homosexual males." *Journal of Acquired Immune Deficiency Syndromes and Retrovirology*, 1992, *4*, 1218–1226.

Baum, M., and others. "Inadequate dietary intake and altered nutrition status in early HIV-1 infection." *Nutrition*, 1994, *10*(1), 16–20.

Baum, M., and others. "Micronutrients and HIV-1 disease progression." *AIDS*, 1995, *9*(9), 1051–1056.

Beach, R. S., and others. "Plasma vitamin B_{12} level as a potential cofactor in studies of human immunodeficiency virus type 1–related cognitive changes." *Archives of Neurology*, 1992, *49*, 501–506.

Beach, R. S., and others. "Specific nutrient abnormalities in asymptomatic HIV-1 infection." *AIDS*, 1992, *6*, 701–708.

Beck, W., and others. "Serum trace element levels in HIV-infected subjects." *Biology and Trace Element Research*, 1990, *25*(2), 89–96.

Beisel, W. R., and others. "Single-nutrient effects on immunological functions: Report of a workshop sponsored by the Department of Food and Nutrition and its nutrition advisory group of the American Medical Association." *Journal of the American Medical Association*, 1981, *245*(1), 53–58.

Bistrian, B. "Physicians Workshop." *Malnutrition in the Hospitalized Patient*, Harvard Medical School Conference, 1994.

Burkes, R. L., and others. "Low serum cobalamin levels occur frequently in the acquired immune deficiency syndrome and related disorders." *European Journal of Haematology*, 1987, *38*, 141–147.

Cathcart III, R. F. "Vitamin C: The nontoxic, nonrate-limited, antioxidant free radical scavenger." *Medical Hypotheses,* 1985, *18*(1), 61–77.

Chernow, B. "Magnesium: A critical nutrient in acute illness." *Malnutrition in the Hospitalized Patient,* Harvard Medical School Conference, 1994.

Chernow, B. "Overview: Micronutrient effects in critical care." *Malnutrition in the Hospitalized Patient,* Harvard Medical School Conference, 1994.

Cirelli, A., and others. "Serum selenium concentration and disease progress in patients with HIV infection." *Clinical Biochemistry,* 1991, *24*(2), 211–214.

Constans, J., and others. "Membrane fatty acids and blood antioxidants in seventy-seven patients with HIV infection." *Rev. Med. Interne,* 1993, *14*(10), 1003.

Coodley, G. O., and others. "Beta-carotene in HIV infection." *Journal of Acquired Immune Deficiency Syndromes and Human Retrovirology,* 1993, 6, 272–276.

Droge, W., and others. "Requirement for prooxidant and antioxidant states in T cell mediated immune responses: Relevance for the pathogenic mechanism of AIDS?" *Klinische Wochenschrift,* 1991, *69,* 1118–1122.

Dworkin, B. M. "Selenium deficiency in HIV infection and the acquired immunodeficiency syndrome (AIDS)." *Chemico-Biological Interactions,* 1994, *91*(2–3), 181–186.

Dworkin, B. M., and others. "Abnormalities of blood selenium and glutathione peroxidase activity in patients with acquired immunodeficiency syndrome and AIDS-related complex." *Biology and Trace Element Research,* 1988, *15,* 167–177.

Elin, R. J. "Magnesium metabolism in health and disease." *Disease-a-Month,* April 1988, pp. 171–209.

Falutz, J., and others. "Zinc as a cofactor in human immunodeficiency virus–induced immunosuppression." *Journal of the American Medical Association,* 1988, *259*(19), 2850–2851.

Favier, A., and others. "Antioxidant status and lipid peroxidation in patients infected with HIV." *Chemico-Biological Interactions,* 1994, *91*(2–3), 165–180.

Fordyce-Baum, M. K., and others. "Nutritional abnormalities in early HIV-1 infection: II. Trace elements." *International Conference on AIDS,* 1989, *5, 467.*

Fuchs, J., and others. "Oxidative imbalance in HIV-infected patients." *Medical Hypotheses,* 1990, *36,* 60–64.

Gogu, S. R., and others. "Increased therapeutic efficiency of zidovudine in combination with vitamin E." *Biochemical and Biophysical Research Communications,* 1989, *165*(1), 401–407.

Gogu, S. R., and others. "Protection of zidovudine (AZT)–induced bone marrow toxicity and potentiation of anti-HIV activity with vitamin E." *Abstracts of the Annual Meeting of the Society of Microbiology,* 1990, *90,* 338.

Greenspan, H. C. "The role of reactive oxygen species, antioxidants, and phytopharmaceuticals in human immunodeficiency virus activity." *Medical Hypotheses,* 1993, *40,* 85–92.

Hatchigan, E. A., and others. "Vitamin A supplementation improves macrophage function and bacterial clearance during experimental salmonella infection." *Proceedings of the Society for Experimental Biology and Medicine,* 1989, *191,* 47–53.

Hemila, H. "Vitamin C and the common cold." *Journal of Nutrition,* 1992, *67,* 3–16.

Herbert, V. "Deficiency in AIDS." *Journal of the American Medical Association,* 1988, *260*(19), 2837.

Hoffman-Goetz, L., and others. "Febrile and plasma iron responses of rabbits injected with endogenous pyrogen from malnourished patients." *American Journal of Clinical Nutrition,* 1981, *34,* 1109–1116.

Hussey, G. D., and Klein. "A randomized, controlled trial of Vitamin A in children with severe measles." *New England Journal of Medicine,* 1990, *323,* 160–164.

Ireland, J., and Romeyn, M.. "Alterations in bone mineral density in HIV-infected men: A new risk factor for osteoporosis?" International Conference on AIDS, 1998, in submission.

Kieburtz, K. D., and others. "Abnormal B_{12} metabolism in human immunodeficiency virus infection." *Archives of Neurology,* 1991, *4,* 312–314.

Kinter, A. L., and others. "The role of anti-oxidants as suppressors of cytokine-induced HIV expression." *International Conference on AIDS,* 1991, *7*(2), 149.

Malcolm, J. A., and Sutherland. "When do low serum levels of trace metals represent a true immunodeficiency state?" *International Conference on AIDS,* 1993, *9*(1), 527.

Mantero-Atienza, E., and others. "Selenium status of HIV-infected individuals." *Journal of Parenteral and Enteral Nutrition,* 1991, *15*(6), 693–694.

Mehdani and others. "Vitamin E supplementation enhances cell-mediated immunity in healthy elderly subjects." *American Journal of Clinical Nutrition,* 1990, *52,* 557–563.

Miller, T., and others. "Is selenium deficiency clinically significant in pediatric HIV infection?" *International Conference on AIDS,* 1993, *9*(1), 306.

Moseson, M., and others. "The potential role of nutritional factors in the induction of immunologic abnormalities in HIV-positive homosexual men." *Journal of Acquired Immune Deficiency Syndromes and Human Retrovirology,* 1989, *2,* 235–247.

Nowak, D., and others. "Ascorbic acid prohibits polymorphonuclear leukocytes influx to the place of inflammation: Possible protection of lung from phagocyte-mediated injury." *Archivum Immunologiae et Therapiae Experimentalis,* 1989, *37,* 213–218.

Odeleye, O. E., and Watson. "The potential role of vitamin E in the treatment of immunologic abnormalities during acquired immune deficiency syndrome." *Progress in Food and Nutritional Science,* 1991, *15*(1–2), 1–19.

Olmsted, L., and others. "Selenium supplementation of symptomatic human immunodeficiency virus–infected patients." *Biology and Trace Element Research,* 1989, *20*(1–2), 59–65.

Packer, L., and Suzuki. "Vitamin E and alpha-lipoate: Role in antioxidant recycling and activation of the NF-kappa B transcription factor." *Molecular Aspects of Medicine,* 1993, *14*(3), 229–239.

Passi, S., and others. "Blood levels of vitamin E and polyunsaturated fatty acids of phospholipids, lipoperoxides, and glutathione peroxidase in patients affected with seborrheic dermatitis." *Journal of Dermatological Science,* 1991, *2*(3), 171–178.

Phuapradit, W., and others. "Serum vitamin A and beta-carotene levels in pregnant women infected with human immunodeficiency virus–1." *Obstetrics and Gynecology,* 1996, *87*(4), 564–567.

Picardo, M., and others. "Vitamin E, polyunsaturated fatty acids of phospholipids, lipoperoxides and glutathione peroxidase status in HIV seropositive patients." *International Conference on AIDS,* 1991, *7*(2), 287.

Rivers, J. M. "Safety of vitamin C ingestion." *Annals of the New York Academy of Sciences,* 1987, *498,* 445–454.

Sappi, C., and others. "Relative decrease in antioxidant status during evolution of HIV infection: Effect on lipid peroxidation." *International Conference on AIDS,* 1992, *8*(3), 132.

Semba, R. D., and others. "Maternal vitamin A deficiency and mother-to-child transmission of HIV-1." *Lancet,* 1994, *343*(8913), 1593–1597.

Singer, P., and others. "Nutritional aspects of the acquired immunodeficiency syndrome." *American Journal of Gastroenterology,* 1992, *87*(3), 265–273.

Skurnik, J. H., and others. "Micronutrient profiles in HIV-1 infected heterosexual adults." *Journal of Acquired Immune Deficiency Syndromes and Human Retrovirology,* 1996, *12*(1), 75–83.

Smit, E., and others. "Dietary intake of community-based HIV-1 seropositive and seronegative injecting drug users." *Nutrition,* 1996, *12*(7–8), 496–501.

Smith, I., and others. "Folate deficiency and demyelination in AIDS." *Lancet,* 1987, *2*(8552), 215.

Suzuki, Y. J., and Packer, L. "Inhibition of NF-kappa B activation by vitamin E derivatives." *Biochemical and Biophysical Research Communications,* 1993, *1,* 277–283.

Tang, A. M., and others. "Effects of micronutrient intake on survival in human immunodeficiency virus type 1 infection." *American Journal of Epidemiology,* 1996, *143*(12), 1244–1256.

Thurnham, D. I. "Antioxidants and prooxidants in malnourished populations." *Proceedings of the Nutrition Society,* 1990, *49,* 247–259.

Watson, R. R., and others. "Alcohol stimulation of lipid peroxidation and esophageal tumor growth in mice immunocompromised by retrovirus infection." *Alcohol,* 1992, *9*(6), 495–500.

Zaloga, G. *Nutrition in Critical Care.* St. Louis, Mo.: Mosby, 1994.

Zeman, F. J., and Ney. *Applications of Clinical Nutrition.* Upper Saddle River, N.J.: Prentice Hall, 1988.

Zheng, R., and others. "Zinc folds the N-terminal domain of HIV-1 integrase, promotes multimerization, and enhances catalytic activity." *Proceedings of the National Academy of Sciences USA,* 1996, *93*(24), 13659–13664.

"Vitamin B_6 and immune function in the elderly and HIV-seropositive subjects." *Nutrition Reviews,* 50(5), 145–147.

CHAPTER 5

•

Other Supplements
That Enhance
Immune Response

In Chapter Four we looked at substances everybody needs and can normally get in their diet, and examined their particular relevance to HIV. In each case we paid special attention to the role of these elements in enhancing immunity, to help us respond to and battle the virus.

In some cases we were concerned with *physiologic* replacement—making sure these substances were as present as they should be, in the range seen normally in states of good health. In other cases we looked at the value of *pharmacologic* replacement, or supplementation—giving ourselves more than a healthy body would usually get from its diet. We were trying to ensure, in these cases, that greater amounts of these substances than are normally found would be present and available for a specific medical effect—in this case, for fighting the virus and its progression.

But vitamins, minerals, and trace elements are not the only supplements used to fight the HIV virus. Others are commonly in use against HIV. And although they have different mechanisms of action, in each case they are used for their contribution to, or role in changing, the immune response.

These substances can be bought in health food stores.

Using these substances will take you one step further: rather than simply supporting your body by optimizing your nutrition, you will deliberately alter your internal environment, to make it less friendly to the virus.

You've already started in this direction if you're pushing your antioxidant vitamins. In fact, two of the treatments we'll talk about here are antioxidants.

You may choose to go further still, trying things that haven't yet made it into the medical community—or won't. Some of those more controversial therapies will be discussed later in this book. They are not all entirely benign.

For now, though, let's look at some simple, safe things you can do for yourself, beyond what you do with your vitamins.

Special Antioxidant Treatments
•

We reviewed the basic actions of antioxidants, including their activity against free radicals, in Chapter Four. Now let's get a little more specific.

Within the cells in which the virus lives, there are reactions that produce peroxide and superoxide molecules—creating free radicals in the cellular environment. Under normal circumstances, this may represent a form of immune protection, making the environment unfriendly to invaders. Cytokines, for instance, are known to stimulate these reactions, increasing the supply of free radicals in immune cells in response to infection. In the setting of HIV, however, free radicals help trigger the growth of the virus.

The body has several systems for reducing these free radicals, or reactive intermediates as they are called. One is based on a molecule called cysteine, and another on a molecule called glutathione. These two systems are complementary. Within the cell, in the absence of cysteine, glutathione levels are markedly reduced.

Certain enzymes drive the reactions that permit glutathione to deactivate free radicals within the cells. In the presence of more of these enzymes, glutathione's activity increases.

Glutathione is also important for the clearance of many prescription drugs. Some medicines are broken down by stages in the liver. At certain points in that process, they become toxic and can harm us. Glutathione inactivates these harmful by-products and breaks them down further, into substances that are harmless and are eventually excreted.

It is thought that the commonly seen reactions to trimethoprim-sulfamethoxazole (the prescription drug Bactrim) in people with HIV are due to the presence and circulation of its toxic intermediate products, whose further breakdown has been stalled in the liver because of low glutathione levels.

Glutathione is severely reduced in HIV. In addition, cysteine cannot get across the cell membrane when antioxidant activity is impaired and oxygen intermediates remain reactive. Since cysteine levels affect glutathione levels, this becomes a vicious cycle. The cell heats up with free radicals and is severely stressed.

It is in this setting that HIV replication picks up. The virus creates an atmosphere of oxidative stress, enhancing the generation of free radicals within the immune cell that is its home. This atmosphere activates that part of the HIV virus's generative material that directs its replication. When the cat's away, the mice will play.

So it becomes important to understand this process, in order to affect it. Put as simply as possible, we can increase the activity of glutathione by feeding it extra enzymes to help drive its reactions. We can increase the amount of glutathione by increasing cysteine levels in the cell. And we can increase the amount of cysteine in the cell by increasing the amount we deliver to the body. And none of these interventions will harm us.

So here are two supplements that can increase the amount of glutathione in our bodies.

Superoxide Dismutase (SOD)

Superoxide dismutase is an enzyme that is normally found in the body. Its function is to help drive the antioxidant reactions of glutathione. We can increase its presence, and hence its availability, by supplementing our intake.

Recent studies suggest that the presence of HIV within the cell causes SOD deficiency. In order to promote its reproduction, the virus itself increases oxidative stress, depleting both SOD and glutathione within the cell. In the process, free radicals such as peroxide are formed. They damage the cell, while increasing HIV replication. Of the cells that die as a result, there is current concern that naive T cells—those that remain capable of changing to recognize a new invader or infection—are particularly at risk.

SOD supplementation has already been used to help deter the effects of aging, some of which are also the result of oxidative stress. You will find it listed in vitamins marketed to the elderly. It is currently under study for treating HIV. We don't know the exact amount that's best. Until we do, I recommend one pill, containing 2,000 units, three times a day. Ideally it's taken on an empty stomach.

N-Acetyl Cysteine (NAC)

Intracellular cysteine levels can be enhanced, and glutathione levels increased, by taking N-acetyl cysteine.

NAC has been studied extensively in relation to HIV. Research results are mixed, but it's been shown to inhibit inflammation, and with it the burst in HIV replication commonly associated with immune activation. Its dampening effect on inflammation may help ameliorate the wasting syndrome. It helps protect the virus-invaded cell from death, and the consequent release of its viral load.

There remains a lot of controversy about the benefits of NAC. Clearly, it helps block HIV-associated damage to T cells growing in culture. T cells are more able to resist the effects of HIV-induced oxidative stress. Less HIV virus is made. There may even be a trend toward less apoptosis, or programmed T-cell death, although some papers disagree. But that may not be the whole story. Some studies, for instance, show that HIV reproduction may be slowed by NAC in T cells, but actually increased by NAC in monocytes and macrophages. So it's hard to interpret the data. And the real task is to understand NAC's effect on HIV replication and cell survival, not in a dish on a laboratory bench but within a living person.

Living people are much more complicated than culture dishes. Many of the interactions between systems are interrelated, as are our bodies' effects on HIV. So what we need to know is whether taking NAC will help us to stay well.

A study published in 1997 has trumpeted the fact of statistically significant increased survival after thirty-two weeks on NAC. The study itself is badly flawed. It lumps together placebo-controlled study time and treatment-by-choice study time; it bases its conclusions on only a fraction of the people who started out in the study; and it clearly reflects investigator bias. So although I like the premise, I can't rely on its claims. Still, the publication of this and other research does suggest that NAC is more likely to do you good than harm.

Until we have better information, I cautiously recommend it.

Again, this is the bottom line: viral proteins stress the cell; free radicals result; generation is activated; HIV is replicated; and NAC may help block this process.

Researchers suggest that part of the effect of NAC against the virus takes place by means of different, as yet unknown, mechanisms.

Based on the amounts used with good effect in study subjects, I recommend 300 to 600 milligrams a day. That's 150 milligrams two to four times a day.

Cell Membrane Components

Earlier in this book we spoke about cytokine release and its effect on loss of weight and lean body mass. To review briefly, these factors are released by, and act on, immune cells, to permit an acute immune response that is targeted to protect against abrupt and overwhelming illness.

The presence of HIV in immune cells spurs a low level of chronic release, which is enhanced by the presence of any other infection that requires an immune response. This is what triggers and sustains the wasting process.

The mediators of this process—cytokines, leukotrienes, and prostaglandins—are specific in their actions. Even a small change in their structure can also change their function. Ideally, it can make them less effective.

These substances are formed from what is known as the arachidonic acid cascade—a complex series of reactions that originates from a fatty acid found in the cell membrane. That fatty acid is called arachidonic acid.

Arachidonic acid is taken up from our diet and incorporated

into the cell membrane. But if we eat a lot of another fatty acid—eicosapentanoic acid—we can replace it, in some measure, on the membrane. So when immune response is activated, the body builds its factors for immune response from a different building block. The molecules produced are different, without the same inflammatory effect.

The source for this different fatty acid, omega-3, is fish oil. In fact, it's hard to eat enough of this to maximize its impact. Studies show that it takes eighteen grams a day—more than half an ounce of fish oil—to reverse the wasting process. That's a lot to ask of anyone, even someone with an appetite. And it makes your mouth taste fishy.

But most people tolerate lesser amounts. You can start with three grams a day and build up to six as tolerated. Most of my patients take six grams.

And if you take it, that's enough. You don't ever have to remember the names of those molecules again.

Other Disciplines
•

Many people fighting HIV look to other philosophies and approaches to choose what supplements they eat. Herbal treatments, mostly not prescribed by their doctors, are part of their nutritional program.

Two books on HIV and AIDS discuss these approaches simply and at length: *The HIV Wellness Sourcebook: An East/West Guide to Living Well with HIV/AIDS and Related Conditions,* by Misha Cohen, and *Treating AIDS with Chinese Medicine,* by Mary Kay Ryan and Arthur D. Shattuck. These books are included in the References for this chapter.

I am not trained in these disciplines. And since there are still few data to support their suggestions, I can't give you advice. I must leave that to you.

REFERENCES

Aukrust, P., and others. "Increased levels of oxidized glutathione in CD4+ lymphocytes associated with disturbed intracellular redox balance in human immunodeficiency virus type 1 infection." *Blood*, 1995, *86*(1), 258–267.

Aukrust, P., and others. "Markedly disturbed glutathione redox status in CD45RA+CD4+ lymphocytes in human immunodeficiency virus type 1 infection is associated with selective depletion of this lymphocyte subset." *Blood*, 1996, *88*(7), 2626–2633.

Baker, D. H., and Wood. "Cellular antioxidant status and human immuno-deficiency virus replication." *Nutrition Reviews*, 1992, *50*(1), 15–18.

Baruchel, S., and Wainberg. "The role of oxidative stress in disease progression in individuals affected by the human immunodeficiency virus." *Journal of Leukocyte Biology*, 1992, *52*, 111–114.

Cayota, A., and others. "In vitro antioxidant treatment recovers proliferative responses of anergic CD4+ lymphocytes from human immunodeficiency virus–infected individuals." *Blood*, 1996, *87*(11), 4746–4753.

Cohen, M. *The HIV Wellness Sourcebook: An East/West Guide to Living Well with HIV/AIDS and Related Conditions.* New York: Henry Holt, 1998.

Endres, S., and others. "The effect of dietary supplementation with omega-3 polyunsaturated fatty acids on the synthesis of interleukin-1 and tumor necrosis factor by mononuclear cells." *New England Journal of Medicine*, 1989, *320*, 265–271.

Fuchs, J., and others. "Oxidative imbalance in HIV infected patients." *Medical Hypotheses*, 1991, *36*, 60–64.

Hellerstein, M. K., and others. "Interleukin-1-induced anorexia in the rat." *Journal of Clinical Investigation*, 1989, *84*, 228–235.

Herzenberg, L. A., and others. "Glutathione deficiency is associated with impaired survival in HIV disease." *Proceedings of the National Academy of Science USA*, 1997, *94*, 1967–1972.

Jensen, G. "Fish oils and structured lipids." *Malnutrition in the Hospitalized Patient*, Harvard Medical School Conference, 1994.

Kameoka, M., and others. "Intracellular glutathione as a possible direct blocker of HIV type 1 reverse transcription." *AIDS Research and Human Retroviruses*, 1996, *12*(17), 1635–1638.

Raju, P. A., and others. "Glutathione precursor and antioxidant activities of N-acetyl-L-cysteine and oxothiazolidine carboxylate compared to in vitro studies of HIV replication." *AIDS Research and Human Retroviruses*, 1994, *10*(8), 961–967.

Roederer, M., and others. "Cytokine-stimulated HIV replication is inhibited by N-acetyl-L-cysteine." *Proceedings of the National Academy of Sciences USA*, 1990, *87*, 4884–4888.

Ryan, M. K., and Shattuck, A. D. *Treating AIDS with Chinese Medicine.* Berkeley: Pacific View Press, 1994.

Shatrov and others. "HIV type 1 glycoprotein 120 amplifies tumor necrosis factor-induced NF-Kappa B activation in Jurkat cells." *Aids Research and Human Retroviruses*, 1996, *12*(13), 1209–1216.

Staal, F. J., and others. "Antioxidants inhibit stimulation of HIV transcription." *AIDS Research and Human Retroviruses*, 1993, *9*(4), 299–306.

Von Schacky, C., and others. "Long-term effects of dietary marine omega–3 fatty acids upon plasma and cellular lipids, platelet function, and eicosanoid formation in humans." *Journal of Clinical Investigation*, 1985, *76*, 1626–1631.

Westendorp, M. O., and others. "HIV-1 Tat potentiates TNF-induced NF-kappa B activation and cytotoxicity by altering the cellular redox state." *EMBO Journal*, 1995, *14*(3), 546–554.

CHAPTER 6

•

Improving Your Appetite

Now that the first part of your database is built, you know where you stand and what your goals should be. You see your own patterns of eating and have set goals for improving them. You've established your priorities and identified problem areas to work on.

You know what foods, and how much of them, you should eat. You know how to supplement those foods, to ensure the proper intake of micronutrients. You know how to monitor your performance, for starters, by watching your weight. You're ready to build your own program.

But now it's time to consider another crucial aspect of your nutrition: the desire to eat.

HIV's Effects on Appetite

•

Knowing what's enough, and deciding to eat enough, don't always get you there. You also need to *want* to eat enough. This is harder for people who are HIV-positive; infection with HIV carries with it a real threat to appetite.

We have seen that HIV-positive people who are ill, particularly people with active secondary infections, eat less than people who are HIV-negative. But we also know that even healthy, asymptomatic people with HIV tend to eat less than their HIV-negative counterparts. In this case, the differences are subtle.

This means that, even if you feel terrific, you may still be eating less. And this may be the first time you've realized it.

So it's important to monitor your appetite, as well as what you do with it. First of all, you can take special care to get enough nourishment, if you know special care is in order. Also, this may alert you to look for other symptoms; an early infection may announce itself by a sudden loss of interest in food.

There are many ways in which appetite is affected in HIV. Some effects are caused by infection with the virus, others to the results of that infection, others to our body's way of fighting that infection, and others to the methods used in its treatment. Still others result from the additional infections that can accompany HIV, particularly in advanced stages.

We've discussed some of these already in Chapter Two. We'll review them here.

The Effect of HIV Itself

As we have seen, we respond to the presence of HIV by chronically activating our immune response. This response is valuable in the setting of an overwhelming, acute infection. The body attempts to eradicate that infection aggressively and quickly. Life itself may hang in the balance; the temporary loss of appetite that results from immune activation is of minimal concern to the body, which is fighting to survive.

But because we can't get rid of HIV, that type of response smolders on throughout the life span of our infection, and hence throughout our life. The effects are not as dramatic as they are at initial activation, but they last much longer. No matter how subtle they are, the result is that we want to eat less, and less often.

The Effect of Secondary Infections

Secondary infections and their treatments can compromise our appetite further. Our own immune response to these secondary infections is increased to acute levels and increases anorexia. This response of immune cells leads not only to their increased production but also to their activation. Cytokines, factors that influence appetite and metabolism—what we eat and what we do with it—are produced in large quantities by these activated cells. This is why we don't feel like eating when we have fevers or night sweats; all of these symptoms are signs that our system is using cytokines to fight an invader.

Medicines

Prescription medicines, and some herbal remedies, can reduce appetite. This can be especially true when they are first started, before your body has adapted to them.

Many of the medications commonly used against HIV cause anorexia or nausea. AZT, or zidovudine, is one example. Chemotherapy regimens can be another. Other medicines can alter the absorption of your food.

Others, chiefly antibiotics, eliminate bacteria normally present in your gut. A healthy body relies on these bacteria for proper absorption of nutrients, or conversion of substances within the gut into their active form before they are absorbed.

Conversely, when they are not properly absorbed, some nutrients can cause bacterial overgrowth; the result can be bloating, extra gas, or an inappropriate sense of fullness.

Mouth, Throat, and Esophageal Lesions

Herpes, thrush, and other infections or ulcerations can make the act of eating painful. Painful swallowing can leave us afraid to eat, and fear can override hunger.

If salivary glands don't produce well, the resulting dryness in the mouth (xerostomia) will make chewing and swallowing difficult. The more work it is to eat, the less we want to eat.

Malabsorption

The effects of HIV, as well as other intestinal infections, on the gut wall can cause us to absorb nutrients less efficiently. Fats, in particular, can be malabsorbed. When this happens, undigested remnants in our gut can make us feel full, or even nauseated, until they are eliminated. Fatty acids—the inadequately absorbed breakdown products of fats—can act as irritants, resulting in increased contractions of the gastrointestinal tract. This is perceived as abdominal cramping. Bacteria normally present in the gut can feed on nutrients that are not properly absorbed and increase in number; that bacterial overgrowth may result in increased amounts of gas released as a product of their digestion.

Like the elderly, people with HIV often have reduced amounts of acid available in the stomach to help them digest their food. This can also increase discomfort.

Enlargement of the Liver or Spleen

If the abdominal organs enlarge, due to infection, infiltration, or an inappropriate immune response, they can press against the gut. The body may not differentiate the cause of this pressure; we may think we are full when we're not.

In some cases, particularly if organ enlargement is rapid, this may cause abdominal pain, depressing appetite further.

Diarrhea

Diarrhea can be caused simply by HIV's direct infection of the intestinal lining. More commonly, it is due to other organisms' taking advantage of weakened immune defenses in a gut wall already damaged by HIV. Whatever its cause, diarrhea results in abdominal discomfort. Frequently, episodes are stimulated by the act of eating itself; we tend to compensate, often unconsciously, by eating less, or less often.

In some cases, diarrhea can be a result of too much vitamin C. This is rarely a problem in the dosage range I've recommended in this book. Amounts of four to ten grams, though, can loosen stools—especially if your body isn't used to such doses. And many people who take more than ten grams a day will have diarrheal symptoms.

Certain prescribed medicines may trigger diarrhea, too. This is especially likely to be a problem at first, when your body's just getting used to them.

Lactose Intolerance

We have seen that HIV infection of the gut wall changes its architecture and function. One result is the reduced presence of lactase, an enzyme needed to break down milk sugars. In its absence, those sugars are undigested and remain within the gut. They are broken down further by bacteria living in the gut. These bacteria may multiply when their food source is increased. They create gas as a byproduct of digestion and are responsible for a feeling of fullness, or bloating, that makes us less hungry.

Changes in Taste or Smell

Because HIV itself can alter the way things taste—due to its effects on your taste and smell receptors—foods you previously loved may now give you less pleasure. They may taste bland or actually different.

You can experiment with this for yourself by brushing your teeth with a commercial toothpaste, and then drinking orange juice. After your taste buds have been damaged by sodium laureth sulfate, a common ingredient in commercial toothpaste, they can no longer taste sweetness to the same degree. Most of us unconsciously avoid this surprise by drinking our orange juice first, or by waiting awhile after we brush our teeth.

Fortunately, taste and smell receptors can recover from such an assault, and the effect from our toothpaste is brief. Even when they are damaged beyond repair, these receptors are rapidly replaced. But if illness or medications make the damage permanent, we lose much of the pleasure of eating.

Your sense of smell, normally a vital part of your appetite, may be less responsive as well.

Depression

People who are depressed often show disturbance in appetite. While increased appetite can also be a manifestation of depression, decrease is much more common. In HIV infection, where there are already multiple assaults on the appetite, this can be as significant a problem as the depression itself.

Fatigue

When you're really tired, your appetite suffers too. While it's true that you can feel tired just because of illness, fatigue can often be a result of pushing too hard. If you don't listen to your body, pacing yourself to make the most of the energy available to you, your body will not want to eat.

•   •   •

Remember, these are only potential effects, and they are subject to treatment. The more we understand, the more we can intervene.

What You Can Do to Improve Your Appetite

Once you recognize these threats to your appetite, you can start to find ways to counteract them. Here are some simple approaches.

Timing Your Meals

Often, the most important key to maintaining your interest in food is adapting to the rhythm of your body.

Some people find that the morning meal is best for them. Poor absorption can cause the undigested remnants of that first meal to make them feel full later in the day. If that's so for you, try to get as many calories into that first meal as possible. And try to enjoy it. Eat the foods you like when you can eat.

For other people, especially if the liver or the spleen is enlarged, a better approach is to eat often, in lesser amounts. There's no rule restricting you to breakfast, lunch, and dinner. Six or eight small meals a day can give you just as many calories and just as much protein.

Timing your meals around exercise can help, too. Some of us are ravenous after a workout; others lose interest in food for the next hour or two. If you watch your own patterns of hunger, you can eat when your body most wants to.

You'll have to tinker with this a little. Explore different schedules, different ways to get the food in. Be sensitive to changes in your appetite at different times, and adjust your eating patterns to fit. Attune yourself to your body's requests for food, and give in to your instincts. Most of all, don't give up trying.

Food Cravings

Sometimes we feel an urge for a specific food. In the past, eating that food may have provided something we needed in our diet. From that point on, our body associates that need with that particular food. Or a craving may simply result from changes in hormone levels, or levels of neurotransmitters—the chemicals used by nerve and brain cells to communicate. Women may crave chocolate, for instance, at or around the start of menstruation, when certain hormones are at a low point.

Normally, when we crave a specific food, that food is highly spiced or flavored, or is rich in fats or sugars. Pizza, potato chips, clam dip or pickles, bacon or double chocolate cake—foods you might normally want to avoid—become highly desirable. And the craving may last only briefly.

Be alert to fluctuations in your desire for food and quick to act on them. And every time you crave some special food, even for a moment, give in to that and have it. Do it right away, while the urge is strong.

If you have recurrent cravings for some foods, you may want to keep them in the refrigerator, so you can get them the minute you want them.

Enjoying Comfort Foods

Comfort foods are foods you find pleasure in even when you're not hungry. These are often foods that trigger memories for us, conscious or otherwise. Maybe it's the butterscotch pudding your mother used to make. Maybe it's hominy grits, or apple pie. For me, Campbell's chicken noodle soup does it every time. For my kids it's mashed potatoes or hot dog casserole.

Comfort foods make us feel safe, remind us of times we were cherished and loved, and give off a scent that triggers warm and happy memories like nothing else can do. They feed us doubly—both with calories and with contentment. Whether they fit into our formal diet plan or not, they are a crucial part of our nutritional armament.

Be sure you always have some of these in the house. When you want nothing else to eat, they may still, often, look tempting.

Adjusting to Medications

Notice if poor appetite, or the symptoms that induce it, are associated with the medicines you take. If these are temporary medicines, or if symptoms resolve within a week or two, it shouldn't pose much of a problem. But some of these medicines must be taken for a long time. And giving them up, in order to eat more, isn't usually productive; remember, if disease is active and unopposed, absorption and proper use of nutrients are impaired. You have to fix the car, as well as fill the gas tank.

There are ways to help your body tolerate these medicines, by adjusting the way in which they are prescribed. We'll talk about that more in Chapter Thirteen. But you can make improvements yourself, even without your doctor's help.

When taking medicine on an empty stomach is not specifically prescribed, try taking your pills with food or just after eating. Split them up: take your vitamins separately, for instance.

A water-based vitamin E preparation may be more tolerable than an oil-based one. If you can't keep food down at all, there are sublingual, or under-the-tongue, preparations of some vitamins. You will note, though, that dosages are smaller in these preparations.

Pay attention to the medicines you buy over the counter, too. Aspirin and ibuprofen, for instance, may cause stomach pain, nausea, or heartburn. If this is so for you, try to do without them.

A recent study begun in New York to look at the possible benefits of aspirin in HIV was halted before completion, because aspirin was shown to lower glutathione levels. (We discussed glutathione in Chapter Five. It's a substance the cell uses to reduce the state of oxidative stress in which the virus thrives.)

One would assume that other anti-inflammatory drugs, such as ibuprofen, might have the same effect. Acetaminophen, or Tylenol, also requires glutathione if it is to be broken down without toxic by-products.

That doesn't mean you can't take these medicines, if they help you to feel better in other ways. You have to take something for fever or pain sometimes. And interestingly, ibuprofen has been shown to dampen the inflammatory effects of cytokines in rats. So there may be some compensatory benefit. But be alert for the indirect impact of these medicines on your appetite, if they make you uncomfortable. Make sure the net effect is positive.

If you are protecting your glutathione reserves by supplementing with NAC and antioxidants, as suggested in Chapters Four and Five, I recommend acetaminophen first. And if aspirin or ibuprofen don't upset your stomach, it's okay to take them too.

Mouth, Throat, and Esophageal Lesions

If you have thrush or herpes, your doctor will have prescribed medicines to fight them. There are also medicines that soothe or numb the pain. You can buy liquid antacids like Maalox or Mylanta without a prescription and swish them around in your mouth. Kaopectate will work in the same way.

Sucrets and other anesthetic lozenges help numb a sore throat before eating. Artificial saliva preparations like Oralube or Mouth Kote can ease the pain of a dry mouth. Drinking liquids freely with your food will help you chew and swallow.

Cold foods are soothing and are better than warm ones when your mouth or throat is sore. Chewing ice can help. Avoiding highly spiced foods helps too.

Avoiding Malabsorption

Reducing the fat in your diet may help you avoid the fullness and cramping associated with fat malabsorption. Again, there's a role here for eating your main meal first.

Addressing Diarrhea

If diarrhea is triggered by eating, try taking your antidiarrheal medicines half an hour to an hour before you eat. Also, eat as much as you can when you do eat; in this case larger, less frequent meals will initiate fewer episodes.

Don't push the vitamin C. One to three grams a day should be okay; more may exacerbate diarrhea.

Avoid fatty foods. The BRATT diet—bananas, rice, applesauce, tea, and toast—favored by pediatricians for kids with diarrhea, is especially easy to digest.

The use of Gatorade or other electrolyte-balanced sports drinks will help replace molecules lost from your blood because of diarrhea.

Lactose Intolerance

Watch out for milk products. Don't deny yourself ice cream if it's your favorite food, but be on guard for its effects on your body and your appetite, and adjust your intake accordingly. If milk products give you discomfort, try Lactaid or other commercial products that aid lactose digestion. You can also buy special milk products made for people with lactose intolerance. These have special bacteria added to provide what's needed to break down milk sugars.

Changes in Taste and Smell

Susan Schiffman of Duke University reports on a study in which people with HIV with disturbances in taste or smell were given foods with flavor enhancement. These were commercial flavor additives made for the food industry. Green pea flavoring was added to green peas, for instance; pork, roast beef, and other flavors were added to other foods. As Dr. Schiffman's earlier research has shown with elderly nursing home residents, who also had a reduced or altered sense of smell or taste, appetite and food intake increased in subjects with HIV.

What is particularly promising about this study for people with HIV is that workers reported an improvement in weight as well. This was a small study, and lean body mass was not measured. However, the results match those shown by Dr. Schiffman in studies with thousands of elderly subjects—studies that, in addition to weight gain, showed improved absorption of foods with flavor supplementation.

Thus it is possible that enhancing the taste of food not only helps us to eat more, but may actually help us to absorb what we eat, and hence use what we eat, better.

This work is still very new. But it does hold promise. It may be worth a try, even for those of us cooking at home, if altered taste and smell are a part of our appetite problem. Commercial flavor additives are sold in large quantities and are, therefore, somewhat impractical for home use. But buyers' clubs might consider serving as purchasing agents.

You may also want to explore this approach more simply, by increasing the amount of your favorite spices or the sugar or salt in your food. In fact, this may be why people with HIV often crave high-sugar snacks and foods that are heavily spiced.

Sugar in the Diet

There is controversy over the use of sugar. Many people who refuse or avoid standard treatments for HIV, trying to control their illness through natural means only, feel that high sugar intake should be avoided. It's felt that sugar in the diet increases the likelihood and intensity of yeast infections such as oral thrush.

If you don't take medicines to fight yeast infections, this may well be true. A higher concentration of sugar in the saliva probably makes it easier for untreated fungal infections to grow and thrive. But it seems to me that avoiding processed sugar carries with it a high price—one that is significantly more costly than that of taking medicine to protect against fungal infection.

People with HIV need calories. Quantity, as well as quality. And we need to eat things that we'll absorb. Simple sugars are among the things the body absorbs most easily. And simple sugars are what the body must make from most of the foods absorbed anyway, to satisfy energy requirements and protect protein stores. It's when we run low on sugars that we start breaking down proteins to provide for our energy needs.

And, as we saw in Chapter Two, the HIV-infected body does not break down fats well, to convert them to sugars for energy. So the body spends sugars preferentially—and when it runs out it must spend proteins to make more.

I am much more concerned with maintaining protein stores—our lean body mass—than I am about avoiding medicine for fungal infections. And I'm much more concerned that people eat what tastes good, getting pleasure from their food along with calories.

There are so many sacrifices, so many adaptations, that we must make to honor our bodies and stay healthy with HIV. It seems to me excessive to give up more than we have to.

Depression and Fatigue

These indirect threats to your appetite will be addressed in Chapter Seven.

• • •

There are other ways to improve your appetite or reduce the symptoms that attack it, which you can work out with your doctor. One of the most interesting is marijuana or medical marijuana derivatives. Marijuana and its effects on appetite will be discussed in Chapters Eight and Twelve. Other appetite enhancers are also available by prescription; we'll talk about them later in this book as well.

REFERENCES

Little, A. C. "Appetite, food intake and nutritional status among AIDS/ARC patients." Unpublished study, 1990, Berkeley, personal communication.

Schiffman, S. "Taste and smell in disease." *New England Journal of Medicine,* 1983, *308*(21–22), 1275–1279, 1337–1343.

Schiffman, S. "Anorexia and dysgeusia in the elderly." *Malnutrition in the Hospitalized Patient,* Harvard Medical School Conference, 1994.

Schiffman, S. S., and Warwick. "Effect of flavor enhancement of foods for the elderly on nutritional status: Food intake, biochemical indices and anthropometric measures." *Physiology and Behavior,* 1993, *53,* 395–402.

Ullrich, R., and others. "Small intestinal structure and function in patients infected with human immunodeficiency virus (HIV): Evidence for HIV-induced enteropathy." *Annals of Internal Medicine,* 1989, *111,* 15–21.

CHAPTER 7

•

Improving
Your Environment

There are other factors that directly and indirectly affect the way you get your food, and therefore your nutrition. Some of them involve access to food, some the means of preparing it, and others the state you're in when you receive it.

How You Get Your Food
•

If you're able to buy and prepare your own food, you're ready to go. You know what you want, and by now you know what's good for you. Make the most of the energy available for the task.

Shopping for Food

Make a list: include foods you love and foods that offer natural nutrition. Be sure to include foods from all the basic groups we talked about in Chapter Three.

Prioritize your shopping, so that if you tire, you will have gotten the essential things first.

Prioritize your spending, too. Again, start with the things you love most and the things you need most. Spread the money a little thinner, if you need to, on the rest of your purchases and on impulse buying.

Ideally, you should be able to open the refrigerator or the cupboard and see something that appeals to you at once and that can be eaten while you still want it.

Often, you can find good deals on fruits and vegetables that are just at, or almost past, their prime. Realize that some of their vitamin value may be lost. But if you are taking supplements, you should be okay. And fresh foods are especially satisfying.

Pay special attention to your list of comfort foods. Be sure you always have some of these in the house. When you want nothing else to eat, these may often still look tempting.

When Others Shop for You

If others are doing your shopping for you, you need to educate them.

If possible, make out a list. Again, list the foods you love and the foods you most need, paying special attention to protein, good sources of calories, and diversity. Draw from the food groups discussed in Chapter Three.

Ask your shoppers, as well as your food preparers, to be careful about greasy foods or any other foods that make you uncomfortable. Tell them what spices and flavorings you like.

Your shoppers may be friends or family members. If so, enlist them in your battle—they may not know what's good for you, but they want what's good for you.

If you have an attendant who does your shopping, be specific in your directions. Don't be afraid to hurt anyone's feelings by expressing your preferences. One of the things you can do for yourself and for others is to give clear instructions.

Insofar as you can afford it, ask for the brands and the types of food you like best—snacks, especially. If money is a problem, be sure your shoppers understand how important protein is. Tofu, or soy protein, is a cheap and healthy protein source and is easily digested. So are fresh eggs.

Most people will be happy to learn from you what you now know. They want to do a good job, too, and they will be excited to feel they are a part of your health and improvement. Some will even want to read this book along with you, so they can better understand their contribution to your continued health.

Success is addictive; and praise, when well earned, is the best drug in the world. So even if your friends, or your partner or family members, or whoever does your legwork are a little miffed at first by your taking charge here, they will learn. And you will have made them your allies.

Preparation of Food
•

Food, once purchased, must be properly prepared. If you have a working kitchen, this shouldn't be a problem.

Methods of Cooking

Don't overcook fruits and vegetables, or much of their nutritional value may be lost. If you can, use the cooking water in soups, or in sauces, for cooking your pasta or rice. That way, vitamins that have been transferred to the cooking liquid will still be part of your nutrition. If you use your cooking liquids in this way, do so at once; bacteria multiply quickly in cooled, unrefrigerated vegetable or fruit broths.

Don't *undercook* meats, fish, or poultry. It's okay to eat beef or lamb medium rare, as long as the center of the meat is hot; but pork and poultry must be well cooked to be safe. This includes duck, which is sometimes incompletely cooked on purpose for better flavor.

There's a simpler way to be sure that baked or roasted meats, fish, and poultry are fully cooked. Place a skewer, or a thin knife, in the fleshiest part of the meat; if it comes out smoothly, and the juice that runs out is clear and not red, you will know that it's ready to eat.

If you like beef or lamb rare, buy a meat thermometer. A temperature of 140 degrees in the deepest part of the meat should offer safety, without compromising flavor or texture.

Long, slow cooking of meats or stews may reduce some of their vitamin content. Still, if this kind of cooking produces foods you enjoy, don't deny yourself. It's important to like what you eat. The vitamins that are not destroyed, but have leached into the sauce, will still be available to you. And one of the reasons vitamin supplements are so important is that they allow you to eat foods the way you like them, by making up for vitamins lost.

Cut away any bruised, softened, or darkened portions of fruits and vegetables before you eat them.

Consider cooking vegetables without peeling them. Much of their vitamin content is found in their skin. Even if you don't eat the skin, you'll get more vitamins this way. And the cooked skin will peel away easily.

If you add salt, do so when you eat rather than in cooking. This will help preserve vitamin content.

Cooking is often uneven in microwaved food. Be sure any microwaved food is hot throughout, before you eat it.

Pay attention to your food's appearance. Bright colors, such as those found in beets or red and yellow peppers, make a stew or casserole look more appetizing. Placing an assortment of different foods on your plate with a balance of color, texture, and flavor can boost your appetite.

We know from research on smell and taste receptors that they adapt quickly to a given flavor; thus if you can eat first one food, then another, the taste of the first food will be stronger when you come back to it. Also, if you fill up quickly, you will have gotten a little of everything first.

Avoiding Infection from Food

Fresh fruits and vegetables eaten raw should be well washed to avoid infection from surface bacteria. One way to reduce the chance of infection is to add two drops of tincture of iodine — available at pharmacies — to a sinkful of water. You can wash fruits and vegetables in this first, and then rinse them well with clear water. Two drops are plenty; you want the antiseptic effect, but you don't want to oversupplement your iodine intake, as this may affect thyroid regulation.

Wash the vegetables you plan to cook, too.

Meat, fish, and poultry should be refrigerated quickly, both before preparation and after eating. When raw meat, fish, or poultry is cut or handled on a kitchen surface, that surface should be washed well as soon as you or your helper are finished. Your iodine-treated sink water is good for this. Poultry, in particular, can be teeming with diarrhea-causing bacteria when it's raw.

Hands should be washed, too—*always* before preparation; after preparation; before and after handling meat, fish, or poultry; before touching any other food; and even before serving.

Bacteria in the food are not your only concern; you also don't want to acquire someone else's germs as she or he prepares your food. Many people can carry infections that don't bother them if their immune system is fully competent. You are more at risk.

Don't leave food out after cooking. Clean up and put food away as soon as your meal is finished. Especially watch out for egg, meat, or poultry and mayonnaise combinations, which can breed salmonella.

Have the courage to throw food away if it's been in the refrigerator too long. If you think it might be old, then it's old. Even if you cook contaminated food long enough to kill the germs, there may be toxins from bacterial growth that can cause food poisoning.

Don't eat anything that's moldy.

Don't eat raw meat or raw fish. Sushi made just before eating from fresh, *cooked* fish is acceptable; otherwise avoid it. Steak tartare (made from raw beef) is not safe for you; toxoplasmosis is a real concern for people with HIV and can be acquired from raw beef.

When you reheat leftovers, reheat them fully. Don't refreeze what's been defrosted. If food has been defrosted, use it quickly.

Don't eat anything that even hints of tasting spoiled. Watch out in particular for purchased, prepared, homestyle dishes. You don't know how long they've been sitting there before you buy them. The risks are greater for you than for the average consumer.

If there are expiration dates listed for freshness, respect those dates. Be aware that many stores and supermarkets illegally sell out-of-date foods at a discount to get rid of them. This may offer an acceptable level of risk for healthy people, but it's too much risk for you.

If you don't have access to a refrigerator, don't buy perishable food—especially meat, fish, or poultry—that you can't consume in a day.

Avoiding Infection from Water
•

An area of real concern is avoidance of infection from the water we drink. While bottled or filtered water may be a luxury for some, for people with HIV it can be a lifesaver. Organisms that live in water, and make it through the filters and disinfection procedures of your local water supply, may also make it past your immune system, to set up housekeeping in your gut. This may show up as diarrhea. Or, if your own immune system can control the invaders now, they may show themselves only later, at a time when you are less equipped to fight them. Cryptosporidium is the parasite of greatest concern, although there are others. It can also be found in well water.

Infection with cryptosporidium may also be seen in people who are HIV-negative. In most cases, though, infection is short, and the organism is completely cleared. In the presence of HIV, eradication is harder. As a result of HIV and AIDS immunosuppression over the past decade, cryptosporidial infection has been recognized as a cause of illness all over the world.

Cryptosporidium oocysts are tiny and can pass undetected through the filters of your local water supply. They can pass through many home filters, too. I recommend drinking bottled water—if possible from a bottler who screens closely for cryptosporidium. Distilled water is also likely to be safe.

If you prefer to use a filter at home, be sure to get one with adequate cryptosporidium filtration. You'll find a list of bottled water and filters that are considered relatively safe for you in Appendix XI. That appendix also reviews the best ways to avoid cryptosporidium infection.

If it costs too much to pay for safe water or a filtration system, boiling water is a good alternative. Just remember, ice cubes and water used to wash raw food should also be boiled for protection.

Cryptosporidium is not sensitive to chlorine, so it can be acquired from public swimming pools. Be careful not to swallow water if you swim. And watch out for wave pools in amusement parks. It's hard not to swallow water when it's coming at you.

Feeding Programs

Keeping food fresh and safe is especially hard for people who don't have kitchen facilities. If you are one of these people, you should try hard to qualify for a feeding program. In many major cities there are feeding programs specifically for people with HIV. These programs deliver the food fresh and cooked. If you don't try to save it without refrigeration, but eat it when it comes, you'll do well.

Here in San Francisco we have Project Open Hand. This remarkable organization delivers hot meals and bags of groceries to people with symptomatic HIV disease.

Delivery starts on the day it is requested. Meals for the homeless are delivered to the street corner of their choice at a predetermined time on a daily basis. An Open Hand food bank allows people to shop for their own free food, if they are able; others receive a bag of groceries a week.

Menus are designed to satisfy ethnic and cultural preferences, as well as special nutritional needs. Client preferences and complaints receive immediate and painstaking attention.

Every client has an opportunity to consult with and be followed by a dietician specializing in HIV nutrition. Where indicated, supplements are provided to those with evidence of wasting. Those who still lose weight can be referred to a specialized clinic for HIV, for basic wasting interventions and for experimental programs when all else fails.

Meals are delivered by volunteers. Every penny received from contributions goes directly to the provision of food.

It's a privilege to be involved with an organization like this. Other programs around the country look to it as a model.

In our travels around the country to talk to people with HIV, my friend Bruce and I have met many of the women and men who dedicate themselves to making such programs work. Because of these people, the programs are remarkable. There's a personal feeling to them, and a quality of sharing that transcends the provision of food.

Each program has its own flavor. Some are part of family service programs, or drug rehabilitation efforts. Some perform the important task of bringing people together to eat as a family. And others, like Project Open Hand, specialize in bringing food to people who are homebound. Almost all offer nutritional counseling, adapted to the values and culture of the city and the people that they serve.

You can find out if there's an HIV feeding program in your town by calling your local AIDS service organization. The discharge planning or social service departments of your local hospital will be able to direct you, too. In addition, you'll find a list of HIV-associated feeding programs in major cities in Appendix X.

Even in places where there is no specifically designated HIV feeding program, there are "Meals on Wheels" programs that deliver foods to shut-ins. While the nutritional focus may not be as precise, it is often possible to request certain special diets. A high-protein, high-calorie, low-fat diet should meet your needs well.

The Importance of Shelter
•

A special problem not well addressed in our country is the problem of maintaining nutritional and basic health status in people with HIV who lack shelter.

HIV in the Homeless

Responding to HIV infection is difficult under the best of circumstances. For those who are homeless, the problems are infinitely greater.

Exposure carries with it its own threats to the immune system. Tuberculosis is much more common. Illness is more frequent and harder to cure when people are cold and tired. Proper nutrition is almost impossible when you have no place to prepare or store your food. The dangers of rape and violence are magnified. Access to birth control, even simple barrier protection, is limited. Access to medical care is much more difficult.

Every person with HIV needs dignity and respect, food and shelter, clothing and medical care. The societal and economic implications of allowing sick people to exist in our culture, without these basic requirements, are overwhelming. Programs like Project Open Hand at least make a start at dealing with the problems our governments have not properly addressed.

If you are among the homeless, you need to hook up with social services and try to find shelter. This is often more easily said than done. But one good strategy is to be vocal about your problems. You can request assignment to a social worker in your city, for starters. You can register at a clinic for medical care. In major cities, there may be drop-in centers for the homeless. If not, you can learn where to go for help by contacting your local AIDS society.

Often, your break comes when you are hospitalized. In order to discharge you, a hospital has to show that you have a place to go to and adequate social supports. Thus, you have the resources of their discharge planners and their social service department at your disposal.

When you're in the hospital, they *want* you on public assistance if you have no money; otherwise they don't get paid for your care. So they're willing to do the highly skilled work of getting you that assistance. Unless you are willing to go back to the street, they *have* to help you; if you don't have a place to go, they must keep you. And that's expensive.

Thus hospital social workers and discharge planners can be your best allies. They can plug you in to welfare and Medicaid, refer you to a clinic for outpatient medical care, set you up for feeding programs, and give you a fresh change of clothes. But they are overworked, and you will have to ask.

Hospitals are legally required to arrange at least temporary housing before they let you go. If you need it and request it, your social worker or discharge planner can often get you placed on a waiting list for a drug treatment program. These people can refer you to clinics that will help you fight your habit while you wait for placement. They can get you assigned to a city or county social worker. Often they can refer you to free programs that provide the medicines you need.

And if you know they have to do it, they will do it. Ask them. This is one of the best and most elemental examples of what people with HIV can do for themselves.

If You Have Shelter

If you have a place to live, try to organize it so it supports you.

Medical equipment should be kept, when possible, in one room, so that the rest of your home retains a sense of normalcy. If it's dark inside, open the shades or use lights freely. Make sure it's warm enough.

Fill your home with things that make you happy—photos of

people you love, for instance. I know that, in my apartment, I need my shells and rocks around me.

Open the windows regularly, or get someone to do it for you, so the air smells fresh and clean. If you respond to fragrance, add it—with air fresheners, scented candles, potpourri. Health food stores sell an air freshener called Orange Mate, or Lime Mate, made entirely from the essence of the fruit and peel. Its scent is light and fresh, but it will neutralize sickroom smells and brighten stale air for days. Perfumed soaps, kept out in the bathroom, will fill the room with fragrance.

Avoid smoking cigarettes in the house—apart from any direct effect, you don't want to live with the smell of stale tobacco smoke.

Avoid loose-lying rugs, tangled phone cords, or other things on the floor that could cause you to trip and fall.

Do everything you can to avoid clutter. It's depressing. If you can't keep things orderly yourself, apply for an attendant.

Bright colors, warmth and light and air, mementos, fragrance, simplicity, and order—all these things can help make your home a place of healing.

Other Challenges
•

The dangers to our health posed by fatigue or emotional distress can also be confronted.

Fatigue

Even when you're really weary, you can sometimes compensate by husbanding your energy—shopping for, cleaning, and preparing food when your strength is at its best—so you can eat without effort during down times. You can even eat in bed if you need to. And often, just eating a little will give you an extra lift.

Much of the problem of fatigue is that it's self-perpetuating. The longer we stay in bed, the harder it is to get up. There is actual deconditioning, a loss of muscle strength, that results from disuse. You have to balance this, then—not pushing yourself to the point of exhaustion, but pushing just a little when you can. Even lying in bed, you can exercise your arms and legs.

Anyone who is too tired to make her or his own food should qualify for a community feeding program.

Depression or Confusion

When you're too sad to eat or you just can't seem to care enough to make your food, it's time to get help from others.

Finding emotional support from people who care for you is a start. Friends can help. Support groups play a real role here, too. Studies have shown that women with breast cancer who attended a support group not only felt better, but lived longer—a lot longer. We are less disabled by our pain when we know we're not alone. We'll talk more about the importance of support groups later in this book.

More practical support can come in the form of feeding programs, which at least remove the effort of preparing food. We've addressed the help they can offer already. But overcoming true depression often takes more than that. If you're depressed and unable to function enough to take care of your needs, it's time to ask for help.

We'll talk more about this when we talk about what you can do with your doctor. There are medicines and treatments that can help you take hold of your life again. It's also possible to talk to people who are trained to help you work this through, at the same time. But the critical thing is to seek help early, before you're too immobilized to do so. And you will be the first one to know when that is.

If you find you are sad and listless for two weeks or more; if you find you're not eating because you don't care; if you're not getting out of bed; if you don't want to answer the phone or the door; if you're turning away from family or friends; if you think life is really this bad, and it's going to be this way forever; if you're thinking of killing yourself—it's time to stop listening to your body and start asking for help. When your body thinks like that, *your body is wrong.*

If your pain, or the danger of suicide, is even more acute, call the hot line first and the doctor second. But reach out while you can. Suicide is rarely a reasoned decision, but rather an impulsive response to suffering that is too great to be borne alone.

Much of the time these feelings are based in a chemical imbalance and respond well to medications—medications without major side effects or danger of addiction—that can help you correct what is an incorrect view of your circumstances. These medicines won't take away your problems, but they can leave you with the strength to address them.

Confusion and memory loss, so frightening when they appear, are often features of clinical depression. And even when they're not—when they directly reflect HIV's effects on the brain—there are still ways to treat or reverse them.

You can't deal with this by yourself. And you must deal with it. If you simply stop eating, you will simply stop living. You will become a victim of your illness, rather than the guardian of your health that you've worked so hard to become.

None of these conditions—exhaustion, depression, confusion, memory loss—are things to be ashamed of. And in almost every case, none of them need be permanent. Ask for help quickly; don't wait until you are too overwhelmed to do so.

Loneliness

When we're healthy, we live in the world—going to work or school, playing with friends or strangers, following our recreational interests. All of these things put us with other people.

We have stresses or victories at work that we share; we have dinner with friends; we have love affairs; we have sex. The richness and complexity of life is shared with others.

But when you're tired, you cut back on such activities. And if you're also weak and homebound, you lose access to all of these pleasures. When life is constricted by the limits of strength, one major problem is the loss of human interaction.

None of us were made to be alone all the time. In fact, the loss of companionship has been shown to be associated with immune suppression and a greater tendency toward illness.

Take a look at what's available to you. If you have friends, let them know you want company. In particular, try to share a meal when they come by. If you're a member of a church or synagogue, ask for a regular visitor. If you don't have these supports, look for others.

Many AIDS organizations have volunteers who provide emotional support. They can drop in to visit or just hang out. This is not charity; these volunteers find enormous reward in the work they do. Many of them are HIV-positive themselves and feel that time so spent contributes to their own health and survival.

Some of my patients who volunteer as companions tell me that this is the only time they really relax. They are too busy, or place too many demands on themselves, to watch TV, play Scrabble, or enjoy other activities for their own sake. Often the first step to understanding their own need for recreation is to share it for the sake of someone else.

If you are homebound, and have a social worker or case manager, inquire about the possibility of attendant care. Medicaid will often cover this. It's nice to get your bed made or your dishes done, but the company is even more important.

Loneliness can often be eased by the presence of a pet in the house, too. This has been shown to improve life, and prolong health, in shut-ins. And it gives you a chance to feel useful again, providing care for another being.

Choose a pet that will not require more care than you can manage. Dogs and cats are the most common choice. If they require too much work, birds or small mammals (guinea pigs, gerbils, or hamsters) can provide company.

Be sure your pet is not a source of infection. If you have or are getting a cat, for instance, have it checked for toxoplasmosis. Use cedar shavings, which make less dust than commercial cat litter, in the litter box. Make sure the box is big enough so that you only have to clean it once or twice a week. Wear a mask when you do so. Birds and small mammals should also be checked for infections.

You may have a pet already. If not, consider adopting one, so you can know you are saving a life.

REFERENCES

Blaney, N. T., and others. "A stress-moderator model of distress in early HIV-1 infection: Concurrent analysis of life events, hardiness and social support." *Journal of Psychosomatic Research*, 1991, *35*(2–3), 297–304.

Bridgman, S. A., and others. "Outbreak of cryptosporidiosis associated with a disinfected groundwater supply." *Epidemiology and Infection*, 1995, *115*(3), 555–566.

deAbramowvich, B.L., and others. "Detection of cryptosporidium in sub-terranean drinking water." *Revista Argentina de Microbiología*, 1996, *28*(2), 73–77.

Jacobsburg, L. B., and Perry. "Psychiatric disturbances." *Medical Clinics of North America*, 1992, *76*(1), 99–106.

Keusch, G. T., and others. "Cryptosporidia: Who is at risk?" *Schweizerische Medizinische Wochenschrift, Journal Suisse de Médecine*, 1995, *125*(18), 899–908.

MacKenzie, W. R., and others. "A massive outbreak in Milwaukee of cryptosporidium infection transmitted through the public water supply." *New England Journal of Medicine*, 1994, *331*(3), 161–167.

McAnulty, J. M., and others. "A community-wide outbreak of cryptosporidiosis associated with swimming at a wave pool." *Journal of the American Medical Association*, 1994, *272*(20), 1597–1600.

Nieminski, E. C., and others. "Comparison of two methods for detection of giardia cysts and cryptosporidium oocysts in water." *Applied and Environmental Microbiology*, 1995, *61*(5), 1714–1719.

Spiegel, D., and others. "Effect of psychosocial treatment on survival of patients with metastatic breast cancer." *Lancet*, 1989, *2*(8668), 888–891.

Srp, F., and others. "Psychosocial issues of nutritional support." *Nursing Clinics of North America*, 1989, *24*(2), 447–459.

Staats, J., and others. "Effect of neuropsychiatric signs and symptoms on homeless persons with AIDS in a group residence." *International Conference on AIDS*, 1989, *5*, 388.

CHAPTER 8

•

Sex, Drugs,
and Exercise

As you probably realize by now, living well with HIV and fighting its progression can be a full-time job. And no one can do it but you. You are the one who will choose how much effort to give it, and how much change you are willing to make.

For some people, the renewed love for life they experience when a potentially life-threatening illness is diagnosed makes such changes easy and welcome, particularly if they know it will help them do better. For others, change may still be quite difficult.

At the Center for Attitudinal Healing in Tiburon, California, where I worked as a facilitator during my residency training, there are ongoing support groups, run for and by people with serious illness. The members of my group—chiefly people living with cancer or HIV—had a name for other, healthy people. They called them "the temporary immortals"—people who had not yet faced any direct threat to their lives, whose concerns and life issues were therefore, they believed, more superficial.

All of us—facilitators and members—grew quite close. We often preferred one another's company. Our concerns seemed

more valid; our longings less frivolous; our ability to see and respond to real pain and real joy more substantive; our relationships
more authentic. We felt we were wiser. Certainly I learned more in
those two-hour group meetings than I ever learned in ten years of
college.

All of us are going to die one day. Some of us know it. And that
makes decisions, hard choices, much simpler. We don't want to
throw life away.

So if you are ready to look, really look, at your life, and at the
results of the choices you make, then you can really take charge.

You control or can learn to control other facets of your
lifestyle, beyond what you eat, that will help maximize your nutritional status. They concern attitudes and behaviors that are at the
very root of how we live, or even who we consider ourselves to be.
Sex is one of them. Our choice of mood-altering drugs, including
alcohol and cigarettes, is another. Our commitment to fitness and
exercise is another. In each of these categories, HIV infection may
give us a chance to rethink our priorities.

Remember, anything that speeds replication of the virus speeds
the circumstances that favor wasting. Any new infection, on top of
HIV, triggers the changes in nutrient use that lead to wasting. Any
added stress you subject your body to will promote viral production, put you at risk for infection, and directly threaten your nutritional status.

Sexual Behaviors
•

Much has been written about practicing safe sex, or safer sex, in
order to avoid HIV infection. Issues that are particularly relevant
to people who are already HIV-positive have received less attention.

Many people who are HIV-positive feel that sex is no longer an
option for them. Their concern about infecting their partner over-
whelms their conscience, and sometimes their desire. But now that
we can extend survival, and perhaps live out our whole life, we
need to address the quality of that life more than ever. Physical intimacy, as Paul Volberding says, "is as essential to well-being as
proper nourishment." Dr. Volberding suggests that people with

HIV may in fact have a greater need for such intimacy than most people, because they have often had to make do with less; and that sex is "too primal, too pleasurable, and too central to human identity for most people to give up."

The question, then, is not whether to have sex but how to do so — how to maximize the pleasure and minimize the risks of sexual activity to your partner and yourself.

Of course you don't want to risk passing the virus to someone you love or make love to. But in many of the acts that might raise this concern, you are at great risk as well.

To begin with, we know that the virus progresses much faster in the presence of another infection. So if you are already HIV-positive, getting herpes or gonorrhea or chlamydia or hepatitis B — all transmitted in unprotected sex — can speed your progression to AIDS, or increase the severity of your infection at any stage. Gonorrhea, in any orifice, can be asymptomatic, but deadly in its stimulation of the virus. Syphilis can be hard to eradicate in people with HIV. Genital warts, or condyloma, are also of special concern, as these are caused by papilloma virus. Several strains of papilloma virus — not always the same ones that lead to venereal warts — can cause the cells to lose their internal controls and proceed to cancer. Often this can happen even when warts themselves are not found.

Unprotected Anal Sex

We think of the danger of condyloma especially in women, where cervical cancer can result. We now know that the same risks apply to any receptive partner, and that anal carcinoma is much more likely in a person who has been sexually exposed to papilloma virus. Risk factors include a history of receptive anal intercourse, a CD4 count below 500, and a history of high-grade cervical intraepithelial neoplasia on a women's pap smear. People with these risk factors should be tested annually by anal pap smear and referred for further workup if pap smears are abnormal.

Unprotected anal intercourse carries other risks, as well. Many of the organisms that cause diarrhea in people with HIV are easily controlled in people whose immune system is healthy. They can carry these germs — *you* can carry these germs — and not know it. If you don't have them, you don't want to get them.

Some of these agents are hard to get rid of, even in healthy people. Others are harder to treat in the setting of HIV. But healthy people, positive or negative, can keep them suppressed, and not suffer diarrhea or other symptoms.

So if you are not already carrying any of these parasites—cryptosporidium, for instance, or microsporidium—you can acquire them through anal contact and not know you have them.

Your immune system, however, pays an immediate price for that control. The virus spreads faster with immune activation, and your body's efforts to control the invasion of another parasite can result in increased HIV replication.

And, most concerning of all, you are risking your health *later*. No matter how high your CD4 count is now, there may come a time when it's low. If you don't have other stressors, you can go on just fine. But if you do—if you are chronically carrying organisms your body can no longer suppress—those organisms will cause diarrhea. You may never be able to fix it. And HIV replication will increase as a result of your body's attempts to clear those organisms.

In advanced stages of HIV, cryptosporidium and microsporidium are incredibly hard to treat. They are among the most common, the most direct, and the most drastic precipitants of wasting.

Often we just can't make headway. So we have to resort to expensive nutritional treatments, trying to make up for nutrients lost, and to regimens that control diarrhea mechanically. But we still can't block the metabolic changes, in response to infection, that foster the wasting syndrome.

If you already have these infections, there are things you can try with your doctor. But if you don't have them, *you don't want them.*

Acquiring New Strains of HIV

It's also important to understand the natural history of the HIV virus itself once it's made its way into your body. HIV has a remarkable capacity to mutate, or change. That's why vaccines are so hard to design and why antiretroviral drugs used separately, or drugs used in combination at subtherapeutic doses, will always lose their power over time. The virus studies its environment, figures out what stops it, and redesigns some of its offspring to survive in that same environment. As it gets smarter in successive generations, it evolves into more virulent forms. Some of these forms can cause groups of your cells to run together (syncytium-forming strains), so that many cells at once can become infected.

You may be able to stop, and can certainly delay, these changes in your own body's HIV population. But to do that, you need every weapon you can get. You can avoid speeding progression by not acquiring, during unprotected sex, those forms of the virus that are already more sophisticated and harder to fight than the strains you currently carry. This is more true now than ever, as many people with HIV are using multiple, very strong antiretroviral combinations. Even if their viral load is undetectable, some virus is still present; it is part of a long chain of viruses that have been working to exist in the presence of those very strong drugs. If some of that virus comes into your body, it will carry with it the genetic memory of how to survive despite some of the strongest weapons we have against HIV. And those weapons are likely not to work for you. So even in the presence of excellent treatment and suppression, even in the absence of detectable viral load, unprotected sex with an HIV-positive person carries grave risks regardless of your own HIV status.

This is one of the reasons, I think, why it becomes so important for all of us to develop the art of gratitude. This reprieve we've been given, with better drugs and better monitoring and more political clout to promote better access, is not an infinite gift. It's a second chance, an opportunity, to live out a full life. It's not a guarantee. And as so many of us feel healthy again, and begin to express that health in a renewed sexuality, we must not be careless with it. If we are we will throw it away.

We already have documentation of transmission of multidrug-resistant HIV from one person to another. And Daniel Berger in Chicago, who uses genotypes to follow HIV-resistance patterns in a selected group of patients, reports a change in genotype for some of those patients—with the new appearance of viruses resistant to drugs that these people have never seen. When questioned, these people report a return to patterns of unprotected sexual intercourse. A rigorously designed study will be needed to support these data, but the implications are clear. For these people, precious weaponry has been lost. And progression can be much more vicious and unrelenting. No matter how healthy you or your partner feel, or how encouraging your lab tests are, you need to put a rubber on it.

So, all HIV viruses are not created equal. You're stuck with yours. You don't want somebody else's.

Unprotected Oral Sex

It's also important to look at other means of transmission, or infection. Statistics tell us that HIV is transmitted most frequently by receptive anal intercourse. That makes oral sex look much safer, and it probably is. But those statistics are affected by the way we compile them.

If you've had seven thousand acts of unprotected oral sex prior to documented infection, and one act of receptive anal sex, your means of infection will still be documented as receptive anal sex. Thus thousands of cases of HIV transmitted by oral sex are hidden within the statistics. Given this method of statistical reporting, we actually have no way of knowing how many instances of HIV transmission have occurred through oral sex. So unprotected oral sex, while it doesn't carry as much risk as unprotected receptive anal sex, is not as benign as it seems.

Even if your partner is also HIV-positive, there are grave risks for both of you with unprotected sexual intercourse. If you're going to do it, put a rubber on it first.

Right now, there's a lot of political debate in the HIV community about these issues. After years of being careful, people start to let their guard down. Here in San Francisco, the reported use of condoms for oral sex is low—even among those activists who dedicate their time to fighting HIV.

Gay men with HIV have lost more than friends and lovers to HIV, more even than their own health. They have lost the expression of a way of life that was fundamental, in the past, to their culture. As they become accustomed to living with their illness, and to the fear of coinfection, they rebel. Even receptive anal sex, without a condom, is increasing. And as symptoms resolve and the certainty of death recedes because of new treatments, it's more tempting to let go of the discipline that we practiced for so long. This may be especially true now, when our hopes are higher, but the price is too. Survival can be purchased, but at the cost of so much regimentation and self-control. Sometimes we just get sick of it. Sometimes we just say "screw it." Sometimes we do.

Many activists believe the time has come to settle for preaching relative risk. They don't think everyone will settle for constant barrier protection, any more than they will settle for abstinence. So these activists concentrate on urging condoms for the riskiest behaviors—receptive anal intercourse, receptive vaginal intercourse, sex during menstruation—and *avoiding oral-anal contact.*

I agree. If you're not willing to use rubbers, you are better off with oral sex than with any of these other behaviors. If you do have unprotected oral sex, at least be careful not to take ejaculate, or the fluid that precedes it, into your mouth. Other precautions, offering partial protection, include not douching, which disturbs the balance of vaginal secretions; not brushing or flossing your teeth before oral sexual activity, to reduce the risk of infection through irritated tissue; aggressive prevention and treatment of gum disease; and avoiding open sores in the mouth or on the genitals. That way, your risk is lower.

But your risk remains.

Good Sex, Healthy Sex
•

What then, can people with HIV do to permit themselves a satisfying sexual lifestyle? To begin with, they can educate themselves. Often, they will also educate their partners. It's particularly critical to talk about these matters—not just to run through the classic "Let's talk, I have HIV" script, but to discuss the mechanics of sex as well. Positive or negative partners have as much to gain or lose as you do and may not know as much. You can reassure them.

Table 8.1 gives a rough estimate of the degree of risk of HIV transmission from unprotected sex. The risks of protected sex are quite different. While it's true that condoms have a 3 to 12 percent failure rate for pregnancy protection, the rate of HIV transmission is lower than the rate of pregnancy per encounter. Thus, while not entirely risk-free, a condom used correctly is almost foolproof.

Note that this table deals only with the risk of HIV transmission. Warts, herpes, and other infections must also be considered. No form of sexual activity without barrier protection is entirely safe.

TABLE 8.1.
•
Relative Risk of HIV Transmission During Sex Without Barrier Protection.

Activity	Participation	Degree of Risk	Added Risks
Penile/Anal Sex	Receptive	++++	Ejaculation++
	Insertive	++	Skin breaks+
			STDs+
Penile/Vaginal Sex	Receptive	+++	Ejaculation++
	Insertive	+	Menstruation++
			Skin breaks+
			STDs+
Penile/Oral Sex	Receptive	++	Ejaculation++
	Insertive	+	Skin breaks+
			STDs+
			Mouth lesions+
Vaginal/Oral Sex	Receptive	0	Skin breaks+
	Insertive	+	STDs+
			Mouth lesions+
Fingering or Fisting	Either	0[a]	Skin breaks+
Sex Toys	Either	0[a]	
Mutual Masturbation or Kissing	Same	0[a]	Skin breaks+
Bites	Receptive	+	

[a]It's important not to share sex toys without disinfecting them before they are used on the other partner. It's also important to remember that rough sex, by finger, fist, sex toy, or masturbation, can increase susceptibility to HIV transmission during less safe forms of sexual activity that may follow.

Proper condom use is easy to learn. Here are some things to pay attention to:

1. Put it on inside right, with the rolled part on the outside like a roll-up stocking cap.
2. Squeeze the reservoir at the tip, so there's no air bubble that may burst.

3. Use a water-based, not an oil-based, lubricant. Consider one with nonoxynol 9, or another additive that helps to kill HIV. Adding lubricant to the penis itself before putting on the condom may increase sensation.
4. Remove the penis immediately following ejaculation, holding the end of the condom to keep it from slipping off.
5. Rinse off, and use a fresh condom before inserting again.

For women, there's a new female condom. Simple rules for insertion and proper use are as follows:

1. Unwrap gently.
2. Use a water-based lubricant on the outside, on the rings, and on the vagina.
3. Tilt your pelvis forward, as if you were putting in a tampon.
4. Squeeze the ring at the closed end and insert.
5. Put your finger inside the open end and ease the condom back until it's stopped by the cervix and can't go any further. Make sure the closed end is past the pubic bone, by feeling for a hard bone in front with your finger, from inside the condom. The open end of the condom should extend about an inch outside the vagina.
6. Make sure the condom isn't twisted. If your finger moves easily in and out of the open end, you're okay. If not, gently take the condom out and reinsert it.
7. Until you and your partner get used to the condom, guide the penis gently into place by hand at the time of penetration.
8. After ejaculation, squeeze and twist the open end shut, and gently remove the condom. Use a fresh one for repeat penetration.

A female condom may be inserted up to eight hours before sex. It should never be used with a male condom, as it may not stay in place and the male condom may break.

An appealing product for women, called Janesway, was displayed at the National Conference on Women and HIV in May 1997. It's actually a pair of bikini underpants, with a detachable latex portion that covers the outside of the vagina and goes all the way inside to permit penetration. It's pretty, easy to use, and unobtrusive. Best of all, it's in place already, so foreplay need not be interrupted.

As this edition goes to press, Janesway is seeking funding for government testing in order to bring it to market. You can contact them for an update at 707–823–1446, or by e-mail at janesway@pacbell.net.

Recreational Drugs
•

In the discussion that follows, we'll be talking about studies of various types, designed to assess the effects of drug use on HIV progression. Some of these studies are done on cells grown in culture (in vitro) in the lab. Some are done on animal models; these are designed to approximate conditions in humans. Some are actual human studies, designed with varying levels of control. You will find a description of the methods used for these studies, and an appraisal of the reliability of results from each type, in Appendix V.

Those of us who drink a glass or two of wine with our dinner or smoke an occasional cigarette may not think of ourselves as drug users. But these, and most other recreational drugs, can have an impact on HIV. We'll go through them one at a time.

Alcohol

When we looked at antioxidant vitamins in Chapter Four, we spoke of in vitro studies with vitamin E and vitamin C. HIV-infected cells grown in the lab (in a nutrient broth called a culture medium) showed reduced viral replication, or production, when either of these vitamins was added.

In similar studies, the addition of alcohol to the culture medium resulted in a burst of viral production. At least in the culture dish, alcohol is food for the virus. The virus needs an environment of oxidative stress to trigger reproduction. Alcohol provides that environment.

We know from experience with chronic alcoholics that long-term use changes immune response, making people more susceptible to, and less resistant to, infection. We know that chronic alcohol use predisposes people to tuberculosis and bacterial pneumonia.

We know that, in cell studies, MAC—mycobacterium avium complex, a common infection in people with HIV and low CD4 counts—grows much more rapidly with the addition of alcohol to the culture medium. In other studies, uninfected cells exposed to alcohol and then to HIV were much more susceptible to HIV infection than uninfected cells not so exposed.

One interesting study took cells from healthy donors, both before and after giving them alcohol to drink. HIV was introduced into all the cultures. Cultures of cells taken from donors after they drank alcohol showed much higher rates of HIV production than did their cells before alcohol.

We know that in animal studies the addition of alcohol to drinking water resulted in less production of CD4 (T-helper) cells and CD8 (HIV-fighting) cells. In particular, immune cells and activity in the gut wall were decreased, reducing immune defenses within the gastrointestinal tract. We also know that resistance to cryptosporidium, a common cause of diarrhea in AIDS, was reduced in mice with AIDS that were fed alcohol.

We know that alcohol injures lymphocytes and reduces their production. In one study, cells from healthy donors and people with AIDS were treated with alcohol. Lymphocyte production was suppressed in both groups with high doses of alcohol; but in the cells from donors with AIDS, suppression occurred with low doses of alcohol as well.

We know that in animal studies both normal and AIDS-infected mice have reduced levels of zinc and vitamin E when they are given alcohol in the diet.

So we can suspect, then, that the following are true:

- Alcohol may increase our susceptibility to secondary infection, in particular MAC and cryptosporidium.
- Alcohol may contribute directly to vitamin E and zinc deficiency.
- Alcohol may damage our immune barriers in the intestine.
- Alcohol increases HIV replication.
- Alcohol may increase susceptibility to HIV infection.
- Alcohol may increase the rate of progression to AIDS.

These assumptions are based on animal or in vitro studies. They are not as conclusive as studies done on people would be. But those are just not going to happen. I think we have to go with the information we have. And I think it's a dangerous drug.

If you are drinking, and if you can stop, you should do so. If you're not going to stop, at least recognize the danger—and be sure to take vitamin E.

Another thought ventured by alcohol researchers is that alcohol, by reducing inhibitions, makes safer sex practices less likely. There have been retrospective, observational studies on this. Essentially, you are thought to be more at risk if your behaviors are already borderline. That's one important point in favor of alcohol education—so that young people, newly experimenting with sex, will be better protected while they get their good habits in place.

One study evaluated HIV status in patients presenting for alcohol rehabilitation and found that more than 10 percent were HIV-positive. Another study looked specifically at the effect of alcohol abuse on sexual practices in women. The researchers reported that alcohol intake was most likely to lead to unsafe sexual practices in women who were single, had started having sex young, had drunk five or more drinks at one time at least once in their life, and were aware of the dangers of HIV. Thus HIV risk-reduction counseling alone does not appear to offer sufficient protection for these women. The authors concluded that HIV risk-reduction counseling should be accompanied by interventions to reduce levels of alcohol use.

Studies of gay men have shown that alcohol abuse or dependence correlates with increased risk-taking behavior. The authors of one review suggest that proximity to available partners at the time of intoxication may be a predisposing factor. In other words, you may be less likely to have unsafe sex with strangers if you get drunk alone at home than if you do it down at the bar. It's hard to believe someone had to do a study to figure that one out!

Given the importance of alcohol and the bar and nightclub scene to the singles culture—both gay and straight—alcohol is thus doubly dangerous. It supports viral replication and attacks common sense.

So do the best you can with this one. It's better not to drink. If you do drink, take your rubbers with you. And take your antioxidants. Remember, also, that chronic alcohol abuse in men leads to testicular atrophy, reduced sexual desire, and poor sexual performance.

Cigarettes

Cigarette smoking results in 400,000 deaths per year in the United States. Users trying to stop cigarette use report more difficulty, more intense cravings, and more severe withdrawal symptoms than users trying to stop heroin, cocaine, alcohol, or marijuana. This difficulty is compounded by the ready availability and relative social acceptance of nicotine addiction, in a country with enormous bias against those who use illegal drugs.

Smoking has adverse effects on the heart, blood vessels, skin, and lungs. It is a risk factor for many types of cancer, as well as strokes, heart attacks, migraine headaches, chronic bronchitis, and emphysema. It reduces our ability to build or maintain weight. It makes us look wrinkled and old before our time. It makes us smell bad.

Smoking also increases oxidative stress. It has been associated with an increased risk of acquiring HIV infection.

One in vitro study showed that some of the substances in cigarette smoke increased viral replication by twenty times within the cells, releasing seventy times as much antigen outside of the cells. What gets in your blood from your smoking, then, may stimulate growth of the virus.

If you smoke heavily, you leave your lungs less able to defend naturally against bronchitis and pneumonia. And particularly if you have had pneumonia, or have any chronic lung problem, you will recover more fully if you stop.

Studies done on HIV-negative people have shown that less weight and lean body mass is gained, per calorie eaten, when people smoke. So there may be a direct effect on your nutritional status, too.

Like the issue of barrier protection, though, there may be limits to how much you'll do without. If you're currently smoking cigarettes, and also drinking alcohol, I'd start by getting rid of the alcohol.

Amphetamines ("Speed")

Studies suggest that amphetamine danger is especially associated with intravenous use, as we would expect. This is because of the associated dangers of injecting contaminants and of using dirty needles. Sexual indiscretion, moreover, seems to be greater in this population. One British study of women amphetamine users states that, in the six months reported, over 80 percent of subjects had engaged in unprotected sex.

But much of the concern about speed is over its nutritional effects. Anorexia is a well-known and sometimes sought-after effect. Speed is, after all, what was once used in diet pills. Many people who use speed say they do so to get thin. But with HIV, when you lose weight you lose protein. You're breaking your nutritional bank.

Another concern is exhaustion, after the high is over. You're less able to fight off infections when you're worn down.

There are no studies on the specific effects of methamphetamine on viral progression. The indirect effects we've discussed, though, are of real concern to people with HIV.

MDMA, or Ecstasy

MDMA is an amphetamine derivative that has become fashionable in the 1990s. It is said to have a mild psychedelic effect, and to make people feel happy and loving. Normally it's used collectively as a party drug, in what are called rave parties. It deserves special mention here because of the danger of its rise to lethal levels when taken with ritonavir, or Norvir. This protease inhibitor will be discussed more fully in Chapter Thirteen. The makers of ritonavir warn that most people on ritonavir will have two to three times the expected level of MDMA, and 3 to 10 percent of people can have levels rise to ten times the normal amount. One death has already been reported from MDMA with ritonavir.

Heroin and Methadone

Heroin use has been associated with multiple immune abnormalities. It appears that these are largely associated with IV use, however. Because heroin is usually taken by injection, the reported changes in immune status may have to do mainly with lifestyle, with infection through shared needles, or with damage from injecting substances used to cut heroin.

Methadone is used in maintenance programs for heroin addicts, to keep them from needing to inject heroin. It lasts longer, gives less of a high, and can be taken orally.

Some studies suggest that methadone does not affect immune status, although this is controversial. In fact, there even appears to be some improvement in immune function when IV heroin users are switched to a methadone maintenance program, according to other studies. This supports the idea that it is chiefly the lifestyle, and the means of delivering the drug, that lead to immunosuppression in narcotic addicts.

Studies also show that the use of opiates by injection results in less concern about sharing needles or unsafe sexual practices. People who frequent shooting galleries are more likely to use other people's needles, or the house works, and are more likely to exchange unprotected sex for drugs. Especially at risk are younger users, people with psychiatric diagnoses, victims of incest and rape, and those who are homeless. Thus social vulnerability and a history of sexual abuse, injection drug use, or mental illness all increase the risks of unsafe drug and sexual practices in this group.

People who work with heroin addicts report that their appetite and food intake are decreased. Nausea is a common side effect of heroin and can occur after injection. The relative inactivity induced by heroin's high contributes to reduced intake. And during periods of withdrawal between injections, the addict's attention is focused on getting more drugs, not on eating.

Heroin addiction is a special problem in pregnancy. On the one hand, fewer complications are seen during pregnancy itself when methadone maintenance is instituted. However, the newborn can suffer from severe withdrawal at birth when its addicted mother has been maintained on methadone.

One study looked at people with and without HIV, during and after heroin detoxification. Most nutritional measurements were within normal range for both groups. Immune function was reduced in both groups. Both groups showed improvement in lean body mass after detoxification.

Malnutrition is often associated with heroin. Retrovirus-infected mice given morphine showed decreased body weight. In the presence of malnutrition, the immune changes normally seen (reduced CD4 and CD8 cells) were exacerbated.

The consensus, however, is that the malnutrition seen with heroin use is not a direct effect, but rather a part of the social picture associated with drug addiction. Poverty, unemployment, the use of other drugs, and illness resulting from existing malnutrition, due largely to poor diet, are thought to be contributing factors.

If you are pregnant and addicted to heroin, I think that what we do know, so far, argues for methadone maintenance. It does leave the job of withdrawal to the baby, at birth; but the reduction of stressors during pregnancy and the possibility of a more organized lifestyle—with better medication compliance, more and regular medical follow-up, and the likelihood of better nutrition—may be worth it. This is especially true now that we have learned that zidovudine (AZT) given to the mother during pregnancy greatly reduces the chance of HIV transmission to the baby: those mothers who are in methadone maintenance programs have access to regularly scheduled medical care, including zidovudine. I would rather see an infant go through narcotic withdrawal at birth than increase its risk of contracting HIV.

Cocaine

Appetite is reduced during a cocaine high, and energy expenditure is greater. So it's a direct threat to getting enough food to meet your energy needs.

Like alcohol, cocaine has been shown to reduce the number of lymphocytes available for immune response in the gut wall. This can permit chronic cryptosporidium or giardia infection. Protein malnutrition can exacerbate this. These organisms disrupt your absorptive capacity and cause diarrhea.

Studies in mice show that the pattern of cocaine's immune suppression in the gut is similar to the effects of HIV—fewer antibodies, fewer CD4 cells, and fewer CD8 cells. Taken together, the effects of cocaine use and HIV are more pronounced. When mice are fed a low-protein diet, simulating HIV malnutrition, immune suppression is dramatic and severe.

Other animal studies have shown reduced body weight with cocaine administration.

One study took cells from healthy, HIV-negative subjects and exposed some of them to cocaine. Both the exposed and the unexposed cells were then infected with HIV. Cells pretreated with cocaine showed much higher rates of HIV replication. This has been shown as well in another study, where cells also infected with cytomegalovirus (CMV) showed increased HIV replication in the presence of CMV, and even more with the addition of cocaine.

HIV infection itself is more likely to spread to those who are uninfected, or to those who are infected with a less resistant virus, because of the social patterns of cocaine use. As with heroin, there are gathering places, or crack houses, where crack cocaine may be purchased and smoked. Unsafe sharing of needles for injection of cocaine or other drugs is common, and unprotected sex is frequently exchanged for this highly addictive drug.

Thus it is possible that cocaine does more than reduce intake and increase energy expense. It can also increase the danger of infection with HIV, and can increase its progression once a person is infected.

Marijuana

Marijuana is a different matter. It is used, and bought illegally, as a recreational drug. It is estimated that 20 percent of people of child-bearing age use it or have used it; I suspect that figure is on the low side.

Marinol (dronabinol, a marijuana derivative with similar effects) is not only available, but is "indicated" (proven useful and recommended for the treatment of HIV wasting). Such an indication for a drug is politically very powerful, as it means that insurers can no longer consider it experimental, and cannot deny payment—though they can do their best to limit its use by slowing down the approval process and requiring proof of its applicability to the case of a given patient. Patients on MediCal (the California equivalent of Medicaid) can get it paid for by the government. And that's appropriate: it's a powerful appetite enhancer.

Many people living and thriving with HIV swear by the use of inhaled marijuana for the relief of nausea and for appetite enhancement, helping them to eat enough to fight the wasting process. Certainly it has proven itself as an appetite enhancer, as well as an antinausea drug; that's why dronabinol is marketed as a legal version. But many people with HIV feel that inhaled marijuana is superior to dronabinol. They report a quicker onset of effect, which they can titrate for just the relief they need, less sleepiness and confusion, and better tolerability than with an oral drug when nauseated.

Efforts to test these claims have been stonewalled by the federal government, which first required that marijuana for testing come from within the United States, and then refused to supply it or approve the trials. Five years have passed, during which time proposed studies have been modified repeatedly in response to stated reasons for refusal. All requests have been refused. Currently, research proposals have been submitted again, despite a comment by the National Institute on Drug Abuse that they could not imagine why anyone would consider testing such a toxic substance.

The tide of public opinion is turning, however. In a blistering editorial in the *New England Journal of Medicine,* Jerome Kassirer urged a less hysterical and politically driven approach. Medical societies and physicians' groups have lobbied for the right to study marijuana.

The government's latest response is to authorize a one-million-dollar, eighteen-month review of existing studies on marijuana—despite the fact that virtually no studies have been done since the last such review, in 1982, which recommended further research for potential medical value. So we'll wait a little longer.

While scientists have been trying to study marijuana, patients have concentrated on getting it. Initially, HIV activists worked to pass laws permitting importation of drugs approved in other countries, for personal use. The formation of buyers' clubs made it possible for people to band together to do this as a cooperative venture, and this practice continues today. Laws were passed, however, exempting marijuana from this law.

Buyers' clubs continued to sell marijuana, illegally, to those with diagnoses considered appropriate for its use. Even in states that recognized the legitimate interests of people with HIV, cancer, and glaucoma and left these clubs alone, federal authorities cracked down. Marijuana was confiscated, and principals were charged. In addition, the files of those patients, including letters of diagnosis from their doctors, were seized.

Since that time, voters in Arizona and California have passed laws legalizing marijuana for medical use. These laws stand in opposition to federal laws, which make it illegal for any physician to prescribe or recommend it. General Barry McCaffery, a retired army general appointed by the Clinton Administration to head the Office of National Drug Control Policy, has since sought to block medical use of marijuana by threatening to revoke the license of any physician who recommends or advocates its use.

In January 1997, a group of physicians and physicians' organizations filed suit against the federal government for violation of their First Amendment rights. In February, a physician in Placerville, California, was the focus of a government inquiry, based on his recommendation of marijuana for medical reasons. In May 1997, an injunction was obtained to halt the federal government's attempts to punish physicians for recommending marijuana in California.

Here in San Francisco, the Department of Public Health has worked hard to bring order out of this chaos. A uniform letter has been drafted for doctors' referrals to buyers' clubs. Plans have been established to monitor these clubs. Medical review boards have been established to evaluate the appropriateness of applications. Confidentiality, chiefly to protect referring doctors, has been ensured by off-site filing of records and telephone verification of referrals. Clubs monitor their product for quality control, to avoid herbicidal or fungal contamination. Often, the herb is grown to order for clubs that respect the importance of delivering an uncontaminated product.

While state laws appear to protect patients in those two states, people with HIV in other states must consider the risks of breaking the law. Jail is not a good place to get your HIV care. And physicians must also be careful.

It's important also to remember that we don't really know what marijuana does. We know that it makes people feel better and helps them to eat more. But we still don't know whether it helps to build lean body mass. And we haven't been able to evaluate its effects on the respiratory system, because we haven't been allowed to study it.

My own experience with patients suggests that marijuana works better when you smoke it than when you eat it. The resulting increase in appetite lasts longer when you smoke it. People placed on Marinol who aren't used to its effects get sleepy, and the time they have to eat—before they get sleepy—is shortened. I'll go over this material in detail in Part Three.

The early, well-publicized studies on marijuana in the 1970s, which purported to show a negative effect on immune status, used amounts far in excess of what recreational smokers, or wasting patients with prescribed medication, would actually use. With rational use—two or three pills or joints a day—I know of no significant effects on immune status.

There can be drawbacks, however, to using marijuana. Certainly if you have asthma or other acute or chronic lung ailments, there can be additional irritation from smoke inhalation. In addition, if you don't qualify for the diagnosis of wasting and can't get this by prescription, and if you are not a member of a buyers' club, you may be at serious legal risk.

Marijuana is also criticized for reducing ambition and memory retention. These are appropriate criticisms, and they could be made against many of the drugs doctors prescribe, when used by people who have less to gain than the function they lose. On balance, though, looking at marijuana medically rather than sociopolitically, this is a good drug for people with HIV.

We'll talk more about the use of marijuana and dronabinol in Chapter Twelve, when we look at medical interventions for the wasting syndrome.

We'll also talk more about buyers' clubs in Part Three. A representative list of buyers' clubs can be found in Appendix IX.

It's important that your doctor proceed carefully, if she or he wants to help you. She must not put herself at risk; there are others who will need her help in time.

Needle-Exchange Programs

Throughout the world, needle-exchange programs have been an important tool in preventing the spread of HIV. Since the first program was initiated in Amsterdam in 1984, the practice has spread to include most of Western Europe, as well as Australia and Canada. These programs have been shown to reduce needle sharing, reduce HIV transmission by 15 to 33 percent, reduce transmission of hepatitis B and C by six to seven times, and increase referrals to drug rehabilitation programs.

The United States is the only country in the world that bans the use of federal funds to provide for needle-exchange programs. Six government-funded reports have urged the adoption of a needle-exchange policy. These recommendations have met with no response.

A recent article in *Lancet* attempted to count the cost of this refusal. Based on infection rates for injection drug users, their partners, and their children, it estimated that five to ten thousand infections with HIV could have been avoided so far, and that five to eleven thousand more could be prevented by the year 2000. The cost of treating those first five to ten thousand patients, even in 1994 dollars, was estimated to be $244,000,000 to $538,000,000. There's no way to estimate the costs of treating the second wave.

This is another example of government reluctance to admit that what exists—a large segment of our citizens who are going to use drugs whether we approve or not—is not going to go away by telling it to just say no. To substitute disapproval for action, when so many lives are at stake—and so many more will be, as infections breed new infections—is a terrible waste of our nation's health and welfare. And we will pay the price.

If you are using injection drugs, please take this danger seriously. Get fresh needles and use them every time, if you can. If not, clean your works with bleach. And never, never share your needles. This is to protect you, as well as people who are not infected. You don't need what they have, either.

Exercise
•

The role of exercise in HIV is now under study and holds great promise.

Part of the reason for the loss of lean body mass seen in people with HIV is their reduced activity. The body compensates for its increased resting energy expense by reducing its active expenditure. Thus, when you're sick, you don't want to work out. And a muscle that's not used will waste.

But we know that the process of wasting begins very early. And we know there's only a finite amount of lean body mass that you can afford to lose. Studies have shown an actual increase in lean body mass with the institution of a progressive resistance exercise program in healthy, asymptomatic people with HIV.

In one study, twenty-four men with AIDS, who had recently had pneumocystis pneumonia but were now without symptoms, were randomly divided into two groups. All were tested for muscle strength and stamina at the start of the study. Twelve of them worked out on a progressive resistance exercise machine three times a week for six weeks. At the end of just six weeks—eighteen workouts—those men had greater strength, greater endurance, and *increased lean body mass*.

Multiple studies since then have borne this out. People with HIV can build up their lean body mass with progressive resistance exercise alone. And, as we'll see when we look at anabolic therapies in Chapter Twelve, we can also get much more out of anabolic therapies if we work out.

Studies reported in 1997 show us that:

1. Intensive progressive resistance exercise alone led to greater than 4 percent increases in lean body mass in only eight weeks in 7 Massachusetts patients.
2. Increased intensity of progressive resistance exercise was predictive of greater lean body mass in 152 Washington, D.C., patients receiving nutritional supplements and no anabolic therapies.
3. Progressive resistance exercise in combination with anabolic steroids, micronutrient supplementation, and a high-protein diet led to substantial gains in lean body mass in 29 Texas patients.
4. Progressive resistance exercise in combination with oxandrolone led to greater increases in lean body mass than the use of oxandrolone alone in 16 San Francisco patients.

So, just at the time you find out you're infected, just when you're loaded with drive to do something about it, long before you have symptoms—we now know you can add to your energy bank by building your muscle mass. Even later on, after an active illness, you can do so when you're feeling well. Weight lifting, machine workouts, even a personal trainer if you can afford it—all these can help you prepare for the fight.

Studies are currently assessing the value, or danger, of exercise in people who are actively ill. Until we have more answers, I think you should listen to your body, letting it rest when it wants to rest. If you feel up to exercise, though, and if it doesn't wear you out, then it's probably good to do it. The emotional benefits and release of tension are substantial. And there may be a more concrete benefit, as well.

My patient, Pat, who suffers from great fatigue as a result of an active chronic secondary infection, reports that doing what he can every day makes him able to do it the next day. When he skips a day, he loses ground. For him, this has been a way to turn his discipline and commitment into energy for living.

There isn't much written about aerobics. We know that people with HIV who did aerobics responded better, with less depression, to the disclosure of their HIV infection. We know that knowledge of their diagnosis in controls who were not exercising resulted in a loss of immune cells at the time of notification, apparently in response to their distress. And we know that those who had done aerobics—again, for just a short while—did *not* suffer the same reduction in immune cells. So it seems to make sense that the emotional conditioning we receive from regular aerobic exercise should help us to do better physically. There have been no nutritional or body composition studies to confirm this, though.

If you feel good, do it. If it feels good, keep doing it. If you still have the energy after your weight lifting or machine workout, I can see no reason not to run.

If aerobics or running consistently make you tired, however—or if you feel ill—it's okay to hold back. The important thing, if you're not at top form, is to push yourself only a little. You don't want to wear yourself out.

We know that marathon runners lose T cells after a run. You don't have to stress yourself to the point of exhaustion. And cardiac conditioning is less important for you now than building muscle mass.

Dancing is good for you, too, if you feel up to it. The more you move your body in different ways, the better you'll know your body. And the more it will be able to tell you, and the louder it will speak.

The human brain has far more inhibitory neurons—nerve cells whose job it is to screen out unnecessary stimuli—than excitatory neurons, whose job it is to get your attention. When something stays the same, your mind forgets it. Right now, for instance, you don't notice that the clock is ticking or the refrigerator's running. And now you do notice, because I mentioned it.

It works the same with body information. If your body only moves in certain ways, in chunks of muscle groups that don't know they can move separately from each other, pretty soon you don't know you can move with greater variety, through more dimensions. If you don't feel the interplay of different muscle groups as they move or exercise, you will forget to differentiate them. If you tighten up around a back that hurts, or walk with small, rigid steps to avoid foot pain, your back will forget that it can flex or arch, or your legs will forget that they can stride freely. The less you use your body, the less it will be able to tell you.

We only remember what touches our senses. We only remember the parts of our bodies that move or the parts that are touched. So move your body playfully. Enjoy the exercise you do, and use it for building awareness.

There's also a role here for yoga, tai chi, or other exercise disciplines that keep your body aware of its movement potential.

Massage is good, too. Partly for the passive exercise and release of tension it offers—but also because, if your edges are touched, you will know where they are and will feel them. If your muscles are reminded of their separate form, by the movement or pressure of hands, your mind will be able to find those muscles. And if you find them, you'll know how to use and relax them. You'll know when you feel good, and where. You'll know when you hurt and will consciously adjust your body to relieve that pain.

• • •

So, in summary, your lifestyle will influence your nutritional status. Your sexual practices can affect it, both directly and indirectly. Sex is good, and safer sex is safer. If you use recreational drugs, you should carefully consider their effects on nutrition and health, *and you should particularly avoid alcohol.* Injection drug use is risky, but less risky when you use clean needles and don't share. Exercise can enhance your well-being and help you gain lean body mass. Movement keeps your body aware and more likely to keep on moving. Massage and other movement therapies can relieve stress and tension and improve your own body awareness. Attention to all of these aspects contributes to homeostasis, to reducing the burden of stress, and to keeping your body in balance.

REFERENCES

Bagasra, O., and Forman. "The biological role of cocaine in the development and expression of AIDS." *International Conference on AIDS*, 1989, *5*, 677.

Bagasra, O., and Pomerantz. "Human immunodeficiency virus type 1 replication in peripheral blood mononuclear cells in the presence of cocaine." *Journal of Infectious Diseases*, 1993, *168*(5), 1157–1164.

Bagasra, O., and others. "Effects of alcohol ingestion on in vitro susceptibility of peripheral blood monocytes to infection with HIV and of selected T-cell functions." *Alcoholism: Clinical and Experimental Research*, 1989, *13*(5), 636–643.

Bagasra, O., and others. "Alcohol intake increases human immunodeficiency virus type 1 replication in human peripheral blood mononuclear cells." *Journal of Infectious Diseases*, 1993, *167*(4), 789–797.

Bermudez, L. E. "Effect of ethanol on the interaction between the macrophage and mycobacterium avium." *Alcohol*, 1994, *11*(2), 69–73.

Bermudez, L. E., and others. "Exposure to alcohol up-regulates the expression of mycobacterium avium complex proteins associated with bacterial virulence." *Journal of Infectious Diseases*, 1993, *168*(4), 961–968.

Brown, L. S., and Siddiqui. "Relationship between cocaine use and HIV disease progression in injecting drug users (IDUs)." *International Conference on AIDS*, 1991, *7*(1), 337.

Caetano, R., and Hines. "Alcohol, sexual practices, and risk of AIDS among blacks, Hispanics, and whites." *Journal of Acquired Immune Deficiency Syndromes and Human Retrovirology*, 1995, *10*, 554–561.

Calabrese, L. H., and LaPerriere. "Human immunodeficiency virus, exercise and athletics." *Sports Medicine*, 1993, *15*(1), 6–13.

Casella, P., and others. "Absence of effect of risk behavior on progression of HIV-disease among male Brazilian sex workers." *International Conference on AIDS*, 1993, *9*(2), 702.

Chen, L. H., and others. "Effects of chronic alcohol feeding and murine AIDS virus infection on liver antioxidant defense systems in mice." *Alcoholism: Clinical and Experimental Research*, 1993, *17*(5), 1022–1028.

Clapper, R. L., and Lipsitt. "A retrospective study of risk-taking and alcohol-mediated unprotected intercourse." *Journal of Substance Abuse*, 1991, *3*, 91–96.

Coates, R. A., and others. "Cofactors of progression to acquired human immunodeficiency syndrome in a cohort of male sexual contacts of men with human immunodeficiency virus disease." *American Journal of Epidemiology*, 1990, *132*(4), 717–722.

Darke, S., and others. "Benzodiazepine use and HIV risk-taking behavior among injecting drug users." *Drug and Alcohol Dependency,* 1992, *31*(1), 31–36.

Edlin, B. R., and others. "Intersecting epidemics: Crack cocaine use and HIV infection among inner-city young adults." *New England Journal of Medicine,* 1994, *331*(21), 1422–1427.

Ferrando, S. J. "Substance use disorders and HIV illness." *The AIDS Reader,* 1997, *7*(2), 57–64.

Fineberg, H. V., and Wilson. "Social vulnerability and death by infection." *New England Journal of Medicine,* 1996, *334*(13), 859–860.

Friedman, L. N., and others. "Tuberculosis, AIDS and death among substance abusers on welfare in New York City." *New England Journal of Medicine,* 1996, *334*(13), 828–833.

Gibert, C. I., and others. "Body composition and frequency of muscle building activities in HIV-infected men." *Nutrition–HIV Infection, Second International Conference,* 1997, *13*(3), P-31, 286.

Gordon, S. M., and others. "The response of symptomatic neurosyphilis to high-dose intravenous penicillin G in patients with human immunodeficiency virus infection." *New England Journal of Medicine,* 1994, *331*(22), 1469–1473.

Hutchings, D. E., and Dow-Edwards. "Animal models of opiate, cocaine, and cannabis use." *Clinical Perinatology,* 1991, *18*(1), 1–22.

Kall, K. I. "Effects of amphetamine on sexual behavior of male IV drug users in Stockholm: A pilot study." *AIDS Education and Prevention,* 1992, *4*(1), 6–17.

Kassirer, J. P. "Federal foolishness and marijuana." *New England Journal of Medicine,* 1997, *336*(5), 336–337.

Klee, H., and Morris. "HIV-related risk among young amphetamine users." *International Conference on AIDS,* 1993, *9*(2), 820.

Lafeuillade, A. "HIV cofactors in the course of AIDS." *Presse Médicale,* 1992, *21*(30), 1426–1430.

Lai, P. K., and others. "Activation of human immunodeficiency virus in human myeloid cells by cocaine." *International Conference on AIDS,* 1990, *6*(3), 138.

Lake-Bakaar, G., and Rao. "Alcohol and HIV disease progression in intravenous drug addicts." *International Conference on AIDS,* 1989, *5*, 812.

LaPerriere, A. R., and others. "Exercise intervention attenuates emotional distress and natural killer cell decrements following notification of positive serologic status-1." *Biofeedback and Self-Regulation,* 1990, *15*(3), 229–242.

Larrat, E. P., and Zierler. "Entangled epidemics: Cocaine use and HIV disease." *Journal of Psychoactive Drugs,* 1993, *25*(3), 207–221.

Lopez, M. C., and Watson. "Effect of cocaine and murine AIDS on lamina propria T and B cells in normal mice." *Life Sciences,* 1994, *54*(9), 147–151.

Lopez, M. C., and others. "Alteration of thymic cell subsets by cocaine administration and murine retrovirus infection in protein undernourished mice." *Thymus,* 1992, *3,* 171–181.

Lopez, M. C., and others. "Modification of spleen cell subsets by chronic cocaine administration and murine retrovirus infection in normal and protein-malnourished mice." *International Journal of Immunopharmacology,* 1992, *14*(7), 1153–1163.

Lopez, M. C., and others. "Modification of thymic cell subsets induced by long-term cocaine administration during a murine retroviral infection." *Clinical Immunology and Immunopathology,* 1992, *65*(1), 45–52.

Lotz, M., and Seth. "TGF beta and HIV infection." *Annals of the New York Academy of Sciences,* 1993, *685,* 510–511.

Lurie, P., and Drucker. "An opportunity lost: HIV infections associated with lack of a national needle-exchange program in the USA." *Lancet,* 1997, *349,* 604–608.

Maas, U., and others. "Infrequent neonatal opiate withdrawal following maternal methadone detoxification during pregnancy." *Journal of Perinatal Medicine,* 1990, *18*(2), 111–118.

McEwan, R. T. "Sex and the risk of HIV infection: The role of alcohol." *British Journal of Addiction,* 1992, *87,* 577–584.

McLachlan, C., and others. "The effects of methadone among injecting drug users: A review." *British Journal of Addiction,* 1993, *88*(2), 257–263.

McManus, T. J., and Weatherburn. "Alcohol, AIDS and Immunity." *British Medical Bulletin,* 1994, *50*(1), 115–123.

"Medical marijuana: Reports from February AIDS grand rounds." *Synopsis, Minutes of the Community Consortium's Business Meeting,* March 1997, pp. 3–7.

Northfelt, D. W., and others. "Anal neoplasia: Pathogenesis, diagnosis and management." *Hematology/Oncology Clinics of North America,* 1996, *10*(5), 1177–1187.

Ostrow, D. G., and others. "Recreational drugs and sexual behavior in the Chicago MACS/CCS cohort of homosexually active men." *Journal of Substance Abuse,* 1993, *5*(4), 311–325.

Peterson, P. K. "Cocaine potentiates HIV-1 replication in human peripheral blood mononuclear cell cocultures: Involvement of transforming growth factor-beta." *Journal of Immunology,* 1991, *146*(1), 81–84.

Peterson, P. K., and others. "Cocaine amplifies HIV-1 replication in cytomegalovirus-stimulated peripheral blood mononuclear cell cocultures." *Journal of Immunology,* 1992, *149*(2), 676–680.

Pillae, R., and others. "AIDS, drugs of abuse and the immune system: A complex immunological network." *Archives of Toxicology,* 1991, *65*(8), 609–617.

Poet, T. S., and others. "Stimulation of natural killer cell activity by murine retroviral infection and cocaine." *Toxicology Letter,* 1991, *59*(1–3), 147–152.

Remien, R. H., and others. "Cessation of alcohol and drug use disorders in an HIV sample." *International Conference on AIDS,* 1989, *5,* 754.

Romeyn, M., and others. "The role of exercise in oxandrolone — Mediated repletion of HIV-1-associated wasting," *International Conference on AIDS,* 1998, in submission.

Roubenoff, R., and others. "Feasibility of increasing lean body mass in HIV-infected adults using progressive resistance training." *Nutrition–HIV Infection, Second International Conference,* 1997, *13*(3), O-15, 271.

Salvato, P. D., and others. "Anabolic steroid use in HIV/AIDS patients." *Nutrition–HIV Infection, Second International Conference,* 1997, *13*(3), 0–03, 268.

Schechtel, J. "Risky business." *AIDS Care,* 1997, *1*(2), 25–28.

Spence, D. W., and others. "Progressive resistance exercise: Effect on muscle function and anthropometry of a select AIDS population." *Archives of Physical Medicine and Rehabilitation,* 1990, *71,* 644–648.

Starec, M., and others. "Immune status and survival of opiate- and cocaine-treated mice infected with Friend virus." *Journal of Pharmacological Experimental Therapy,* 1991, *259*(2), 745–750.

"Symptoms of substance dependence associated with use of cigarettes, alcohol and illicit drugs, United States, 1991–1992." *Morbidity and Mortality Weekly Report,* 1995, *44*(44), 831–839.

Varela, P., and others. "Nutritional assessment of HIV-positive drug addicts." *European Journal of Clinical Nutrition,* 1990, *44*(5), 415–418.

Vering, A., and others. "Heroin abuse and methadone substitution in pregnancy." *Geburtshilfe Fräuleinheilkunde,* 1992, *52*(3), 122–147.

Volberding, P. "Sex in the age of AIDS." *AIDS Care,* 1997, *1*(2), 19.

Wang, Y., and Watson. "Ethanol, immune responses, and murine AIDS: The role of vitamin E as an immunostimulant and antioxidant." *Alcohol,* 1994, *11*(2), 75–84.

Wang, Y., and others. "Ethanol-induced modulation of cytokine production by splenocytes during murine retrovirus infection causing murine AIDS." *Alcoholism: Clinical and Experimental Research,* 1993, *17*(5), 1035–1039.

Wang, Y., and others. "The effect of alcohol consumption on nutritional status during murine AIDS." *Alcohol,* 1994, *11*(3), 273–278.

Watson, R. R., and others. "Modification of lymphoid subsets by chronic ethanol consumption in C57B1/6 mice infected with LP-BM5 murine leukemia virus." *Alcohol and Alcoholism,* 1992, *27*(4), 417–424.

Watson, R. R., and others. "Resistance to intestinal parasites during murine AIDS: Role of alcohol and nutrition in immune dysfunction." *Parasitology,* 1993, *107*(Supplement), S69–S74.

Weinstein, M., and others. "Period of risk for drug use and sexual behavior among black teenage crack users." *International Conference on AIDS,* 1990, *6*(2), 483.

Westerburg, V. S. "Alcohol measuring scales may influence conclusions about the role of alcohol in human immunodeficiency virus (HIV) risk and progression to acquired immunodeficiency syndrome (AIDS)." *American Journal of Epidemiology,* 1992, *135*(7), 719–725.

Wilke, G., and others. "Influence of methadone maintenance on lymphocyte subpopulations in HIV infected patients." *International Conference on AIDS,* 1991, *7*(2), 386.

EPILOGUE

•

Your Personal Program

Time to recap: you've finished Part II of your assessment; you've identified threats to your nutritional status; you know not only what to eat, but how to do it right. Organize what you've learned, first, by circling the subheadings in Part II of your nutritional assessment that require special attention. Then list the changes, the interventions you'd like to make for yourself, based on the problems identified. Prioritize them: critical ones first, important ones next, fine-tuning last. And see how much change you can make.

- You need to eat. Enough calories, enough protein. Enough variety to get natural nutrients.
- You need to like what you eat.
- You need to take additional vitamins, minerals, and trace elements.
- Consider aggressive supplementation with antioxidant vitamins.
- Consider SOD, NAC, and omega-3 fatty acids.
- Consider alternative treatment modalities.

- Adjust your mealtimes and medicine times to best support your appetite.
- Adjust your seasonings and choice of foods to adapt to changes in taste and smell.
- Pay attention to how your food is provided and prepared.
- Take special precautions to avoid infections from your food or its preparers.
- Apply for a feeding program if needed.
- Do everything you can to ensure you have adequate shelter, and make it as nice as you can.
- Address fatigue, depression, confusion, and loneliness as soon as you recognize them. Reach out for help right away.
- Find and join a support group.
- Use barrier precautions whenever you have sex.
- Evaluate the drugs you use for recreation, if any. If they're bad for you, try to do without.
- Exercise, within the range of your capabilities.
- Consider massage and movement therapies.
- Try to change one habit at a time.

Check your list every now and then, to monitor your progress. Redo the form in three months. See how your behaviors, and your results as measured in weight and energy, have been affected. Reassess and prioritize your goals.

Realize how much you can do, every day, for yourself. And notice that you've taken charge.

PART III

•

What You Can Do with Your Doctor

•

CHAPTER 9

•

Choosing a Doctor

You are about to begin one of the most important relationships of your life.

Now that you are HIV-positive, you stand at the beginning of a time of profound change in your life. Like the toddler years, or adolescence, or old age, this change marks the beginning of a whole new stage of personal, emotional, and spiritual growth for you.

Much of your time and effort will be spent adapting to and strengthening yourself in response to that change. While there is much you can do for yourself, you will need the help of others to do more.

Your doctor can be an important part of that help. She or he will be your monitor while you are well, your resource as you guard your health, and your protector during times of illness. You will work together on the changes you must make to stay well, and rejoice together at your successes. You and your doctor will form a partnership, with a common goal. Each of you will be invested in your progress.

You may be ill now. If not, there may be times of illness in the years ahead. During those times, the bond between you and your doctor will deepen. The shared success of recovery can deepen it still further. You will come to know each other well. You will build trust together. Each of you will affect the other deeply.

Psychiatrists who have studied the doctor-patient relationship have observed that a good one can be more than important; *it is an independent factor in improving outcome.* Call it a placebo effect; they do. But if it works, it works. And anything that can help you to do better deserves your close attention.

If you've just been diagnosed and don't yet have a doctor, you have a unique opportunity to look at the kind of doctor, and the kind of relationship, that's best for you.

Even if you already have a doctor, you need to look at how the two of you work together and what she or he has to offer you over the years to come.

What to Look for in Your Doctor

•

Take a moment to think about the qualities you value in a doctor, and about what makes a doctor the right one for you. Consider, also, these attributes.

Absence of Prejudice

To start with, you need a doctor who is not biased against people with HIV.

Especially in rural areas and small communities where AIDS has not yet made inroads, people may still be fearful when it presents and critical of behaviors that can lead to infection. This prejudice can extend to include anyone with HIV, regardless of the means of acquisition.

HIV-positive people often choose to go back to the homes of their childhood to be with their families or childhood friends. Friends and family may let go of old biases quickly, as they are emotionally invested. So even if the larger community is not supportive, the closer community can be. The fear and ignorance that surround that community will have little direct impact.

You must be certain, though, that your doctor does not share such biases. You need a doctor who will be objective and on your side. Whether you live in a rural town or in San Francisco, you can't get proper care from someone who is fearful of AIDS or overwhelmed by the demands of its care, or who thinks you deserve what you got.

A Good Fit

Each person has her or his own set of biases and her or his own individual responses to the personality characteristics of others. These must be considered too. Particularly if you don't trust doctors, it's important to choose one whose style won't antagonize you.

Some of us are playful and like to laugh a lot. For some patients, this is a good coping mechanism. To others, such behavior may seem callous or unfeeling.

Some people want their doctors to be forceful or directive. For them, such a doctor makes them feel safer. They want to feel taken care of and like to be told what to do. Others may resent this style. It can trigger their own issues around control and power. It may be perceived as a threat to their autonomy.

These people will often do better with a doctor who can take a back seat, treating and advising, where appropriate, according to the patient's own schedule. As long as a doctor lets you know the impact of your preferences and continues to be sure to do no harm, this can also be a good working strategy.

For some patients, a level of denial is an important part of their coping style. Full disclosure of potential problems can provoke more anxiety than they are ready for. For these people, a doctor who is thorough but gentle—and less forthcoming—will be a better choice than one who is blunt and straightforward.

Others, though, need to know everything up front. Their anxiety is reduced once they face all the facts. They can feel more in control. In fact, they feel safer retaining control, if they know they'll get an argument when their doctor thinks they're headed in the wrong direction. They may mistrust doctors who *don't* tell them everything, in the plainest possible terms. These patients will do well with a straight shooter who is loyal to them and not afraid to take them on.

The concept of personal space is important, too. Each of us has our own acceptable degree of intimacy. We aren't comfortable when we move too far out of that range. You can tell where you stand on this continuum by looking at the level of closeness you choose in your social relationships. People generally come together for pleasure with people whose intimacy needs aren't too different from their own.

If a doctor seems cold and distant to you, or if you feel invaded or crowded, your notions of acceptable space may be different. A little of this is okay and may actually be beneficial for both of you. If the difference is too great, though, it can threaten the development of a good working relationship.

Involvement

If you prefer to keep people at a distance, there may be benefit to reconsidering this preference, in this particular relationship.

Doctors are trained to be detached. The culture in which they live, throughout the long years of medical school and residency training, prizes toughness and aggression; encourages selfishness, to ensure self-preservation; uses gallows humor, to defend against the suffering around them; and rewards technical competence, erudition, and showmanship far above compassion and concern. The more unusual the disease, the more interesting the case. And the patient, we are taught, is the one with the disease.

I don't agree with this. To me it seems we are all a part of this disease, and of every form of human suffering. And I would want a doctor who thought so too.

To your doctor, you want to be a person, not a case. You want her or him to care about your problems, even if they're not medically exotic. You want her or his interest in you to be based on what you feel, and what you need to make you better—not just on intellectual excitement. You want the kind of doctor who is in it for the pleasure of relieving suffering, of making things better. You want encouragement. You want a friend and advocate. There is much to be said for working with a doctor who likes to get involved.

Commitment

You can get excellent care from intelligent, well-trained doctors, regardless of their personal feelings about the importance of the HIV epidemic. But I have to suspect that your care will be better, more thorough, and perhaps more aggressive if both of you feel the urgency of fighting HIV.

Commitment to *your* care is necessary, too. You don't want to invest time building a relationship with a doctor who will discharge you if your insurance or economic status changes. You want someone who's there for the long haul.

Willingness to Teach

This one isn't easy. You will have to do your part.

Doctors are under increasing pressure to provide care quickly, in order to lower the costs of medical care. Costs are further controlled by supervisors and case managers employed by insurance companies or program administrators. These are often the same administrators who hire doctors and pay them their salaries.

Cost control is obtained by reviewing documentation about patient care, and deciding on the basis of that documentation whether treatment is appropriate. Documentation requirements increase yearly. The additional time required to fill out all those forms further reduces the time that can be spent on direct patient care. So for your doctor, time is incredibly tight.

But no matter what the time constraints, you have to understand your care.

First of all, you will be educating yourself as much as you can on your own. Much of the direction for your homework will come from your own case and treatment. You have to know where to start. Second, you have to be sure, in an era of such hurried medical care, that nothing important has been missed. For that you have to understand not only what your doctor is doing, but why.

No matter how tight your doctor's schedule is, there must be time, every visit, for explaining. If your doctor likes to teach and to have you share in management decisions, your insistence on this will be respected. If not, you are at a disadvantage.

In my office, we keep a current HIV file in the waiting room. Newsletters, faxes, and the newest reports on HIV are placed there on arrival at our office. Patients and their friends are encouraged to come early, to catch up on the latest news.

Often, they get to information before I do, and I hear the news from them—well in advance of my weekend reading sessions.

If my appointments are running late, their waiting room time is better spent. And we get a head start on education, once it's their turn. Despite our time restrictions, our knowledge base keeps growing.

Willingness to Learn

Another response to the time crunch is your doctor's increasing need for focus. The body of knowledge affecting HIV care is complex and dynamic. Because the disease itself is so new, a timely understanding of new approaches is critical to providing state-of-the-art care. There just isn't time to spend on side trips.

You have more time to look around. New approaches, originating outside traditional medicine, alternative treatments of interest to you and the HIV community, practical tips passed from patient to patient on maintaining and improving the comfort and quality of life or on accommodating to the demands of treatment, opportunities in the community for social support, political actions having an impact on HIV—you can gather all this information and share it with your doctor.

You want to be in charge of your care. Some doctors will not be used to this in a patient. You may not agree with their approach to treatment, and you will have to say so.

The more open your doctor is to your participation, the more you will participate in your care. If you choose a doctor who is not dogmatic and controlling, but is open to your input, everybody wins.

Knowledge Base

Regardless of personal characteristics, your doctor must have a good grasp of medical information. Studies have shown that doctors who have taken care of HIV patients before do better than those who have not. Those doctors were reported to also see patients more often, order diagnostic tests earlier, and treat sooner and more aggressively. Thus it's not clear whether they do better because they know more or because they try harder. But either way, you'll do better with a doctor on your team who knows what she or he is doing and does more of it.

HIV medicine is complex and can be highly technical. Knowledge increases daily, requiring frequent changes in management strategy to ensure state-of-the-art care. Controversies rage, because information is incomplete. If you and your doctor are to form your own opinions about the best approach for you, you must both know all the options and the arguments.

And there's more to medicine than book learning. Ideally, you want a doctor who has seen a lot of HIV patients and will recognize the signs and symptoms that signal need for care.

In those parts of the country where demand for HIV medicine is still low, care is often managed by infectious disease (I.D.) specialists. These women and men have had extra training, beyond their internal medicine specialization, in diseases caused by infection. The greater part of their work is done in acute care hospitals.

In areas where most doctors are not comfortable with the demands of HIV management, I.D. specialists are the logical choice. The spectrum of patients they care for is narrowly defined, so they can keep current on new developments. They will have seen and cared for HIV patients before. Their reputation is based on their ability to manage complex I.D. problems. No I.D. practice worth its salt will refuse, or feel overwhelmed by, the care of an HIV patient.

In parts of the country where HIV is more common, the bulk of patient care is often managed by primary care specialists—internists and family practitioners. There are advantages to this model of care, also.

These doctors are accustomed to caring for people with chronic conditions, over time. They are more likely to consider the non-infectious aspects of HIV. They may pay more attention to comfort, for instance, and to emotional status. They are experienced in pain control, value preventive care, and in some cases understand the importance of maintaining good nutritional status. They are likely to be detail-oriented. Much of their practice is office-based, focused on keeping people active and healthy in spite of their underlying conditions. The people who choose these specialties often do so because they value the rewards of long-term relationships with patients.

Thus, internists and family practitioners who are experienced in HIV can provide excellent care, often with greater breadth and vision than an I.D. specialist has been trained for. It's important to be sure, though, that they have the requisite knowledge, interest, and experience with HIV to give you the care you should have.

Interviewing Your Doctor

Providing good primary care for HIV patients is hard work. Many doctors avoid it because of rigorous academic demands and the importance of detail. Those doctors who avoid it when they can will do it poorly when they can't. They just don't have the experience.

It's possible to get good care from your doctor even when her or his HIV experience is limited. But it requires much dedication and study. In a general medical practice, where many illnesses need attention, that requires a high level of interest.

So you need to get a sense of your doctor's familiarity and comfort with HIV. Here are some of the questions to consider:

- Have you cared for HIV and AIDS patients before? How many?
- Do you welcome HIV and AIDS patients to your practice?
- Are you interested in HIV care? For instance, have you attended conferences or workshops focused on HIV?
- How do you keep up to date on new developments? Do you read journals or attend hospital conferences?
- Are you aggressive in your approach? How often do you monitor CD4 counts and viral load?
- Do you change your management when counts go down or viral load goes up?
- Are your patients on combinations of drugs to directly fight HIV? How do you choose these combinations?
- Do you prescribe medications to protect against secondary infections? Do you do this according to a schedule? Which infections do you try to avoid in this way?
- Do you monitor nutritional status? Do you use medical treatments and interventions when nutritional competence is threatened?
- Do you ever use enteral (through the gut) or parenteral (through the vein) nutritional supplementation for your HIV-positive patients?
- Do your patients work with a dietician?
- Are any of your patients involved in research trials? Do you yourself promote this involvement?
- Are you affiliated with a university or a residency teaching program?
- Do you, or does someone in your office, know where to refer patients for appropriate social services?
- Are you willing to follow patients who initiate alternative therapies on their own?

Obviously, you can't interview this person as if she or he were seeking a job. And you can't afford to be offensive—particularly when this doctor may in fact provide your care. But a first meeting, to get to know the doctor and evaluate her or his level of expertise, can yield essential information.

You will find out a lot about attitude, too. Doctors are generally not thrilled about the interview process and may tend to be guarded; demanding patients are a lot more work. But some doctors actually appreciate a healthy concern about your health care needs. If you find this, it's definitely worth extra points.

If You Already Have a Doctor
•

There's much to be said for time in the building of a bond. If you've been with your doctor for a long while, and you both love and trust one another, you have a head start on finding an ally. Consider that bond as you review the attributes we've discussed above.

If your doctor's technical competence is spotty, you can talk about that. Your doctor may be willing to refer you to a specialist to manage that part of your care. You two can learn and strategize together, based on the recommendations of the specialist. But be sure, no matter how much there is that's worth keeping, that you add HIV expertise to the current mix.

If in fact you're unhappy with your current doctor, the best time to change is during times of health. Don't wait for a crisis to make the change. First impressions are crucial; your new doctor will think of you as sicker than you are, if she or he meets you at your worst. If you are relatively healthy, now is better than later.

One more thing: when considering a change, check the next doctor out before you say good-bye. Doctors are also nourished by the bond between you and will be hurt at some level by your dissatisfaction. The bond will be weaker if you leave and come back.

Building a Relationship
•

The importance of developing a good relationship with your doctor has already been stressed. Much of this will come naturally if you have found a good fit. You can do more to make it better still.

You have a lot at stake here, so you want to make things work. Recognize that your doctor has a lot at stake, too. In HIV care there is already an element of pressure: time is precious, as you've seen, and the rewards—both in autonomy and in pay—are much less than doctors were taught to expect in the past. Emergencies come up and throw the day off schedule. The one reward that remains unchanged, though, is the sense of pride in a job well done.

Making It Work for You Both

Doctors are immensely rewarded by success: there is no better payment than the feeling that we have done well, that our patients have done well, and that we are trusted and appreciated. Those of us who have chosen to provide long-term care for people with chronic health conditions are usually those who value the deepening of friendship that comes with long-term association. As much as you need support and encouragement, we need it too. Giving it, when appropriate, is a good way of ensuring that you will get it back.

There's a real ego boost to be found, too, in seeing the results of our work. If you do well, we feel validated. I want to send some of my patients out with sandwich-board ads on them, I'm so proud of how they're doing. It's really they who deserve most of the credit, but I get a contact high. And it makes me want to work even harder. So the first thing you can do to ensure high-quality care is to be supportive and appreciative where it's warranted.

When you first see your doctor, try to show a willingness to trust, both in her intent and her competence. If you don't feel this trust yet, that's natural. But as in any relationship, starting with hostility and mistrust will make the other person defensive and engender mistrust in return.

Being Prepared

There will be a finite amount of time available for you at each appointment. Especially because you want to understand what's being done, there's a danger that your appointment will run late. Every time this happens, that time must be withheld from the care of other patients or other responsibilities. If this happens more than once, a doctor will approach your visit with the primary objective of damage control.

You can make your appointments work for both of you by being organized and prepared. If you come in with a list, and bring up all your issues at the start of the appointment, problems can be prioritized and addressed in turn. If you have done your homework and know what you want, your doctor may at first fear that her or his authority is being threatened; but when she sees that you're careful about the time, and that your preparedness actually *saves* time, your involvement will be appreciated.

Being Informed

The primary currency of power for people trained as scientists is knowledge. If you are informed about your condition and about the standard of care at your stage of HIV infection, you will win your doctor's respect. If you understand why you want something done, and can argue for it from a scientific standpoint, you will go a long way toward equalizing the power between the two of you in that room. And if you can do so with grace, it will not be resented.

Let me tell you a little about Keith. Keith tested HIV-positive in 1986. He has followed the research closely. Much of what he has learned comes from a period of activist involvement with Act Up, an association of largely HIV-positive people who value the accumulation of knowledge, as much as they value political activism, in the service of their cause. He's been in multiple research trials testing the effectiveness of new drugs in the care of HIV. His eagerness to learn has won him the respect of his investigators, and they have taught him well.

Keith has also made major changes in his lifestyle to maintain his body's ability to fight the progression of his illness.

When Keith first came to my office, he was considering two new approaches to his care. One was the addition of a new antiretroviral drug to his regimen—one I had never worked with. The other was an as-yet-unproven alternative approach to the maintenance of lean body mass. He wanted my opinion on both.

Fortunately for me, he was not disturbed that he knew more than I did about one of these approaches—as long as I was willing to learn.

Fortunately for Keith, my grounding in the physiological basis of HIV disease was more thorough than his, so I could contribute too.

We have negotiated several changes in his care since then. When I can't be certain of the safety of a treatment he's committed to, he takes responsibility for it—listening to my concerns and arranging for his own medicines and supplies if he still chooses to go forward. He always tells me what he's doing, and I monitor him to ensure that he's not hurting himself.

I have so much respect for Keith's fund of knowledge that I try to do my homework before every visit. His involvement and commitment bring out my best. Together we are building a more aggressive and thorough regimen of care than I could possibly have offered him alone. Because he trusts my intentions, he's not threatened by what I don't know; because he's so hungry to learn, I just can't teach enough.

Keith is more work than a lot of my HIV patients. Because he takes the trouble to educate himself, he's worth it. And more and more of my patients are mirroring his style.

Asking Questions

The best way you can be an equal partner in your care is to understand the basis for it. Much of this you will do on your own. But whenever a change is suggested and you don't know why, you should ask. You need to agree with the rationale for your treatment if you are to accept it.

You can do this without hostility, and with respect for your doctor's time. Once your doctor sees that you're sensitive to her needs or his needs, too, this will be welcomed. When there's time, we love to teach. When you understand and agree with your treatment, you will follow it. Everybody wins.

Doing Your Part

It's hard to be compulsive about every aspect of care if the patient doesn't care as much as we do. So you can earn your doctor's best efforts by putting forth your own.

If you show up for appointments; if you take your medicines (when you've agreed to their prescription); if you invest your own efforts in your care, in the ways we talked about in Part Two; if you honor your own body in the way that you live; if you come in promptly when you start to get sick—then your doctor will respect your commitment and work harder. It's tiring and unrewarding to take care of people who won't take care of themselves. When it's a partnership, it's worth it.

Keeping Track

Sharing in the responsibility for your care will improve its consistency. You have more time, and more at stake, than your doctor. You'll find a flow sheet to copy, and suggestions for what to monitor, in Appendix VI. You'll also find cheat sheets—quick summaries of recommended care at different stages of HIV—in Chapter Eighteen. If you keep your flow sheets up to date, and check your care against those recommendations, you will save your doctor time, and save yourself from the chance of missing something.

As a doctor I get positively competitive when people do this. It's almost a race to recommend a step to them before they bring it up to me.

You will ensure that there are no slipups in your care, if you keep track.

Contributing

You want a doctor who's open to your contributions; doctors want a patient who contributes. Every time you add to our fund of knowledge—about alternative treatments in the community, new trials and medicines, a way to deal with mouth sores, or a good, cheap gym—you help us to help others. Every time you add to our fund of knowledge, you make us better doctors. Your interest is contagious. And we are grateful for it.

Some of my patients bring in papers or information almost every time they come in. This helps me broaden my approach to HIV: it shows me areas to focus on in my own reading, helps me enhance the comfort of other patients, offers me more flexibility in providing care for people whose financial resources are strained, and helps me know when something is currently in fashion that might actually do harm, so I can warn my patients of its dangers.

Papers from patients also go in our current HIV file, once I have determined that they offer nothing harmful.

My patients are important contributors to my education and to the pattern of their care. Because of their commitment, we can consider a broader range of treatment options. We can take into account personal preferences and fighting styles. We can add the option of alternative supports to our own knowledge base.

A Dialogue

Of course, the most crucial part of each of these suggestions is that they foster interaction. We learn, we teach, we discuss and argue. We do it with respect for the demands of time and for each other. We do it without criticism. And as we share our excitement at doing the best job we can together, we build a relationship of two adults — sharing the power and the control, as well as the success of good results. When it works, each of us is nourished by the other and feeds the other's enthusiasm. And, as N. S. Lehrman said in an elegant exploration of the doctor-patient relationship, pleasure heals.

REFERENCES

Adler, H. M., and Hammett. "The doctor-patient relationship revisited." *Annals of Internal Medicine,* 1973, *78,* 595–598.

Barnlund, D. C. "The demystification of meaning: Doctor-patient encounters." *Journal of Medical Education,* 1976, *51,* 716–725.

Lehrman, N. S. "Pleasure heals: The role of social pleasure—love in its broadest sense—in medical practice." *Archives of Internal Medicine,* 1993, *153,* 929–934.

Quill, T. E., and Brody. "Physician recommendations and patient autonomy: Finding a balance between physician knowledge and patient choice." *Annals of Internal Medicine,* 1996, *125*(9), 763–769.

Steinberg, C. "I plan a long-term relationship with my HIV patient: We may work together for the next decade." *HIV/AIDS Clinical Insight,* 1994, *4*(5), 5, 9–10.

Vollhardt, L. T. "Psychoneuroimmunology: A literature review." *American Journal of Orthopsychiatry,* 1991, *61*(1), 35–47.

CHAPTER 10

•

Understanding Your Health Care Plan

Chances are you will not pay directly for most of your medical care. If you are working, you may have insurance through a group health plan. If not, there are other provisions for obtaining the care you can't afford.

Since nobody tests HIV-positive by design, you will probably have your insurance in place at the time of diagnosis. If not, don't despair. There are ways to finance care, insured or not, no matter how little money you have.

Each type of plan has its own advantages and disadvantages. If you are insured through a group plan at work, you need to know what it covers and how to make it work for you. You also may have an opportunity to change your plan; many businesses have an open enrollment period every year, during which time employees can choose from among several options. If you choose wisely, you can maximize your benefits.

Models of Health Care Available
•

Health care plans come in many forms. You may be a member of a health maintenance organization, or HMO. You may have a plan that uses a preferred provider organization, or PPO. You may be part of a staff model plan. Or, if you are lucky enough to have one of the traditional plans most common until the last decade or so, you may have an indemnity plan, which pays by a method called "fee-for-service."

If you are not insured, your health care will be provided by clinics, in teaching hospitals, or in private offices through Medicare or Medicaid.

We'll go through each of these models and explain them. Each has its own distinct features.

Traditional Fee-for-Service

This is the kind of plan everybody had, if they were insured, until about twenty years ago. In some parts of the country it is still offered through employers. People who carry independent insurance or are retired may also have this type of insurance.

With a fee-for-service, or indemnity, plan, you can choose all your doctors freely. You can refer yourself to specialists whenever you choose. You can see a dermatologist for acne, a gastroenterologist for abdominal pain, or a cardiologist for blood pressure management if you wish. While such programs generally will not pay for cosmetic surgery and sometimes disallow routine physicals, almost all other costs are covered.

The plan itself generally covers 80 percent of your medical costs, at the full rate charged by doctors, laboratories, and hospitals; you pay the rest, after paying a yearly deductible. Normally, after a certain amount has been spent, all other costs will be covered. Hospital and emergency room visits are usually covered in full.

Nobody tells you what care you can have, and nobody argues with your doctor about what care you need.

Such a plan makes it possible for you and your doctor to be as aggressive as you please with your care. Except for the bother of filing insurance forms, there is generally no further documentation required. Because of this, however, fee-for-service plans are expensive. Often, premiums can be more than twice those charged for other models. Since people who are rarely ill and don't need much attention will seek a cheaper alternative, the price of fee-for-service premiums is driven up by natural selection; those who are left need comprehensive care and are thus more expensive to insure, so costs are shared throughout the group. And as insurance companies try to move away from this model, yearly premiums increase substantially. Those increases cause more people to go elsewhere, raising costs even further for the people who remain. In the worst case you may have to leave the protection of a plan because you simply can't afford it anymore. If this happens, other plans won't be in a hurry to take you.

Prescription costs, if they are covered, are generally covered at 80 percent, after a deductible is satisfied.

The Benefits.　Freedom of choice, control of access, full coverage. You can choose different doctors regardless of their group or hospital affiliation. Your doctor doesn't mind frequent visits, or spending extra time, because it's paid for. Your hospital doesn't question studies or treatments ordered, for the same reason. You can have your doctor's choice of medicines, without concern for cost, where indicated.

The Drawbacks.　Cost of premiums, cost of your copayment, large yearly premium increases. These plans are already hard to find in some parts of the country. In others they will become harder to find over time. If there is a lifetime limit on costs covered, that limit will be reached more quickly. Fragmentation of care between different doctors who don't coordinate their activities can make care less efficient and lead to unsuspected drug or treatment interactions. You may get more care than you need.

Preferred Provider

This type of plan comes closest to the traditional fee-for-service model. Insurance companies contract with certain doctors to provide your care at a discounted rate. When you go to these doctors, you pay only a small copayment for each visit. You may still go to any doctor you choose, though, for a higher fee.

Hospitals, home care companies, and other providers—physical therapists, for example—also contract to provide care at discounted rates, in exchange for an increased volume of work. When you use them, you will pay either none of your bill or a smaller amount.

When you go outside the plan, though, you will pay a significant portion—say, for instance, 30 percent—of the bill yourself. This includes not only doctor visits, labs, and studies, but even hospital costs. So you pay dearly for the freedom you elect. Also, payment for those out-of-plan services may only be made based on the in-plan, discounted rate; therefore, your 30 percent contribution may, in the end, be closer to 50 percent of out-of-plan charges.

Costs in a preferred provider plan can be further controlled by monitoring the primary physician you are assigned to. If that doctor yields to pressure to keep referrals down, and you want a specialist for something, you will have to either do without or self-refer and pay a larger portion of the cost.

Prescription costs may be covered except for a percentage or a nominal copayment.

The Benefits.   Access to comprehensive care, more control, less expense. The option to move outside the plan if you want a particular expert or a service that's not provided or one your doctor won't agree to.

The Drawbacks.   Copayments required within the plan. Costs outside the plan are substantial. Doctors in the plan are dependent on the insurance company, not on you, for economic survival and may be less accommodating. Payment is at discount rates, so office costs and appointment times must be carefully controlled.

Health Maintenance Organizations

HMOs appear to be the wave of the future. Once a rarity, they now make up a large share of the market—particularly in those parts of the country where health care is highly organized. These are organizations that provide all of your health care needs from within their own network, controlling costs by careful review of expenses and providing care according to rigid standards that are often set from above by administrators.

Cost reduction is your HMO's primary objective. This is accomplished, to begin with, by placing your care under the control of your doctor, or "primary care provider." It's called the gatekeeper concept: the role of your doctor is to manage your case, insofar as possible, in the office—minimizing referrals, laboratory costs, and the use of special studies. Referrals to specialists are rare and subject to strict criteria. If your doctor or your reviewer doesn't think you need something, and you think you do, you're out of luck.

Documentation requirements are massive. Doctors often spend more time reporting on or requesting approval for treatment than they do providing it.

Another way in which costs are controlled is to develop plan-wide clinical pathways for managing specific situations; these pathways are said to direct care efficiently and cheaply. The use of medications and treatments must conform to these plans. New uses for medicines, new treatments or preventive methods, even though they may have been proven effective by recent studies and recommended by experts, will not be approved until they are specifically indicated—that is, blessed by the Food and Drug Administration. More aggressive, hence more expensive, approaches to care will be discouraged, if not disallowed altogether.

Thus you are likely to get good basic care, according to standards agreed upon nationally; but if you want more exacting, more current, or more costly approaches to care, you will have to argue for them. And you still may not get them.

On the good side, HMOs usually provide prescription medicines as part of their benefits, for a small copayment. They are more active in education and prevention in those circumstances where it will save them money. And, except for a nominal payment each time you see your doctor, your medical bills will not increase when the demands of your care increase. The all-inclusive nature of their care can be a real plus to someone who will need a lot of doctoring for not a lot of money.

One advantage of the standards imposed by HMOs is that, while you are not likely to find aggressive or proactive care, particularly when it is costly, you are also less likely to receive inadequate or inappropriate basic care. The potential for poor quality may be reduced when all doctors are held to a common standard.

In an HMO, your doctors are likely to be salaried. Thus they are highly controlled by the expectations of the HMO, including its emphasis on cost control. Also, they may not be paid any more for seeing you once a year than for seeing you once a day. If they are busy—and they will be—they will have a powerful incentive to keep you from showing up too often.

Even if your doctors are not salaried, they will often be paid by the head, or "capitated," on a monthly basis, according to the number of patients they care for—regardless of whether those patients come in regularly or not at all. Thus it is to their advantage to have patients who are healthy, without problems or illnesses that need monitoring.

In HMOs with many HIV-positive members, this inequity is sometimes resolved by establishing a panel of doctors who specialize in HIV. All patients with HIV must choose one of these doctors, usually when they reach a predetermined point (say, a CD4, or T-helper, count of 500). They are knowledgeable about HIV, and therefore more efficient in their plans for care. They are also subject to pressure, overt or economic, to provide that care as inexpensively as possible. Thus you must always be your own advocate for excellence of care.

Switching doctors at a certain point in your infection may cost you much of the investment in time and trust you spent building a relationship with your prior doctor. Once your new care is established, however, you are likely to see the same person much of the time. You have a chance to build, again, the kind of relationship you'll need to carry you both through the bad times.

Also, doctors who specialize in HIV care may well be not only knowledgeable, but committed. You won't have to deal with ignorance or prejudice. You may have to deal with detachment, however. And if you think you need treatment, and your doctor doesn't, your doctor's decision will prevail.

In order to control the high cost of HIV care, nurse practitioners or physician assistants, supervised by a physician, may be used for routine monitoring and care. This may not be a disadvantage, however. These people can spend more time with you than your doctor can. And they are almost always there because they believe in their job. They have time to explain things more fully and to work more closely with you.

In some hospitals, particularly where care is capitated and

doctors are not paid for hospital visits, your hospital care may not even be managed by your doctor. To further control costs, these hospitals or groups have an inpatient manager—a doctor who supervises your care whenever you are hospitalized, returning you to the care of your own doctor upon discharge. While these doctors are likely to be technically competent, they will have none of the personal investment in your care that your own doctor has, and that you have worked so hard to foster. And they work for the hospital or group, so they are primarily concerned with cost control.

Some HMOs are managed on what is called a staff model. This means that doctors are salaried and subject to strict controls on how to practice. In some cases, because of understaffing, you will see different doctors for different visits—especially if the visit is not a routine, scheduled follow-up.

One final warning: when doctors are not salaried, and particularly when they are capitated, many of these plans actually have what is called a risk pool—a sum of money put aside monthly, and paid back to the doctors later if it is not spent on patient care. So you must realize that, in a capitated plan, you face the danger of having your care managed by doctors who make more money by doing less for you.

The Benefits.   Lower premiums, no deductible, a small copayment for visit. Basic competence, efficiency, consistency of care. Medications, if they're on the plan's approved-drug list, are available for a small, standardized fee.

The Drawbacks.   Lack of control, independence, and autonomy. No frills. HMOs are the cheapest approach to care, even when it's not the best. Management is from above and in large part not by doctors. You'll have shorter, more hurried, and less frequent visits, with the associated chance that some things may be missed. Doctors have less time to attend to emotional and social issues. There's a low likelihood of proactive care. In particular, there are tight controls on nutritional therapies. There is also the potential for diversion of the doctors' loyalty to the plan—or to their pocketbooks—instead of to you. The interests of the patient and doctor may be at cross-purposes.

Medicare

Patients covered by Medicare either are over age sixty-five or have been disabled for more than one and a half years. Thus while most of their care is paid for by the government, they have earned it with their social security taxes. Social security is not welfare.

While Medicare payments are lower per visit than those of some insurance plans, most doctors will accept them, and many will accept assignment of benefits. If they do, you will not be expected to pay for your care when it is given; doctors who accept assignment will wait to be paid by Medicare. You will pay a $250 deductible at the start of every year, and 20 percent of costs—at Medicare rates—thereafter.

Hospitals will be reimbursed for your care on the basis of your admitting diagnosis. Whether you stay two days or twenty, reimbursement will be the same for the same diagnosis.

Currently, Medicare controls only the rate of reimbursement and not the method of care. Your doctor may be censured for seeing you too often, but these reviews can be challenged. And you can be referred to any specialist, regardless of his or her hospital or plan affiliation. You may, in fact, refer yourself. Thus, while payment to doctors is reduced, control of care is minimized and autonomy preserved.

If your doctor accepts assignment, you won't have to pay up front. If you also carry secondary insurance, it will pay 80 percent of your 20 percent portion, leaving you with only the small secondary insurance premium and about 5 percent of Medicare fee–based costs.

It is illegal under most circumstances for your doctor to waive payment on the portion of costs that you owe. If you are living on a very restricted income, and request deferment in writing of your share of costs, your doctor may be protected against prosecution for Medicare fraud if she or he doesn't make you pay your portion.

Prescription medications are not covered at all for outpatients. Even intravenous medications, such as those used for infections or for nutritional support, are not covered unless you are hospitalized.

The Benefits. Government-funded medical care, except for your portion. Your portion of costs is reduced by government fee controls. Rates are reduced, but accepted by most doctors. Money is

rarely needed up front for care. Control and autonomy are re-
tained, both for you and for your doctor.

The Drawbacks.   Most important, no prescription benefit. Your
share of costs is still burdensome unless you have a supplemental plan.

Medicare Supplement Plans

There is currently a movement afoot to place Medicare under managed care. Insurance companies offer, and heavily advertise,
Medicare supplement plans. Sometimes they require a small
monthly charge for membership; sometimes there is no such
charge, and your 20 percent share is no longer required; sometimes
they pay for all medicines, if they're on their list of approved drugs,
with only a small copayment required from you.

What the plans don't tell you is that you also give up control.
In exchange for your reduced contribution, you must use only
their doctors, and you will have only those treatments or tests they
approve. You will be assigned to a primary care provider, who will
be pressured to keep costs down and to avoid referrals and costly
studies. Home care, physical therapy, and other ancillary supports
may be rigidly restricted. Your doctor may be capitated and paid to
give you as little care as possible.

In short, these Medicare plans offer cost savings, but at the expense of control. In essence, you're back in an HMO, and your
care is primarily directed for profit. The less you get, the more
everybody makes.

There's a reason for all that heavy advertising—which, in the
end, you pay for. Insurance companies make a lot of money on this
arrangement, because much less is spent on your care.

The Benefits.   Same as for HMOs.

The Drawbacks.   Same as for HMOs.

Medicaid (MediCal in California)

You are eligible for Medicaid if you are disabled or on general assistance; if you have, with some exceptions, minimal assets; and if

your income is well below the poverty line. If you are close to the poverty line, you may qualify by paying a share of costs—an amount that brings your available income down to the level at which you qualify for assistance in your state.

Hospitals will take you, though they'll be anxious to discharge you quickly, to avoid a major loss.

Home care is covered, as are home medicines.

Mental health benefits are so poor that few psychiatrists can afford to see Medicaid patients. Virtually none are seen privately. Community mental health clinics can see only the most disturbed patients.

Payment to doctors is so minimal that it's hard for them to break even. For this reason, many private doctors do not accept Medicaid patients. Most reputable doctors, though, will not discharge a patient who eventually ends up on Medicaid. They just won't make any money.

There are, in fact, private practices that are based on, or welcome, Medicaid patients. Some of these practices are humanitarian, believing that everyone has a right to care regardless of ability to pay. Others are set up to process many patients quickly, counting on volume to cover their overhead. Quality of care and expertise, in these cases, can be spotty.

For patients on Medicaid, the best bet is often a university or teaching hospital clinic. You will probably not have the benefit of an ongoing relationship with a doctor in these cases, but you will be able to count on good technical care, sometimes far better than elsewhere in the community. Also, if you work primarily with residents, they are likely to be accessible and concerned, as medicine is still new to them. And the effort to provide excellent care on a low budget results in a team approach, with dieticians, social workers, nurse practitioners, and other health care providers extensively involved. Thus you are likely to get help in finding—and funding—the things they feel you need.

Some of the best HIV care in the world, for example, is provided at Ward 86, the outpatient HIV clinic at San Francisco General Hospital. Doctors come from all over the world to sit in and see how it's done. Patients seen there get first crack at waiting lists for studies on new drugs and treatments.

For this kind of system to work for you, though, you have to be responsible and proactive. If you miss an appointment, for instance, it may take three weeks to get another one. If you don't ask questions, they won't get answered. If you don't list your questions before you come, there won't be time to remember them. If you don't understand your care, things may be missed as you go from doctor to doctor, from visit to visit.

One way to make the best of this arrangement is to volunteer for studies at a university hospital. The principal investigators on HIV studies are well grounded in HIV care. They attend at HIV clinics, teaching and supervising residents. They are deeply interested in HIV. Generally, they don't do patient care full-time, so they enjoy it. If you can establish a relationship with one of these people, you may get some of the best care available, despite the change in day-to-day caregivers.

Medicines are paid for by Medicaid, though these are restricted to a specific panel of drugs. Newer prescription drugs, and expensive ones, are not covered if there is something else that will do the job. In some circumstances, patients are restricted to a given number of prescriptions per month. You have to pay for pain medication other than codeine, for tranquilizers, or for any of the newer antidepressants.

There is no control exerted by the government over your choice of physicians. The controls are largely economic.

After one and a half years of disability on Medicaid, you may also qualify for Medicare. This improves your access, because reimbursement is better. It also retains your prescription benefit.

The Benefits.   Care provided when you can't afford it, and can't afford or qualify for insurance. Superb and comprehensive technical care available at teaching hospitals, if you do your part. Medicaid provides a safety net, regardless of poverty. Access is available to trials for new treatments. Medications are paid for.

The Drawbacks.   Access to quality care limited in the private sector. Virtually no mental health care available except for the sickest patients. There are long waits and much inconvenience inherent in the clinic setting. The safety net fails if you don't keep on top of appointments.

Managed Care Medicaid

Currently, attempts are under way to convert the Medicaid system to a managed care system—often capitated—as well. This is being done on a countywide trial basis in several areas now, with a view to expanding it nationally in the future.

On the good side, reimbursement is better, so more doctors are willing to see you. On the bad side, cost control is paramount again.

The Benefits. Same as for HMOs.

The Drawbacks. Same as for HMOs.

Indigent Care

If you have no insurance and can't afford medical care, you will still be able receive care at county hospitals. These are generally teaching hospitals, and they are excellent sources of HIV care. Because it is in their interest to get your care paid for, social workers will help you qualify for Medicaid or other programs that will cover you. If you need medicines and can't afford them, they will be provided, too.

The Benefits. Same as for Medicaid.

The Drawbacks. Same as for Medicaid.

Making the Most of Your Options
•

You've seen, in this chapter, what each form of health care plan provides. You know, by now, that you need care. Let's look at how to make that knowledge work for you.

No Insurance

If you have no insurance now, it's time try to get some.

If you're working, see if it's possible to get on a company plan. If not, or if you're unemployed, consider whether you can take a job that provides insurance. If not, the next option is private insurance.

Given your status, no company will be anxious to insure you. But some plans do accept people with preexisting conditions. The catch is that you have to go for twelve to twenty-four months without receiving payment for medical expenses for that condition. Your medicines may be covered by AIDS Drug Action Programs (ADARS) in the interim.

If you're not working, and can't work, consider getting an evaluation for disability. If you are in fact disabled, get it documented by a doctor. This way, you start the clock running for Medicare.

If you're not insured, can't work, and can't get insurance otherwise, start with a visit to an HIV clinic that offers sliding-scale fees. Talk with a social worker, and start the process rolling for obtaining assistance.

Currently Insured

If you have insurance now, take a good look at your plan. Consider the benefits and drawbacks we've discussed.

If your current plan is the only one available, learn what it offers and how it works. Be careful not to waste your medical dollars if you have a fee-for-service plan and pay a significant portion of expenses—especially if there's a lifetime dollar limit for reimbursement.

Be prepared to take charge of your own care, and to argue for what you need if your plan is more restrictive. If your doctor's time is limited by poor reimbursement rates or capitation pressures, find ways to use your appointment time well. Be organized, with questions and requests ready when you go in, avoid unnecessary calls and visits, keep track of your own test results, and monitor your own progress. Be proactive, without being hostile. Doctors respect knowledge and appreciate a shopping list.

If you know you are entitled to a level of care, and can argue for it, you are more likely to get it. If you present a list of problems and proposed solutions, you will simplify the demands of your care. No matter what their financial arrangement, doctors like to do a good job—especially if your preparation makes it easier.

Get to know the office staff. Be considerate. If people are on your side, they will work harder to help you.

And whatever you do, don't give up your insurance.

Choosing a New Plan

If you have an opportunity to choose or to change your insurance, consider the benefits and drawbacks discussed previously. In particular, if you consider changing, ask yourself these questions:

- Can you keep your present doctors?
- Is there a prescription benefit offered? How restrictive is it?
- Is there a clause refusing or limiting care for preexisting conditions?
- What controls are in place limiting aggressive monitoring, antiretroviral therapy, use of drugs for wasting, and prophylaxis?
- Who determines the standard of care? Doctors or administrators?
- How burdensome are documentation requirements before a given type of care can be provided? Will those requirements delay access to care?
- Will your doctors be capitated? If so, how much will they be paid to see you or not see you?
- Is there a risk pool?
- Will it be your doctor who oversees your hospital, as well as outpatient, care?
- Will you be forced to change doctors at any given point?
- Are home care, physical therapy, and mental health care provided?
- Is there any provision for nutritional support, such as costly anabolic therapies or total parenteral nutrition, should the need arise?
- How restrictive is the formulary, or list of prescribable drugs?
- Is there a lifetime dollar limit to what the plan will cover?
- Is there an option for conversion to private insurance if you leave your job? If so, what are the pricing strategies?

If you have a series of plans to choose from, choose with care. Talk to your benefits manager at work or your insurance agent. Know what you are getting. Don't buy a plan you can't afford, in terms of share of cost, but buy the best, most comprehensive plan, with the most room for autonomy, that you can possibly manage. You simply cannot find a better bargain.

CHAPTER 11

•

Monitoring
Your Nutrition

You already understand the importance of maximizing nutritional competence—your body's capacity to maintain the stores it needs; to build, repair, and replace its structures; and to perform all of the tasks necessary to maintain health, strength, and a vigorous immune response.

You are already working to help your body do this, by adjusting diet, daily habits, and your lifestyle.

You've already begun the process of monitoring your nutrition on your own. You've learned how to assess your intake and have adjusted your diet to provide enough calories and protein. You're weighing in once a week.

But there's more you can do to monitor your nutrition, *with* your doctor.

To begin with, you can request a formal nutritional consult. At many teaching hospitals, these are available as a matter of course to clinic patients. The private hospital your doctor uses may offer outpatient counseling as well.

Because the dietician who meets with you may not be familiar with the special nutritional concerns of people with HIV, you may want to take along an HIV-focused form designed for dieticians, to focus her or his attention on these features.

Your own nutritional assessment form, filled out in advance, will help you make the most of this consult.

If your doctor's not an HIV specialist, you may know more than she does about the importance of nutrition. But she will have the tools you need for closer monitoring. Many of the tests we will review are part of normal routine follow-up procedures and will already have been done.

Appendix VI consists of the flow sheet we use in my office. Some of these items will be discussed in more detail in Chapters Thirteen through Fifteen, as they involve monitoring for progression of the virus and searching for secondary infections. In this chapter we'll discuss those labs and studies that advise us specifically about nutritional status.

Monitoring Weight and Lean Body Mass
•

Every time you see your doctor, your weight is recorded. Keep track of it on your own flow sheets. If at all possible, you also want to follow your lean body mass. It can be measured by several techniques.

Anthropometry

Dieticians are trained to do anthropometry—measuring certain parts of your body and using these measurements to estimate how much of your weight is fat, and how much is lean body mass. You have seen some anthropometric formulas in Chapter Three, and you may have used them to estimate your frame size in determining your ideal body weight.

Dieticians will also estimate body fat stores by measuring your triceps skin fold. They use calipers to determine the thickness of the skin midway between your elbow and a point on your shoulder blade.

Another estimate of fat versus lean in body composition is made by determining your body mass index (BMI). Your BMI is determined by dividing your weight (in kilograms) by your height (in meters) squared. If your BMI is greater than 27, you are considered obese; a BMI of more than 24 suggests excess fat. However, BMI is not really helpful for you, because it assumes no wasting process. Your height won't change; if your weight changes, your BMI won't discriminate between lean and fat.

Body density can be estimated, instead, by determining skinfold thickness in several areas and plugging those measurements into equations.

One problem with these measurements is that they are chiefly used to detect overweight, which is not your problem. Also, they are relatively imprecise. They are available, though, at almost any hospital, as part of a nutritional evaluation. This method of estimating lean body mass is more likely to be reliable if the same person does the measurements each time.

Impedance

Bioimpedance analysis (BIA) has become the standard for assessing changes in lean body mass in HIV. Bioimpedance monitors will give a more reliable measure of lean body mass, based on the way an undetectable electric current flows through your body. Since electricity travels through fat at a different rate than through lean body mass, the behavior of that current in your body helps determine your fat-to-lean ratio. They are increasingly used to help guide nutritional care. In my office, we do a bioimpedance analysis on our HIV patients about once every three months. When we're doing research, we do it monthly.

If your doctor's office doesn't have this technology, ask whether it's available through your local HIV feeding program. Here in California, most home infusion companies will offer impedance analysis as part of a free annual nutritional consult. Your doctor or dietician may be able to get it for you that way, too. It's worthwhile to have, as it provides objective information on the results of your exercise and nutritional efforts.

Dual Energy X-Ray Analysis (DEXA)

Until recently, researchers used measurement of total body potassium—which is present in greater quantity in lean tissue than in fat—as a measure of lean body mass. Currently the gold standard is DEXA. This is a radiographic study of your entire body, measuring its density throughout with great precision. Originally used to evaluate bone density in studies on osteoporosis, DEXA is an ideal method for quantitating lean body mass.

If you live near a university that does nutritional studies, and entering these studies will get you serial DEXA measurements, you should try to do so.

One of my patients, Bruce, tested HIV-positive in 1985. Because he's part of a nutritional study at San Francisco General Hospital, he gets a DEXA study about every three months. Bruce saw an immediate increase in his lean body mass this year, beginning only four weeks after starting a daily program of progressive resistance exercise. And it keeps getting better and better. He's thrilled and highly motivated to keep working out. *I'm* thrilled to have access to such costly and exact information that allows me to watch him so closely.

Laboratory Tests for Change in Nutritional Competence
•

We can also follow nutritional status by looking at certain laboratory tests. They can give us an idea of where we stand now and warn us of changes when we are at risk for wasting.

Albumin

Albumin is a protein made by the liver and contained in the blood. It serves as a carrier protein for many active substances in the body, bonding with them and keeping them inactive until free reserves get low, then dissociating to permit their activity in the free state. Because the liver makes albumin in large quantity, it's an excellent marker of nutritional status. The liver has to prioritize; when there's a need to conserve or make other proteins, or the organ itself is injured, albumin levels go down.

Observational studies done at UCLA have shown that *survival in HIV is directly associated with albumin level.*

Albumin has a half-life of two weeks in the body, so blood levels won't show immediate changes. That's why, when you're sick, you need more sensitive markers. But for a quick-and-dirty assessment of nutritional competence, you can't beat it.

Normal values are generally about 3.5 to 5.0 grams per deciliter. I'm happy with anything over 4.0, and I start to worry whenever levels go below 3.7—especially in the setting of infection, or in cases of consistent decline. Any value lower than 3.0 calls for urgent, aggressive intervention.

Albumin is included on every routine chemistry panel. Your doctor will be getting it already. You should check it and record it every time.

I check my patients' levels every three months, and more often when they are ill or at risk. If you're in good shape, you may not need it done this often.

Total Iron Binding Capacity (TIBC)

This is an indirect way to measure transferrin, another protein carried in the blood. Transferrin has a shorter half-life (eight to ten days) than albumin. Because it is replaced sooner, it will show protein wasting sooner than albumin. I use this lab test when my patients are acutely ill or unable to eat. Under these conditions, I need a more rapid indicator of protein loss, so I can begin interventions in time.

TIBC is an inexpensive test, and results are available quickly.

Prealbumin

This is a precursor form of albumin and has an even shorter half-life. Thus it's a very sensitive indicator of changes in protein metabolism. Unfortunately, though, it's a send-out lab test in most hospitals. It doesn't help me to have a more rapid indicator if I get my results four days later. So for this reason I use it rarely—almost always for political reasons, to prove the need for special nutritional intervention to an insurance company or government agency. I don't use it to guide my treatment.

If your doctor is part of a large university hospital and can get this result quickly, it's better than TIBC.

Triglycerides
•

Triglycerides are fats carried in the blood. When metabolism is altered by infection in the ways that promote wasting, more fats are released from fat cells, and fewer fats are used by the liver.

Increased triglycerides are seen at all levels of HIV infection and may reflect the body's reaction to the virus itself. In this case they are often not associated with wasting. But a sudden additional rise can often be the earliest indicator of a new secondary infection, and of the wasting it triggers. It's helpful to catch this and increase your and your doctor's vigilance in looking for subtle early signs of new or worsening infection. When infection is found and treated, triglyceride levels usually drop.

With the advent of combination therapy with protease inhibitors, we now occasionally see dangerously high triglyceride concentrations. Especially with ritonavir, we may see levels of 1,000 to 2,000. At those levels, we must face the danger of incurring pancreatitis.

This is a new finding, and we're just learning how to deal with it. Some of us use antitriglyceride drugs to keep triglycerides at a manageable level. Others look for another protease inhibitor regimen that will pose a lesser risk. In either case, the use of rises in triglyceride levels to signal an occult infection is less productive now.

If your doctor thinks your triglycerides are high because of your protease inhibitor combination, remember: it's critical not to stop that therapy without substituting another powerful regimen. You can't afford to risk resistance while you both think about it. We'll talk more about resistance in Chapter Thirteen.

Another recent development in HIV is the natural aging of well-compensated long-term HIV patients. I see heart attacks and coronary artery bypasses, things we just didn't worry about before. For that reason also, there may be a role for treating significant triglyceride and cholesterol elevations.

Like albumin, triglycerides are also found on any routine chemistry panel. In people with HIV, however, they are often not followed, as the dangers of hyperlipidemia doctors are trained to look for aren't so important in HIV. You may have to ask what your levels are.

Your own attention to this and other values will heighten your doctor's awareness of their importance, over time.

Purified Protein Derivative (PPD) and Controls

This is a test performed annually to look for tuberculosis (TB) exposure. A reaction at the site of injection is regarded as evidence of exposure. People with HIV may sometimes test negative inappropriately, because of an inability to mount the immune response required to react. To differentiate, other testing should be done with controls, or substances people are sure to have been exposed to. Candida (yeast), coccidiomycosis, and mumps are most commonly used as controls. In the case of candida, to which all of us have been exposed, a negative control with a negative PPD suggests anergy—that the immune response itself has failed.

As far as checking for TB is concerned, a negative control with a negative PPD buys you a recheck in seven to ten days; if you're still anergic, you get a chest X ray every year. But in terms of nutrition, anergy is an early indicator of reduced nutritional competence. If you are PPD-anergic—if you don't react to PPD or controls—you can often restore the immune response needed to react by improving nutritional competence.

There is some controversy now over the utility of PPDs, with or without controls, in HIV. Some feel that anergy is common, and therefore likely, and treat only if a chest film is abnormal. Others believe that anyone with a low CD4 count should receive TB prophylaxis, because of the danger of reactivation. TB studies, in fact, suggest that primary infection is more common. I'm still doing an anergy panel, though; I often see reactions to controls, and sometimes to the PPD when controls themselves are negative. In either case, it helps to guide my management.

Monitoring for Results of Impaired Nutrition
•

We've already seen that certain vitamin and mineral deficiencies are common in HIV. In addition, hormone levels may change as a result of wasting or other stresses on the body. Reduced testosterone, for instance, may result in poor retention of lean body mass.

Vitamins and Minerals

We don't routinely check for vitamin levels. The tests are costly, and we're already supplementing in a safe and effective range. There are a few of these, though, that are worth checking for, even if you supplement.

Vitamin B_{12}. Vitamin B_{12} absorption is often impaired in people with HIV. Given the frequency and discomfort of peripheral neuropathy, this can be important. It's important to test for this, even if you supplement your B_{12} intake.

If your B_{12} is low when first checked, it makes sense to supplement it orally. One thousand micrograms a day is a good, high dose. A low level of B_{12} in a patient who supplements may indicate a need for monthly replacement by injection.

Folate. Folate deficiency can also play a part in peripheral neuropathy. Because deficiencies in alcoholics and in the elderly are common, the tests are readily available. Red-blood-cell or RBC folate may be a better indicator of body stores than serum folate. The test must be performed soon after blood is collected, though, so many offices draw serum folate instead.

Magnesium. Magnesium deficiencies are frequent in people with HIV, especially when malabsorption is present. As we discussed in Chapter Four, serum magnesium levels may not reflect tissue stores. For that reason, a high-normal level is not of concern, but a low level should be supplemented. We supplement our HIV-positive patients aggressively, even when they are in the low-normal range. If renal function is impaired, we're careful not to overtreat.

Testosterone

Testosterone is a male sex hormone. Deficiency has been associated with reduced sexual interest and function, loss of vigor, and depression. In the elderly, it has also been associated with poor lean body mass retention and increased deposition of fat.

Many men with HIV disease, especially in its later stages, have low testosterone levels. While this may offer some evolutionary benefit to the species in times of famine (by reducing libido, and hence offspring), this benefit may be at cost to you.

It has been reported that 20 percent of men with HIV are testosterone-deficient. Low testosterone levels often accompany weight loss and wasting; this is probably less a cause than an effect. But research so far suggests that testosterone supplementation may help those who exercise to lay down lean body mass. Improvement in body composition has been shown with supplementation.

There are several studies under way on the use of testosterone in the wasting syndrome. No studies have addressed its effects on wasting in women with HIV.

Ketoconazole (Nizoral), used for fungal infections in people with HIV, and Gancyclovir (DHPG), used to treat cytomegalovirus, can lower testosterone levels.

My office screens male HIV patients yearly for testosterone deficiency. We'll discuss supplementation in Chapter Twelve.

• • •

There are other labs and studies we do to evaluate active wasting. These will also be discussed in Chapter Twelve.

REFERENCES

Bell, S. J., and others. "Nutrition support and the human immunodeficiency virus (HIV)." *Parasitology,* 1993, *107,* S53–S67.

Chlebowski, R. T., and others. "Nutritional status, gastrointestinal dysfunction, and survival in patients with AIDS." *American Journal of Gastroenterology,* 1989, *4*(10), 1288–1292.

Ehrenpreis, E. D., and others. "Kinetics of D-xylose absorption in patients with acquired immunodeficiency syndrome." *Clinical Pharmacological Therapy,* 1991, *49,* 632–640.

Ehrenpreis, E. D., and others. "D-xylose malabsorption: Characteristic finding in patients with the AIDS wasting syndrome and chronic diarrhea." *Journal of Acquired Immune Deficiency Syndromes and Human Retrovirology,* 1992, *5,* 1047–1050.

Friedman, B. "Acquired immunodeficiency syndrome." In G. P. Zaloga (ed.), *Nutrition in Critical Care* (pp. 783–800). St. Louis, Mo.: Mosby, 1994.

Garcia-Shelton, Y., and Neal. "Questions in the management of nutrition in HIV disease." *AIDSfile,* 1994, *8*(1), 8–9.

Grunfeld, C., and others. "Hypertriglyceridemia in the acquired immuno-deficiency syndrome." *American Journal of Medicine*, 1989, *86*, 27–31.

Grunfeld, C., and others. "Circulating interferon-alpha levels and hyper-triglyceridemia in the acquired immunodeficiency syndrome." *American Journal of Medicine*, 1991, *90*, 154–162.

Hecker, L. M., and Kotler. "Malnutrition in patients with AIDS." *Nutrition Reviews*, 1990, *48*(11), 393–401.

Hellerstein, M. K. "HIV-associated metabolic disturbances and body composition abnormalities: Therapeutic applications." *AIDSfile*, 1994, *8*(1), 1–4.

Hellerstein, M. K., and others. "Current approach to the treatment of HIV-associated weight loss: Pathophysiologic considerations and emerging management strategies." *Seminars in Oncology*, 1990, *17*(6), 17–33.

Kotler, D. P., and others. "Body composition studies in patients with the acquired immunodeficiency syndrome." *American Journal of Clinical Nutrition*, 1985, *42*, 1255–1265.

Smith, L. C. "Nutritional assessment and indications for nutritional support." *Surgical Clinics of North America*, 1991, *71*(3), 449–457.

Zeman, F. J., and Ney. *Applications of Clinical Nutrition*. Upper Saddle River, N.J.: Prentice Hall, 1988.

CHAPTER 12

•

The Wasting Syndrome

Our understanding of the processes in our bodies and our lives that lead to wasting has increased dramatically over the last few years. As a result many people with HIV, with the help of doctors and other care providers, have been able to maximize their bodies' response in the fight against progression. Quite a few who had been gravely threatened were still here when the new antiretrovirals came along—and, with that boost, now live and thrive despite their HIV. But in parts of this country and most of the world, the enormous power of an aggressive approach to maintaining nutritional competence has yet to be appreciated. Even in those cities at the center of the epidemic, caregivers may be too burned out or overburdened to properly evaluate and address nutritional status. And in systems where medicine is practiced for profit, the extra cost of doing a good job makes proactive care less likely.

This is particularly a problem because the early phase of wasting is a silent one. If you don't know it's happening, if you don't look for it, you'll miss a critical opportunity to oppose it from the start. It's always easier to keep from getting sick than it is to get well again.

We know that the best time to stop wasting is before, or at least as soon as, it begins. We also know that the processes that set wasting in motion start almost at the moment of infection. So you may need to take the initiative here.

Defining Wasting
•

The formal definition of AIDS wasting syndrome, as described by the Centers for Disease Control is shown in Figure 12.1. While it refers to wasting in the absence of known precipitants other than HIV itself, this distinction is meant to broaden inclusion, rather than to narrow it. No one questions that wasting takes place in the presence of known tuberculosis, for example, or with cryptosporidial diarrhea. Rather, it is felt that people who waste *without* the proven presence of such processes are still just as much at risk as, and require the special care and benefits reserved for, those who carry the diagnosis of AIDS based on other criteria.

So it's important for you and your doctor to recognize that loss of weight or lean body mass deserves as much attention and treatment when we know its cause as when we don't.

FIGURE 12.1.
•

**Centers for Disease Control Definition
of AIDS Wasting Syndrome.**

Findings of profound involuntary weight loss of greater than 10 percent of body weight plus either chronic diarrhea (at least two loose stools per day for greater than or equal to 30 days) or chronic weakness and documented fever for greater than or equal to 30 days (intermittent or constant), in the absence of a concurrent illness or condition other than HIV infection that could explain the findings (e.g., cancer, tuberculosis, cryptosporidiosis, or other specific enteritis).

Source: Morbidity and Mortality Weekly Report, December 18, 1992, p. 17.

It's also crucial to remember that the CDC diagnosis represents a definition of wasting *at crisis stage.* If we know that a loss of a third of our weight or half of our lean body mass is life-threatening, *we can't wait to address it till we're almost halfway there.* This is especially true because of what we've learned about HIV's effects on nutritional competence itself: it is infinitely more difficult to restore lean body mass, once lost, than it is to defend against losing it.

So even if you don't meet the CDC criteria for the wasting syndrome, any evidence of wasting must be aggressively addressed. And you need to look for wasting from the start.

What Causes Wasting
•

We've already looked at how and why wasting takes place in Chapters One and Two of this book. We've seen that the causes are multiple. Anorexia can be profound. And reduced caloric intake is the primary contributor. But prevention or reversal of wasting, with reconstitution of skeletal protein, may require more than adequate intake. Appropriate treatment must be tailored to cause in each case.

Acute precipitants of wasting, then, are secondary infections, manifested by weakness or fatigue, intermittent or constant fever, and loss of appetite; diarrhea, even when not severe and even when no causative organism has been found; and other processes, such as cancer, that initiate systemic symptoms—fatigue, fever, and loss of appetite. Loss of appetite then compounds the problem, as do reduced absorption, altered ability to use absorbed nutrients, and increased metabolic requirements in the face of intense immune stimulation, which speeds heart rate, raises body temperature, and wastes absorbed nutrients, increasing resting energy expenditure by these responses. We are unable to compensate sufficiently to match our energy needs to the energy available from our diet. So we respond to increased resting energy spent by reducing active energy spent. And when we lay low we become deconditioned and lose even more muscle mass. While mechanical problems that impair intake do contribute to wasting, the resolution of these problems is not enough to balance our energy economy.

We have to be on guard for wasting. We have to determine all of its causes and fight them.

Monitoring for Wasting
•

An aggressive and appropriate approach to wasting, then, involves three separate steps:

1. Prevention
2. Assessment and treatment of underlying causes
3. Treatment of effects

Treatment of HIV itself is discussed in Chapter Thirteen. Treatment of secondary infections is discussed in Chapter Fourteen. Close monitoring will help you address each of these stages early and direct the interventions needed to minimize potential damage.

Prevention

If you've followed the recommendations made earlier in this book, you're already monitoring for prevention on your own. You're weighing in weekly and checking your protein and calorie intake every three months. If your weight is dropping or your intake has fallen off, you'll be the first to know.

If in addition your doctor follows your lean body mass by bioimpedance analysis, or if you can get it followed by DEXA through a research study, you're ahead of the game. Changes in lean body mass not only exceed, but *precede* weight loss, and they can thus prompt an earlier search for potential causes.

You are already watching your albumin level, using the flow sheet in Appendix VI. It will float up and down a little bit routinely; but a steady drop, even over two doctor visits or two sets of lab tests, should serve as a red flag.

A significant drop in albumin—three-tenths of a point or more, for instance—or a drop over two consecutive visits should prompt efforts to confirm a change in nutritional status. In most doctor's offices, the simplest way to do this is to check TIBC, or total iron binding capacity. TIBC, as we said in Chapter Eleven, is an indirect measure of serum transferrin, a protein that is degraded more quickly than albumin and is also a predictor of malnutrition and hence disease progression. Because it is used up sooner than albumin, it will show depletion of protein stores more rapidly. Thus it will offer a more immediate indication of changes in nutritional status. If you are followed in a university setting, prealbumin results may be available quickly, and they will be even more sensitive.

Changes in triglyceride levels can be another early warning sign. They indicate immune, hence cytokine, activation. If they rise significantly, you and your doctor need to consider the unannounced presence of another process, and look for causes more carefully. In the age of combination treatment with protease inhibitors, however, triglycerides may increase to very high levels in the absence of infection. If this is true for you, your doctor may even be treating your triglycerides with medication, to keep them low enough to maintain your antiretroviral regimen safely. In either case, triglycerides will no longer serve as a marker for early infection.

You can aid in this effort by paying close attention to specific symptoms and recording them. The more precisely you can tell your doctor what you're feeling, the more focused the search can be.

Assessment and Treatment of Underlying Causes

Once you find early evidence that the process of wasting has begun, you can start to seek its cause. Your doctor will direct that search based on several factors.

Perhaps the most important clues in searching for the source of infection will be the presence of symptoms you've recorded. Even bronchitis, or a case of sinusitis, or a urinary tract infection, can precipitate wasting in people with HIV. If you report facial pain, a chronic cough, or pain when urinating, your doctor will know where to start looking for trouble.

You and your doctor also need to look at the circumstances of your life. If you've been eating tacos from street stands in Mexico, for instance, or if you've had unprotected sexual intercourse, the list of possible infections will be different than it would be without these exposures. If your community reports a recent outbreak of cryptosporidium from the water supply, that will be a factor. If you own and care for a pet or work around animals, there will be other specific organisms you and your doctor should look for.

Another way to direct your evaluation will be to look at your lowest-ever CD4 count. We call this your CD4 nadir. It is this number we use, not your most recent CD4 count, when considering likely causes of infection. This is because the immune reconstitution we now see with powerful combination antiretroviral regimens, although remarkable and exciting, is not a complete reconstitution; there may still be less capacity to recognize, and hence respond to, certain invaders. We'll talk more about this in Chapter Fourteen.

Knowing your CD4 nadir will help to direct the search for a likely cause of infection. Certain infections and other processes tend to appear after a given point in HIV progression. Tuberculosis, for instance, can appear quite early; MAC, or mycobacterium avium complex, will rarely present in people with CD4 nadirs of more than 100. Pneumocystis pneumonia is most often seen after CD4 nadirs have dropped below 200, although it can be found in people with higher counts. Sinusitis can appear, with significant systemic effects, very early. Sinusitis may also be chronic, since infections are hard to clear. Chronic sinusitis can be hard to diagnose clinically, as there may be no localized symptoms. Even if your doctor treats for chronic sinusitis on the basis of clinical suspicion, we often see organisms we would not tend to suspect. This is especially true in advanced HIV infection. Thus, any suspicion of sinus involvement should prompt imaging. Also, since plain films may not be helpful, HIV care providers increasingly rely on limited computerized tomography (CT) scans or CAT scans, to evaluate for chronic sinusitis.

It is especially important to establish a cause for diarrhea when it presents. The most likely offenders will also be suggested by your CD4 nadir.

Monitoring for Relapse

When an infection has been found and treated, it is often worthwhile to request a repeat evaluation after the course of treatment has been completed. Certain infections—sinusitis and stool parasites in particular—may be suppressed but not resolve completely with the prescribed course of treatment. If this is so, it's better to extend or step up treatment while the infection has been partially controlled than to wait for it to reappear full-blown.

If your symptoms are gone, wait a week or so after treatment is finished to retest. Many antibiotics continue to have a partial effect for a few days after discontinuance. This can be enough to give you a negative culture or lab test, but not enough to completely eradicate the infection.

Just as close monitoring of simple, easily obtained nutritional lab values can offer early clues to the presence of an infection, their improvement can be a measure of the success of treatment.

Monitoring for Malabsorption

If you're losing weight, or lean body mass, even though you're keeping up with calories and protein requirements, malabsorption may be a factor. There are ways to test for this.

The D-Xylose Test.   This test measures your ability to absorb sugars.

Xylose is a sugar that is not found in the diet or used by the body. Thus whatever gets into your body will be reflected in serum levels, and what goes in will come out.

The test is performed by feeding the subject a measured dose (normally twenty-five grams) of xylose. Serum levels are measured one and two hours later; they should reflect the body's ability to absorb simple sugars. The two-hour level is the most sensitive. Urine is collected for five hours after administration, and its xylose content is also measured. Since this particular sugar is not used or altered by the body, everything absorbed will be cleared through the urine. Low levels of xylose in serum or urine indicate carbohydrate malabsorption in the small intestine.

Some gastrointestinal specialists do not routinely use this test; in the presence of a known infection, D-xylose tests are more likely to be positive. But that is exactly why we *want* to do the study in HIV. We know that people absorb nutrients less well during a stress to their immune system, but we also know *it is that very combination of malabsorption and infection that can contribute to wasting.* And while HIV-negative people who malabsorb during infections can quickly restore weight and lean body mass once their infection has resolved, HIV-positive patients often cannot.

D-xylose testing is most often performed in an inpatient hospital setting. However, it can also be set up as an outpatient study.

We have a convenient arrangement with our hospital lab. Patients are fed a xylose load and given a urinal bottle when they present for testing. They stay around the hospital and return for blood draws two hours later. At the end of five hours, they return with their urine collection.

This works well for us and is simpler and less expensive for the patient. We do get teased about it, though; people look pretty silly sitting around the hospital lobby, or strolling through the halls, with their gallon jug of urine at their side.

Stool for Fecal Fat, or Sudan Stain. These are tests for steatorrhea, or excess fat in bowel movements due to fat malabsorption. For the first test, stools are collected for twenty-four hours, and the quantity of fat they contain is measured. It's a hard test to do, though; people don't much like collecting stool for twenty-four hours, and lab techs are less than thrilled when samples arrive. For this reason we use the Sudan stain. This is a stain that, when applied to a smear on a microscope slide, helps to estimate the amount of fat in the stool. If levels are high, less fat has been absorbed through the gut wall.

A quick-and-dirty way to look for fat malabsorption is to check your stool in the toilet before flushing. Fat is lighter than water; extra fat in your stool can cause it to float. A 1997 San Francisco General Hospital study of fifty-three subjects with HIV-associated weight loss or diarrhea reported fat malabsorption in 79 percent.

If we know a patient is malabsorbing sugars or fats, it gives us a basis for considering the temporary use of aggressive nutritional interventions to support lean body mass, or to minimize its loss during periods of active infection and wasting. Some of these will be discussed below. We can also tailor the foods we take in to our ability to absorb them. It is on this basis that medical foods, specific supplements for specific problems, have been developed. Medium-chain triglycerides, for instance, may be more easily absorbed if fat absorption is poor.

Monitoring During Treatment for the Effects of Wasting

We'll discuss medical treatments that directly affect the course of wasting later in the chapter. During the course of those treatments, in a period of active weight loss, it's especially important to follow the nutritional laboratory values discussed previously.

Prealbumin, transferrin, and TIBC values are valuable in this setting. They indicate response to medicines or other interventions early and keep you on the mark. You can also monitor the effectiveness of treatment by clinical signs: a reduction in the number of bowel movements, for example, or a return of appetite.

Stabilization or increase in weight is encouraging; improvement in lean body mass, when it can be followed, is a true indicator of success.

Medicines to Counter Wasting
•

Aggressive management is necessary to limit loss of weight or lean body mass during periods of active wasting. You need your doctor's help, as most of the medicines we use are available only by prescription. We'll address these interventions based on their mechanism of action—what they counteract, what they capitalize on, and how they work.

Appetite Enhancers

Appetite enhancers are helpful in combating HIV wasting. They are prescribed to help overcome the anorexia, or loss of appetite, we suffer during periods of active illness.

Megace (Megestrol Acetate).   Megace is an antiestrogen therapy first used in breast cancer. It is a powerful appetite stimulant and has been used extensively in AIDS wasting. Weight gain is impressive, but has largely been confined to fat, with only small gains reported in lean body mass. Placebo-controlled trials suggest that continuing loss of lean body mass may be reduced or halted with Megace treatment.

Megace also lowers testosterone levels in men, by as much as 60 percent. This not only can result in a loss of sexual function but may explain its poor record of lean body mass accumulation. Studies are currently under way exploring the results of testosterone and Megace supplementation, together, in men with HIV. In the first report from the Hellerstein trial, a small gain in lean body mass was seen with dual therapy, but gains were still primarily fat. Megace's potent appetite stimulation may make it a candidate for trials in combination therapy with other anabolics, or with other testosterone-dosing regimens.

One word of warning: adrenal suppression has been reported with long-term use of Megace. Therefore, if it is used for an extended period, abrupt discontinuation should be avoided, and the dose gradually tapered.

People who use Megace have reported an increased sense of well-being. I have found it particularly valuable in male-to-female transgender patients. Penile impotence is not a concern, and the distribution of weight gain enhances female appearance.

Marinol. Marinol, or dronabinol, is a marijuana derivative indicated for treatment of the wasting syndrome. Its active ingredient is tetrahydrocannabinol, or THC—the same ingredient that is active in marijuana. Perhaps because it is eaten rather than smoked, its effects on mental state are somewhat different from inhaled marijuana's. But like marijuana, Marinol increases your appetite and interest in food. Thus it helps counteract anorexia in HIV.

The emotional, mental, and physical changes associated with marijuana smoking are also present, though to a lesser degree: mood can be temporarily improved, creativity liberated, and memory and physical dexterity impaired. People may get sleepy. When these effects are unwelcome, the problem can be solved by giving just one dose at bedtime, as Marinol's effects on mental status wear off sooner than its effects on appetite. Because Marinol lasts a good while in the body, people are still hungry when they wake up— without experiencing the "high" they don't like.

Other patients prefer just one dose in the morning, to get them through a large morning meal.

Treatment normally begins with a dose of 2.5 milligrams twice a day. Some patients do better with more; I prescribe up to 5 milligrams, two to three times a day.

Marinol is a wonderful addition to our arsenal in fighting HIV wasting. It is legal, when prescribed; it has no harmful effects on the body; and it helps people eat who can't otherwise do so. Because it is indicated, or sanctioned by the FDA for use in HIV wasting, insurance companies and Medicaid will pay for it. It is an accepted medical therapy with proven results and should be offered to anyone with HIV-associated weight loss.

Marijuana. We've already talked about marijuana in Chapter Eight, where we considered the effects of drugs used for recreation. Marijuana can have a role in medical treatment, too.

Much interest has been generated in the use of inhaled marijuana for enhancing appetite. People who obtain it illegally for this purpose swear by it and report that its effects are superior to those of Marinol. In particular, it is said that the period of intensified appetite (or "the munchies," as it's called) lasts longer. There are some exciting studies planned to test this hypothesis.

Because of the prevailing bias against marijuana as a recreational drug, however, implementing these studies is proving to be very difficult. A special license is required for researchers who use marijuana in testing. That license is not granted until a legal source has been secured. The only legal source at present is the National Institute on Drug Abuse, or NIDA. NIDA has been slow to approve the use of even small amounts for these studies; so, at present, they are stalled at the planning stage.

Clearly, the problem lies with the potential political impact of providing, from a government agency to some of its own citizens, what has long been considered an evil drug. It's a hot potato. People don't want to touch it.

It's been suggested that NIDA may be particularly hesitant to provide material for such a study just *because* it might work. A successful pilot study, showing statistically significant benefit to people with AIDS, would surely result in applications for much larger supplies of medicinal marijuana, to perform much larger trials. If these trials were also successful, showing that longer life, with better quality, resulted from inhaled marijuana use in patients with

AIDS wasting syndrome, the FDA would have to give it an indication for such use. NIDA might thus find itself in the position of providing truckloads of marijuana—a vastly unpopular move in itself—to a group of people against whom there is also a substantial public bias. The Moral Majority would surely claim a decay in the fabric of America, if America were to find itself in the business of growing marijuana for homosexuals and users of illegal injection drugs. The phrase "Right to Life" would take on a whole new meaning.

This, I think, is a prime example of the need for activism. When a medicine, a treatment that might truly prolong life and health, cannot be obtained ever for study due to fear of political repercussions, it's time to create a few repercussions of our own.

As the second edition of this book goes to press, there are still no studies in process to test the value of marijuana use in HIV anorexia, nausea, or wasting. Men and women with HIV, like those with cancer and glaucoma, continue to use it and are convinced of its value. Two states have legalized its medical—not its recreational—use. In other states, users risk criminal penalties, as do their suppliers. The marijuana they buy is not subject to testing for purity or safety. Out of fear of public opinion, their government has denied them even the right to know if the risks they take are worth it.

Public opinion is changing, however. Doctors, respected medical journals, and medical associations have all attacked the hypocrisy that denies us the opportunity to learn whether something may be good because popular prejudice insists that it's bad. California and Arizona, by decriminalizing marijuana use in opposition to the federal government, have polarized the battle. California courts have issued an injunction against the use of physician harassment as a way to block legalized patient access. The tide is beginning to turn.

Here in San Francisco, the Community Consortium continues to rework its proposed study in response to stated objections as to study design, despite open expression of bias against such testing by the National Institutes of Health. One study has been approved by the state of California

I believe we're heading in the right direction. The needs of the few should not be denied based on political expediency and the prejudice of the many. It is inappropriate to block clinical testing of a substance that may benefit those who are ill. And whatever our beliefs about marijuana, we must not permit the public choice of ignorance over objective information.

Cytokine Blockers

Cytokines, you will remember, are substances made and released by our immune cells as part of the immune response. Taken as a group, their actions result not only in loss of appetite but also in altered metabolism—changes in the way our bodies use the food we eat.

The normal allocation of nutrients to protein synthesis for structural and other proteins is disturbed when cytokines are activated. Fat is made preferentially and spent less; sugars are therefore not spared but spent, leaving only our proteins—our structures, our muscles, our lean body mass—to provide for immediate energy needs. This metabolic dysregulation lies at the very heart of the wasting syndrome. This is, in fact, the mechanism that costs us our lean body mass.

As we have come to understand this mechanism, researchers have looked for ways to intervene. Special attention has been paid to seeking substances that interfere with this part of the immune response, blocking the actions of cytokines that cause us to waste. These are called cytokine blockers.

Since this book was first published, we have learned more about the complex role of cytokines in fighting HIV. While immune activation in response to HIV infection does contribute to progression of disease, and while cytokine release does favor wasting and viral replication, other cytokine actions may help fight HIV. Some cytokines, in particular the interferons and IL-2, have been used as therapy against HIV with good result. In these cases, viral replication has still increased, at least temporarily, and wasting and other systemic effects have still occurred. Nonetheless, in certain patients at certain times, the use of these factors has led to significant, sometimes sustained, increases in CD4 counts without lasting increases in viral load.

Thus the net effect of cytokine release or administration may be positive or negative, depending not only on the particular cytokine but on other variables determined by the host. This means that the effects of suppressing or administering these factors will depend on you—your CD4 status, the adequacy of your antiretroviral combination, and other determinants we don't yet understand. And the studies we've seen, while promising, don't yet tell us anything about clinical outcome.

The basic concepts of avoiding wasting by avoiding or rapidly treating secondary infections remain correct and proven. And the results of cytokine therapies used to fight HIV have been positive only in certain people—all of them people with high CD4 counts and good antiretroviral treatments. For people with CD4 nadirs less than 200, results have been uniformly disappointing and side effects severe. These people should not be offered such treatments, experimental or otherwise. But since there are now reported cases where the net effect of an increase in levels of some cytokines has been positive, I hesitate to use strong cytokine blockers freely. And there are instances where some people may in fact benefit from access to a carefully monitored trial of cytokine administration.

Keeping these complexities in mind, let's review cytokine blockers.

Omega-3 Fatty Acids (Fish Oils). Many of the cytokines and other factors that promote wasting are produced from a specific fatty acid present in the membrane that surrounds the cell. This fatty acid, arachidonic acid, can be partially replaced in the membrane by other fatty acids we ingest. Thus the factors that promote wasting are made in lesser quantities, or they are less effective.

When we eat certain fish oils containing omega-3 fatty acids, we can facilitate this substitution.

The addition of omega-3 fatty acids to the diet has already been discussed in Chapter Five. You don't need a prescription to get them, and they can't hurt you. It takes a lot of them to show significant effect, though; they are weak cytokine blockers. There are others, available only by prescription or currently in trials, that are thought to be stronger in their actions.

Pentoxifylline (Trental). Trental has been shown to inhibit cytokine production. It may have some value when wasting is clearly due to cytokine activation—in cases of overwhelming infection, with tuberculosis, for example, or wherever fever, night sweats, and other systemic symptoms accompany the wasting process. In vitro studies showed reduced HIV replication with Trental. This effect was increased in the presence of didanosine (DDI). In clinical practice, people have reported an increased sense of well-being. However, a trial to evaluate use in patients with AIDS wasting syndrome did not show weight gain.

Thalidomide. Thalidomide was first introduced years ago as a sedative. It was quickly withdrawn from the market shortly thereafter. Babies were born without limbs to mothers who had used it while pregnant.

Since then it has had limited but powerful use in the treatment of leprosy. Leprosy is caused by infection with another TB-like organism. The massive cytokine activation that results is actually harmful to the body. Thalidomide reduces those effects by reducing cytokine levels.

Studies in HIV wasting indicate improvement in cases of massive cytokine activation, with weight gain reported in patients with active tuberculosis and HIV. It is thought to block inflammation without suppressing healthy immune response. One placebo-controlled double-blind trial reported in 1997 that HIV viral load was unexpectedly increased, however, suggesting an enhancement of HIV replication by thalidomide.

Dosing and tolerability studies reported in Vancouver, B.C., in July 1996 revealed a high rate of discontinuance due to side effects, particularly at high doses or when used by people with low CD4 counts. The most common side effects were rash, drowsiness, and peripheral neuropathy. An uncontrolled observational study from the Healing Alternatives Foundation in San Francisco reported weight gain at lower doses (100 milligrams per day), with no increase in baseline levels of the above symptoms. Further studies are ongoing.

Thalidomide shows promise, particularly in cases of aggressive wasting in the presence of unresolved secondary infection. Like the men and women of the Healing Alternatives Foundation study, I found it useful in crisis situations before we had access to other powerful therapies. I am concerned, though, about its potential for stimulating HIV production, and especially about using it in people with high CD4 counts, at least until we better understand the role of cytokines in fighting HIV. In addition, side effects at higher doses are daunting. As we learn more about it, and as it is approved for use in wasting, we should have a more precise understanding of when and how thalidomide should be used.

Anabolic (Androgenic) Steroids

Our understanding of the role of anabolic steroids in maintaining or repleting lean body mass has come a long way in the last few years. These drugs have been used by weight lifters and professional athletes to increase muscle bulk and strength. Prescription for these purposes carries criminal penalties in this country. Athletes are screened and expelled from competition if evidence of use is found. Used frivolously and without supervision, some of these treatments can be deadly, increasing aggression, blood coagulability, heart size, and the risk of cardiovascular disease. Sudden death has been reported. But there has been great interest in their appropriate use in states of wasting or depletion. And we now have proof that they work. We'll look at the case for several in this section.

Androgens increase nitrogen retention, weight, and body cell mass. They help maintain bone density. They may improve or reverse anemia. Supplementation improves desire and other aspects of sexual behavior. Because increased levels turn off the hormones in the brain that stimulate our own sex hormone production, they may result in testicular atrophy and infertility.

Testosterone. We've already looked at the basis for testosterone supplementation for men with HIV in Chapter Eleven. There are studies in process now to further assess the effects of supplementation on lean body mass retention or increase in the wasting syndrome. Men who are routinely supplemented do report increased vigor and higher energy. Sexual desire and performance are also enhanced.

We know that many HIV-positive men and women have subnormal testosterone levels. One study relates it to CD4 counts; another reports that it follows rather than precedes weight loss. We still do see it in healthy men who are recently infected and asymptomatic, though. It has even been suggested that testosterone deficiency may reduce sensitivity to growth hormone.

We also know that supplementation in men, even with middle- to low-normal levels at baseline, can help increase lean body mass. One study showed such increases when 400 milligrams of testosterone cipionate were given every two weeks to men with testosterone levels of less than 450 nanograms per deciliter; exercise habits were not addressed in this group. Marc Hellerstein of San Francisco General Hospital reports supplementing at baseline levels of 500 or even 600 nanograms per deciliter in otherwise healthy men with HIV wasting. And there have been no reports of increased or advancing Kaposi's sarcoma with testosterone administration. We do check a prostate-specific antigen (PSA) before we give it to men over fifty, as supplementation is contraindicated in men with prostate cancer. We also urge recipients to exercise, in order to maximize the anabolic benefit.

Testosterone may be administered by multiple routes. Results differ by route of administration.

Oral formulations: Extensive first-pass effect; liver breaks down most of them before they get to target organs. In order to avoid some of this, they must be chemically altered to resist breakdown. Significant potential for toxicity to the liver (as measured by increases in liver function tests). *Unacceptable safety profile. Not recommended.*

Intramuscular injection: Given every one to three weeks in HIV. Slow release from buttocks injection. High peak, falling to low nadir. Drawbacks: frequent trips to doctor; shots aren't fun. Must be given in oil base for slow release, so volume and viscosity of injection can contribute to soreness.

Scrotal patch (Testoderm): Applied daily. Steadier levels, hence better approximation of natural release patterns. No doctor visits required. Drawbacks: scrotum must be shaved; can't wear boxer shorts; have a funny-looking patch to explain. Falls off without adhesive; leaves a sticky scrotum with adhesive. Expensive.

Skin patch (Androderm): Applied daily. Levels even, though low. No doctor visits. Drawbacks: need two at a time; can get contact dermatitis (polka-dot skin); levels often insufficient. Expensive.

Sublingual tablets: Two to three times a day. Rapid absorption; peaks in twenty to thirty minutes. Episodic release, hence closest approximation of natural physiologic levels. May have less impact on natural ability to make testosterone. Liver function tests actually reduced (improved) in one trial. No doctor visits. Cost not yet determined. Drawbacks; FDA approval still pending as of October 1997; frequent administration.

There are as yet no studies testing the advisability of testosterone supplementation for women with HIV. Ellen Engelson, working in New York with Donald Kotler, reports that testosterone levels in premenopausal HIV-positive women are low even for women, and correlate with deficits in lean body mass. Potential side effects of supplementation are irreversible deepening of the voice and increased body hair (complaints have been registered) and increased libido and clitoral size (no complaints on record). There may also be a reduction in the extended protection against heart disease that premenopausal women enjoy.

Given the possibility of increased vigor, and the fact that women have a greater tendency to put on fat than lean, this might be a reasonable tradeoff if it offered increased energy and lean body mass retention. Studies, at least of physiologic replacement to levels normal for women, are badly needed.

Dehydroepiandrosterone (DHEA). DHEA is a testosterone and estrogen precursor made by the adrenal glands. Release is stimulated by adrenocorticotrophic hormone (ACTH). Levels peak in late teens (for women) or early twenties (for men) and drop steadily thereafter. Low levels have been associated with cardiovascular disease, senile dementia, female obesity, breast cancer, and some autoimmune conditions. The report that DHEA may be reduced in depression is controversial; however, small studies report improvement in major depression with supplementation at low levels. In people whose DHEA is low, supplementation is reported to increase memory and improve mood. It is said to have antioxidant activity as well.

DHEA appears to serve as a balance for cortisol, our body's

major stress hormone, and to modulate the body's response to severe illness. Like cortisol, release is elevated in the setting of acute,
overwhelming infection. In chronically stressed states such as HIV
infection, however, its release is reduced, while cortisol levels remain elevated. This may be because people with HIV show less
DHEA response to ACTH stimulation.

Scientific interest in DHEA has paralleled the growing community interest. HIV-associated malnutrition was recently reported to correlate with an increased cortisol-to-DHEA ratio. It has
been suggested that low DHEA levels may be an independent predictor of HIV progression. And in vitro studies report that it mod-
estly reduces HIV reproduction.

Animal studies have shown improved survival against certain
lethal viruses. Studies in humans report cytokine stimulation (especially gamma interferon and IL-2, so there may be a negative effect
on CD4 counts). It seems to help block the immunosuppressive actions of stress hormones.

Increased libido, but not increased testosterone levels, has been
reported in men following DHEA supplementation; women increase
libido and testosterone levels. There are also reports of increased
body hair in women. The use of massive doses in HIV led to substantial CD4 increases in a few cases in one San Francisco study,
and supplementation was well tolerated; but no sustained improvement was shown as a result of treatment.

Effects on HIV wasting have been contradictory. A French
trial reports increased body cell mass; others report mainly weight
loss or fat loss.

Testing for DHEA level is inexpensive, and we do it in our office. If people with low levels are depressed or fatigue easily, or do
not respond to or qualify for testosterone administration in wasting,
it merits a trial of supplementation. We know it won't hurt you, and
it might actually help. But the definitive word on DHEA isn't in yet.

If you're going to test your DHEA levels and supplement, pay
attention to what you're buying. Buyers' clubs are knowledgeable,
but products labeled as DHEA in health food stores and bodybuilders' stores may contain minimal quantities.

Supplementation in recent trials in people with major depression was at the rate of 30 to 90 milligrams a day.

Oxandrolone (Oxandrin).   Oxandrolone is a synthetic hormone with powerful anabolic properties. Both the liver and the kidney can break it down, so it has a good safety profile. It's been used safely to address malnutrition in people with wasting due to severe alcoholic hepatitis, or liver damage, and is currently indicated to oppose catabolic weight loss in burn injuries and other wasting states. It is also indicated to offset bone pain accompanying osteoporosis. It is currently dosed at 10 milligrams, or four 2.5-milligram pills, twice a day. Studies show that the amount and duration of effect increase with increasing doses at amounts of 5 to 15 milligrams a day, and doses up to 40 milligrams a day for women and 80 milligrams a day for men are under study.

Oxandrolone is also a strong appetite stimulant. Its use results in significant gains of both weight and lean body mass. Its androgenic, or masculinizing, potential is quite low—so if you're a woman, it shouldn't put hair on your chest. People who use it report ravenous appetites and renewed energy and vigor, along with changes in weight and body composition. One trial with forty-four participants has reported weight gain in 75 percent of the participants and body cell mass gain in 94 percent, so it seems that body composition can be improved even in the absence of weight gain.

As with testosterone and other anabolic therapies, there's been a lot of interest in the additive effects of oxandrolone and progressive resistance exercise. At the Andrew Ziegler Foundation, we're just winding up a three-month pilot study looking at oxandrolone for HIV-associated weight loss in women and men. Sixteen subjects were randomized to resistance exercise three times a week plus drug, or to drug alone. Preliminary results suggest, as hoped, that body cell mass increases with drug alone, and increases even more with consistent exercise. Marc Hellerstein at San Francisco General Hospital has completed a formal metabolic trial of combination use of oxandrolone and exercise, with baseline testosterone supplementation. Another study is monitoring weight and lean body mass in people using oxandrolone for longer periods. And there is a very exciting study in progress that looks at oxandrolone-induced changes in the actual structure of muscle cells.

Like other potent and lifesaving treatments for HIV wasting, oxandrolone is costly and should not be used carelessly. But for those whose wasting has not been arrested by more conservative measures, or in circumstances where aggressive therapy or prevention is needed, it's a lifesaver — and one of the most promising additions to our armamentarium.

Nandrolone Decanoate (Deca-Durabolin).   This is an anabolic hormone with strong androgenic properties not yet approved for wasting in the United States. Significant increases in lean body mass have been reported with its use, sometimes despite minimal weight gain. In addition, it may partially reverse osteoporosis. Side effects are hoarseness and increased body hair for women. When used in combination with other androgenic hormones in cycles, poor self-image and deficits in problem solving have been reported. Most of the many recent studies report no behavioral adverse effects, however, when used alone or with testosterone.

There is a trial in process using nandrolone decanoate along with maximal nutritional support — counseling, exercise, protein, glutamine, vitamins, antioxidants, and testosterone. In the first nine subjects enrolled, preliminary results report a mean increase in body cell mass of *almost 14 percent*. While there is no control group that would permit us to compare this with the outcomes of the other interventions, and thus assess the relative contribution of nandrolone to this result, it's exciting to see what is possible when we maximize all aspects of treatment.

Recombinant Human Growth Hormone (Serostim)

Access to growth hormone in 1995 marked a major development in the treatment of HIV. For the first time, we were able to actually reverse, not just halt, the deadly course of wasting. Many of the people who first had access to this drug were able to hang on, despite severe immunosuppression, until protease inhibitor combination regimens were available to bring them back to life.

Growth hormone is not a steroid, but it is highly anabolic. In HIV, sensitivity to natural growth hormone appears to be reduced; this may contribute to the process of wasting. Supplementation with human recombinant growth hormone, however, appears to overcome this resistance. Weight is gained, as is lean body mass. Functional capacity (as measured by treadmill work output) is increased.

With reversal of the wasting process, there may even be a trend toward fewer opportunistic infections.

Growth hormone was first offered at a weight loss of 10 percent from baseline. While this drug has been a real lifesaver for some of the people who have presented to our office close to death from wasting, it seems to work better, with fewer side effects, when used sooner. It is a very expensive treatment and should be used in combination with other less costly strategies to maximize its benefit.

People with glucose intolerance may develop diabetes, so blood sugars should be monitored. Carpal tunnel syndrome, which announces itself by tingling or pain in hands and fingers, is also a possibility. Growth hormone should not be used in people with prior carpal tunnel syndrome (unless it has been surgically treated) or diabetes. Minor side effects may include joint aches and slight swelling, especially at hands and feet. These may resolve, or may respond to reduction of dose.

Growth hormone is given in the form of daily injections. For patients at risk for injection drug use, we have sometimes used directly observed therapy, giving it in the office from Monday through Friday.

Studies are currently under way to assess the usefulness of smaller or less frequent doses for maintenance of effect. One 1997 study reports that six patients maintained or increased their weight and body cell mass three months after goals had been reached and growth hormone discontinued.

Nutritional Supplementation When Extra Help Is Needed
•

During periods of active wasting, it is especially critical to receive the nutrition we need. Even if we can't use it as well as at other times, its absence will make things much worse.

There are ways to get nutrients into our body, even if we're not hungry, even if we can't swallow, even if we can't digest or absorb. These methods have been used, when needed, to carry people through periods of illness for years.

Medical interventions include medical foods designed for specific nutritional purposes; enteral feeding, delivered directly to the stomach; and parenteral nutrition, delivered directly to the bloodstream through a vein.

Medical Foods

These are artificially constituted foods—a meal in a can, so to speak. They are designed to provide precise and specific vitamin, calorie, and protein content. They can supplement our intake, or provide a complete, well-balanced diet if circumstances require it. Small quantities provide maximum calories and protein.

Some of them are specifically designed to be better absorbed, when malabsorption is present. Some are designed for other special circumstances. There even is a supplement designed especially for people with HIV, to prevent or defend against wasting.

If you are using these for diet supplementation, to increase your calorie and protein intake beyond what you can eat, there are some you can buy for yourself. Others will have to be ordered by or through your doctor. If your need for special medical foods can be shown, insurance or Medicaid may pay for it. Proof of malabsorption or significant malnutrition will be needed.

Medical foods are calorie-dense, so you can get a lot by eating a little. They taste better and are less filling if you eat them icy cold. Try to drink one at the end of a meal, when you've only a little more room. If you eat them first, they'll fill you up. Or take a few swallows every couple of hours.

You'll find a list of some representative medical foods, and their individual attributes, in Table 12.1.

Enteral Feeding

Enteral feeding is delivered directly to your stomach. We do this if people can't swallow, or are too sick to eat or too weak to protect their airway, and are therefore at risk of aspirating food into the lungs. People who are temporarily on ventilator support are usually fed in this way.

Enteral feeding is generally used in the hospital setting. Some people with chronic problems but good quality of life receive their nutrition this way at home. Delivery is usually by nasogastric tube, passed from the nose into the stomach. If a long-term need is

TABLE 12.1.
•
Medical Foods.

All of these are made to be eaten, so their flavor and feel are considered. It's okay to choose one of these without expert help.

Carnation Instant Breakfast

Where sold:	supermarkets
Average cost:	$.60 plus milk
Serving size (with skim milk):	9.5 ounces
Calories:	130 plus milk (220 with skim)
Carbohydrates:	28 grams plus milk
Protein:	4 grams plus milk
Fat:	1 gram plus milk

Advantages: Cheap, easily available, broad flavor variety, tastes good. Comes in packages of ten. Lightweight, easy to store until added to milk.

Drawbacks: Milk-based, so lactose intolerance may be a problem. High sugar content; tastes too sweet for some.

Ensure Plus

Where sold:	drugstores
Average cost:	$1.50
Serving size:	8 ounces
Calories:	355
Carbohydrates:	47.3 grams
Protein:	13 grams
Fat:	12.6 grams

Advantages: Available in stores. Concentrated calories and protein, lactose-free.

Drawbacks: High fat content a problem with malabsorption. Can sometimes cause diarrhea.

TABLE 12.1. **Medical Foods.** (continued)

Nutren 2.0

Where sold:	mail order 800-776-5446; drugstores will order
Average cost:	$1.50
Serving size:	8.45 ounces
Calories:	500
Carbohydrates:	49 grams
Protein:	20 grams
Fat:	26.5 grams (75 percent medium-chain triglycerides [MCTs])

Advantages: Available in stores, highly concentrated calories and protein, lactose-free. MCTs improve fat absorption. Gluten-free, so it's okay for people who are allergic to wheat. Tastes less sweet. Three cans meet RDAs.

Drawbacks: Diarrhea still a possibility, because of high concentration of nutrients. Vanilla only.

Peptamen VHP

Where sold:	mail order 800-776-5446; drugstores will order
Average cost:	$5.35
Serving size:	8.45 ounces
Calories:	250
Carbohydrates:	26.1 grams
Protein:	15.6 grams (peptide-based)
Fat:	9 grams (70 percent MCTs)

Advantages: Fancy formula to simplify digestion. High protein content; elemental proteins more easily digested in the presence of malabsorption. Low fat content; MCTs improve remaining fat absorption and further improve tolerance. Six cans meet RDAs.

Drawbacks: *Extremely* expensive. Benefit relative to cost not shown in HIV. Taste not terrific.

TABLE 12.1.	**Medical Foods.**	(continued)

Advera

Where sold:	mail order 800-544-7495; HIV-aware drugstores
Average cost:	$2.50
Serving size:	8 ounces
Calories:	303
Carbohydrates:	51.1 grams
Protein:	14.2 grams (peptide-based)
Fat:	5.4 grams; incorporates MCTs

Advantages: Especially designed for the nutritional needs of people with HIV wasting syndrome. Lactose-free. Gluten-free. A serving contains over two grams fiber, so it fights diarrhea. High protein content; proteins more easily digested in the presence of malabsorption. Patented protein source appears to be gut trophic, promoting healing and regeneration in the gut. Low fat content; MCTs improve fat absorption and further improve tolerance. Omega-3 fatty acids—weak cytokine blockers—make up part of the fat content. Preliminary studies suggest *lean body mass supported, hospital days less* in HIV patients on Advera. Chocolate flavor tastes good. Five cans meet RDAs. In some staes, *paid for by Medicaid if HIV wasting can be proven and doctor applies for authorization.*

Drawbacks: More expensive than standard supplement. Orange Cream flavor generally disliked.

Optimune

Where sold:	mail order 888-678-4644; HIV-aware drugstores
Average cost:	$1.15
Serving size:	30 grams powder
Calories:	120
Carbohydrates:	10 grams
Protein:	17 grams
Fat:	1.5 grams

Advantages: Derived from concentrated bovine whey (the curd-free portion of milk), Optimune contains natural antibodies to organisms like cryptosporidium that can cause diarrhea. Several people in our study reported improvement or resolution of their diarrhea with Optimune.

TABLE 12.1. **Medical Foods.** (continued)

Drawbacks: Expensive per calorie. Lactose-reduced, so many lactose-intolerant people can use it. Other will still have symptoms.

MET-Rx

Where sold:	Drugstores, supermarkets, fitness centers
Average cost:	$1.75 per bar
Serving size:	100 grams
Calories:	340
Carbohydrates:	50 grams
Protein:	27 grams
Fat:	4 grams

Advantages: Low in fat and high in protein, this product is particularly popular with bodybuilders. Comes in vanilla, fudge brownie, peanut butter, and chocolate chip cookie dough flavors; also available in powder form.

Drawbacks: Has not been tested as a medical food.

expected, a tube can be placed through the abdominal wall into the stomach or small intestine by a simple surgical procedure.

Often the enteral food supplied is one of the medical foods discussed above. If gut function is compromised, there are easily digested elemental formulas that deliver nutrients in their simplest form.

Normally, if someone is wasting and can't keep up oral intake, enteral feeding is recommended. If there is malabsorption, however, parenteral nutrition may be needed.

Total Parenteral Nutrition (TPN)

TPN is food delivered directly into the blood. Nutrients are given in elemental form, ready to be used by the body. A special intravenous line is placed to provide access to a large central vein. The pharmacist and doctor determine your caloric, protein, and micronutrient needs and directly deliver essential elements in amounts that will keep the blood in proper balance.

TPN is only given when it is not possible to provide nutrition through the gut. This is usually due to acute problems—bleeding or obstruction in the gastrointestinal tract, constant vomiting, overwhelming infection. With treatment and resolution of the problem or infection, the need for TPN resolves.

In HIV, as in cancer or chronic gastrointestinal disease, there can be a real role for TPN during periods of acute illness or in severe malnutrition. Malabsorption is common during acute infections, and more common with advancing HIV disease. On rare occasions, there is a role for ongoing TPN when diarrhea cannot be successfully treated or controlled. Generally, though, we have more effective—and sometimes less expensive—ways to get the job done.

There's an adage in nutritional therapy that says you shouldn't start TPN unless you'll need it for at least a week. This is absolutely not the case in the setting of HIV. As a matter of fact, on the rare occasions when I resort to TPN, patients are usually acutely ill and turn around within a couple of days. If you need TPN for two days, you should use it for two days—no more and no less.

So What Else Is New?
•

There are many exciting developments in our understanding of the nature of HIV wasting, and of its prevention and treatment.

Osteoporosis and Osteopenia

One of the most extraordinary findings we've come across in our office is the high, almost universal prevalence of loss of bone mass in advanced HIV. We had seen osteoporosis in patients after long-term prednisone use, as might be expected. But we began to suspect that loss of bone mineral density might be more common after a patient broke his foot. To test this premise, we offered bone densitometry to HIV-positive men with CD4 nadirs of less than 100 or a history of AIDS wasting; to date, all subjects have shown moderate loss of bone mineral density, or osteopenia, and almost half have shown severe loss, or osteoporosis. Many of these men are currently quite healthy; many have regained muscle mass and increased their CD4 counts substantially; yet their bone mass is still significantly reduced.

This is to us a revolutionary finding. Until now we have seen no reports of HIV-related osteoporosis or osteopenia in the medical literature. It may be that in the years before HAART, or highly active antiretroviral therapy, we simply didn't look; back then we didn't think in terms of staying well enough to grow old. It does raise important questions now, though, about the maintenance of structural and functional integrity in people who are planning to live a long time.

We need to test this finding in a larger population, using matched rather than historical controls. We need to know to whom it happens, when it happens, what makes it happen, how and if we can prevent it, and how and if we can reverse it. And we need to do this in a hurry, so we can get busy and keep these people strong.

For now, our office recommends bone densitometry on all HIV patients at intake. We can't yet recommend frequency of monitoring thereafter. Anyone with a history of wasting or with a CD4 nadir less than 100 should urgently request such evaluations.

There are treatments currently approved for osteoporosis. They offer only partial reconstitution, and they have not been tested in HIV. There may be a real role for current anabolic therapies as well. And I'm going out of my way to avoid long-term prednisone use whenever possible.

With luck, as we learn more about this process, we'll find ways to predict and prevent wasting of bone as efficiently as we have learned to fight loss of muscle mass. Stay tuned.

Effects of Highly Active Antiretroviral Therapy Including Protease Inhibitors (HAART) on Weight and Lean Body Mass

Several 1997 studies have looked at whether viral load reduction and immune reconstitution restore nutritional competence. Results are controversial. While preliminary reports suggest a trend toward an increase in lean body mass as well as weight, a substantial proportion—20 to 25 percent—of those responding to HAART do not replete lean body mass in the absence of specific nutritional interventions. Thus successful suppression of viral load does not guarantee an end to wasting. Continued monitoring and treatment to ensure nutritional competence are still important parts of HIV management.

Convergent Therapy of Wasting

Much of the newest research is devoted to exploring combined interventions, to maximize and individualize nutritional therapy. Some trials are looking at the results of comprehensive nutritional management; some are combining and/or cycling anabolic interventions; some are assessing the clinical result of aggressive combination regimens, to see if an ounce of prevention, however costly, is cheaper than a pound of cure.

Efficiency of Treatment

There is also interest in reducing unnecessary costs in the use of expensive therapies. Dose reduction, dose cycling, and discontinuance of treatment with careful monitoring are all potential cost savers once acute wasting has been reversed. These are under investigation. Aggressive short-term use of costly treatments like oxandrolone and growth hormone, early in the course of an acute episode of wasting, may also prove cost-effective.

Studies in Women

Women's vitamin status, body fat distribution, and patterns of wasting and repletion are all topics of interest now. There may in fact be differences in the way women waste, and in their nutritional response to infection. As these are thought to result from hormonal differences, it becomes important to study hormonal changes in women with HIV. As in men, testosterone levels are reported to be lower. We need to know about other hormonal changes in HIV-positive women as well, and to understand when they occur in the course of HIV or wasting and how they affect progression.

The Bottom Line
•

So how do we put all this together? It's important to address wasting and its prevention in a careful, stepwise fashion—so we don't do more to our bodies or our wallets than we need to—but it's also critical that we don't give up. If one intervention doesn't work, we try another. If no single intervention gets us where we need to go, we use as many as it takes.

Just as there's a role for convergent therapy in fighting the virus—for multiple assaults on replication at once, attacking at different points in the process of assembly to bring the virus to its knees—there's a role for convergent therapy in wasting. We monitor closely, from the moment we know we're infected. We watch our weight, our lean body mass, our protein stores, even our bones, to maximize structural integrity. We start with the basics, with calories and protein and vitamins, using calorie-rich medical foods if we need to. We support the appetite, use antioxidants, and exercise when we are able. We ensure that hormone levels are adequate, and supplement to optimize their effects. We consider anabolic therapies if other interventions don't get us where we need to go. Perhaps we consider them sooner, at the onset of a period of acute wasting.

When we do use these therapies, we don't wait too long to use them. When they don't work alone, we use them in combination. If enteral or parenteral feeding are needed for a period, we use them too. We keep learning, keep reading, and keep asking questions, so the newest approaches don't pass us by.

If what you need to stay alive and well is everything—medical foods, appetite enhancers, testosterone, anabolic steroids, and growth hormone, even cytokine blockers—all at once, every day, if need be—and if it works and doesn't hurt you and you're willing to put up with the hassle, that's what you should do. Just as we shouldn't waste money, or other precious resources, we should not waste your life.

I've seen people like my friend Bob walk up to the edge of the cliff and look over. I've thought it was too late, that we had lost them. But like Bob and his wife Maria, some of those people were damned if they'd give up. They wanted it all and were willing to work for it. And they did. And we threw everything we had at them and they caught it and *they are with us here today*—with bodies no longer wasted—working out, playing with the kids, loving their partners, enjoying food and sex and a whole new chance at life. That might not have happened. It took a lot of work from all concerned, and there were no guarantees. *But they had a right to life. And they exercised it.*

If you're doing well and not wasting, don't take it for granted. Keep doing all the things that keep you healthy, and watch your status closely. If you're wasting, or if you start to waste, exercise your right to treatment. And do it early, when it works the best. Like Bob and so many others, you have a right to life.

REFERENCES

Arver, S., and others. "Improvement of sexual function in testosterone deficient men treated for one year with a permeation enhanced testosterone transdermal system." *Journal of Urology*, 1996, *155*, 1604–1608.

Bagatell, C. J., and Bremner. "Androgens in men; Uses and abuses." *New England Journal of Medicine*, 1996, *334*(11), 707–714.

Beal, J. E., and others. "Dronabinol as a treatment for anorexia associated with weight loss in patients with AIDS." *Journal of Pain and Symptom Management*, 1995, *10*(2), 89–97.

Berger, D., and others. "Measurement of body weight and body cell mass in patients receiving highly active antiretroviral therapy (HAART)." (In submission.)

Bond, A. J. "Assessment of attentional bias and mood in users and non-users of anabolic-androgenic steroids." *Drug and Alcohol Dependence*, 1995, *37*(3), 241–245.

Bowers, M. "Anabolic steroids in the treatment of HIV-related wasting." *Bulletin of Experimental Treatments for AIDS*, September 1996, pp. 13–21.

Centers of Disease Control. "CDC definition of AIDS wasting syndrome." *Morbidity and Mortality Weekly Report*, December 18, 1992, p. 17.

Christeff, N., and others. "Correlation between increased cortisol/DHEA ratio and malnutrition in HIV positive men." *Nutrition and HIV Infection Second International Conference*, 1997, *13*(3), abstract no. 0–05.

Coodley, G. O., and others. "Endocrine function in the HIV wasting syndrome." *Journal of Acquired Immune Deficiency Syndromes and Human Retrovirology*, 1994, *7*, 46–51.

Coodley, G. O., and others. "The HIV wasting syndrome: A review." *Journal of Acquired Immune Deficiency Syndromes and Human Retrovirology*, 1994, *7*, 681–694.

Croxson, T. S., and others. "Changes in the hypothalamic-pituitary gonadal axis in human immunodeficiency virus–infected homosexual men." *Journal of Clinical Endocrinology and Metabolism*, 1989, *68*, 317–321.

Davey Jr., R. T., and others. "Subcutaneous administration of interleukin-2 in human immunodeficiency virus Type 1–infected persons." *Journal of Infectious Diseases*, 1997, *175*, 781–789.

Dezube, B. J. "Pentoxifylline (Trental, PTX) decreases tumor necrosis factor (TNF) and may decrease HIV replication in AIDS patients." *International Conference on AIDS,* 1993, *9*(1), 492.

Dezube, B. J. "Pentoxifylline for the treatment of infection with human immunodeficiency virus." *Clinics in Infectious Disease,* 1994, *18*(3), 285–287.

Dezube, B. J., and others. "Pentoxifylline decreases HIV replication." *International Conference on AIDS,* 1991, *7*(2), 99.

Dieterich, D. T. "Advances in HIV-associated wasting." *Improving the Management of HIV Disease, International AIDS Society–USA,* 1997, *4*(5), 24–27.

Ehrenpreis, E. D., and others. "D-xylose malabsorption: Characteristic finding in patients with the AIDS wasting syndrome and chronic diarrhea." *Journal of Acquired Immune Deficiency Syndromes and Human Retrovirology,* 1992, *5,* 1047–1050.

Engelson, E. S., and others. "Nutrition and testosterone status of HIV+ women." *Eleventh International Conference on AIDS,* 1997.

Fazely, F., and others. "Pentoxyfylline (Trental) decreases the replication of the human immunodeficiency virus type 1 in human peripheral blood mononuclear cells and in cultured T cells." *Blood,* 1991, *77*(8), 1653–1656.

Fields-Gardner, C. "A review of mechanisms of wasting in HIV disease." *Nutrition in Clinical Practice,* 1995, *10*(5), 167–177.

Fields-Gardner, C. *Handbook on Nutritional Management of HIV and AIDS.* American Dietetic Association, 1997.

Fisher, A., and Abbaticola. "Effects of oxandrolone and L-glutamine on body weight, body cell mass and body fat in patients with HIV infection: Preliminary analysis." *Nutrition and HIV Infection Second International Conference,* 1997, *13*(3), P-12.

Force, G., and others. "Characteristics of change in body composition with efficiency of antiretroviral treatment in AIDS patients." *Nutrition and HIV Infection Second International Conference,* 1997, *13*(3), P-43.

Geusens, P. "Nandrolone decanoate: Pharmacologic properties and therapeutic use in osteoporosis." *Clinical Rheumatology,* 1995, *14*(S3), 32–39.

Grinspoon, S., and others. "Loss of lean body and muscle mass correlates with androgen levels in hypogonadal men with acquired immunodeficiency syndrome and wasting." *Journal of Clinical Endocrinology and Metabolism,* 1996, *81*(1), 4051–4058.

Grunfeld, C., and others. "Growth hormone therapy promotes positive nitrogen balance and weight gain in AIDS." *International Conference on AIDS,* 1992, *8,* B230.

Gunzler, V. "Thalidomide in human immunodeficiency virus (HIV) patients. A review of safety considerations." *Drug Safety,* 1992, *7*(2), 116–134.

Haslett, P., and others. "The emerging role of thalidomide therapy in HIV-infected patients." *Infections in Medicine,* 1997, *14*(5), 393–406.

Heinkelein, M., and others. "Pentoxifylline reduces cytokine release and the ability to stimulate cell surface antigen and HIV-1 expression by CD8+ cytotoxic T lymphocytes (CTL)." *International Conference on AIDS,* 1994, *10*(2), 88.

Hellerstein, M. K. "Pathogenesis of wasting and response to nutritional therapies: Rationale for anabolic treatments." *Oxandrolone Investigators' Meeting,* April 1997, Dallas.

Ireland, J., and Romeyn, M. "Alterations in bone density in HIV-1 infected men: A new risk factor for osteoporosis?" *International Conference on AIDS,* 1998, in submission.

Jacobson, J. M., and others. "Thalidomide for the treatment of oral aphthous ulcers in patients with human immunodeficiency virus infection." *New England Journal of Medicine,* 1997, *336*(21), 1487–1493.

Klausner, J. D. "Treatment with thalidomide in AIDS patients." *International Conference on AIDS,* 1994, *10*(1), 221.

Klausner, J. D., and others. "The effect of thalidomide on the pathogenesis of human immunodeficiency virus type 1 and m. tuberculosis infection." *Journal of Acquired Immune Deficiency Syndromes and Human Retrovirology,* 1996, *11*, 247–257.

Koch, J., and others. "Steatorrhea: A common manifestation in patients with HIV/AIDS." *Nutrition,* 1996, *12*(7–8), 507–510.

Koch, J., and others. "Steatorrhea is nearly universal in patients with HIV-associated unexplained weight loss or diarrhea." *Nutrition–HIV Infection Second International Conference,* 1997, *13*(3), abstract no. 0–06.

Kotler, D. P., and others. "Effect of home total parenteral nutrition on body composition in patients with acquired immunodeficiency syndrome." *Journal of Parenteral and Enteral Nutrition,* 1990, *14*, 454–458.

Kotler, D. P., and others. "Enteral alimentation and repletion of body cell mass in malnourished patients with acquired immunodeficiency syndrome." *American Journal of Clinical Nutrition,* 1991, *53*, 149–154.

Kovacs, J. A., and others. "Sustained increases in CD4 counts with intermittent interleukin-2 therapy in HIV-infected patients with greater than 200 CD4 cells/mm3: Results of a randomized, controlled trial." *New England Journal of Medicine,* 1996, *335*, 1350–1356.

Krentz, A. J., and others. "Anthropometric, metabolic, and immunological effects of recombinant human growth hormone in AIDS and AIDS-related complex." *Journal of Acquired Immune Deficiency Syndromes and Human Retrovirology,* 1993, *6*(3), 245–251.

Landman, D., and others. "Use of pentoxifylline therapy for patients with AIDS-related wasting: Pilot study. *Clinics in Infectious Disease,* 1994, *18*(1), 97–99.

Laudat, A., and others. "Changes in systemic gonadal and adrenal steroids in asymptomatic human immunodeficiency virus-infected men: Relationship with the CD4 cell counts." *European Journal of Endocrinology*, 1995, *133*, 418–424.

Lederman, M. M. "Host-directed and immune-based therapies for human immunodeficiency virus infection." *Annals of Internal Medicine*, 1995, *122*(3), 218–222.

Leinung, M. C., and others. "Induction of adrenal suppression by megestrol acetate in patients with AIDS." *Annals of Internal Medicine*, 1995, *122*(11), 843–845.

Lovejoy, J. C., and others. "Exogenous androgens influence body composition and regional fat distribution in obese postmenopausal women: A clinical research center study." *Journal of Clinical Endocrinology and Metabolism*, 1996, *81*(6), 2198–2203.

Macallan, D. C., and others. "Energy expenditure and wasting in human immunodeficiency virus infection." *New England Journal of Medicine*, 1995, *333*(2), 83–88.

Makonkawkeyoon, S., and others. "Thalidomide inhibits the replication of human immunodeficiency virus type 1." *Proceedings of the National Academy of Science USA*, 1993, *90*(13), 5974–5978.

McCutchan, A., and others. "Evolution of pituitary-testicular axis dysfunction in HIV/AIDS." *International Conference on AIDS*, 1993, *1*, 460.

Melchert, R. B., and Welder. "Cardiovascular effects of androgenic-anabolic steroids." *Medicine and Science in Sports and Exercise*, 1995, *27*(9), 1252–1262.

Mendenhall, C., and others. "A study of oral nutritional support with oxandrolone in malnourished patients with alcoholic hepatitis: Results of a Department of Veterans Affairs cooperative study." *Hepatology*, 1993, *31*(1), 564–576.

Mendenhall, C., and others. "Relationship of protein calorie malnutrition to alcoholic liver disease: A reexamination of data from two Veterans Administration cooperative studies." *Alcoholism: Clinical and Experimental Research*, 1995, *19*(3), 635–641.

Merenich, J. A. "Evidence of endocrine involvement early in the course of human immunodeficiency virus infection." *Journal of Clinical Endocrinology and Metabolism*, 1990, *70*, 566–571.

Mole, L., and others. "A pilot study of pentoxifylline in HIV infected patients with CD4+ lymphocyte counts less than 400 cells/mm3." *International Conference on AIDS*, 1993, *9*(1), 488.

Mulligan, K., and others. "Anabolic effects of recombinant human growth hormone in patients with wasting associated with human immunodeficiency virus infection." *Journal of Clinical Endocrinology and Metabolism*, 1993, *77*, 956–962.

Mulligan, K., and others. "Growth hormone treatment of HIV-associated catabolism." *International Conference on AIDS,* 1993, *9*(1), 500.

Muurahainen, N., and others. "Trends in weight and body cell mass changes in HIV-infected men." *Nutrition,* March 1997, *13* (3).

Nemechek, P. M., and others. "Maintenance of body cell mass and phase angle after discontinuation of human growth hormone." *Nutrition and HIV Infection Second International Conference,* 1997, *13*(3), abstract no. P-1.

Oster, M. H. "Megestrol acetate in patients with AIDS and cachexia." *Annals of Internal Medicine,* 1994, *121,* 400–408.

Pharo, A., and others. "A comprehensive program to reverse/prevent wasting syndrome in HIV/AIDS patients." *Nutrition and HIV Infection Second International Conference,* 1997, *13*(3), P-14.

Poles, M. A., and others. "Oxandrolone as a treatment for AIDS-related weight loss and wasting." *Infectious Disease Society of America,* September 1996.

Poretsky, L., and others. "Testicular dysfunction in human immunodeficiency virus-infected men." *Metabolism,* 1995, *44*(7), 946–953.

Rabkin, J. G., and Ferrando. "DHEA and HIV illness." *The AIDS Reader,* January–February 1997, pp. 28–36.

Reus, V., and others. "Dehydroepiandrosterone (DHEA) and memory in depressed patients." *Neuropsychopharmacology,* 1993, *9*(2S), 66S.

Reyes-Teran, G., and others. "Effects of thalidomide on wasting syndrome in patients with AIDS. A randomized, double-blind, placebo controlled clinical trial." *International Conference on AIDS,* 1994, *10*(2), 65.

Romeyn, M., and others. "Osteoporosis in AIDS: A preliminary report." (In submission.)

Salehian, B., and others. "Pharmacokinetics, bioefficacy, and safety of sublingual testosterone cyclodextrin in hypogonadal men: Comparison to testosterone enanthate. A clinical research center study." *Journal of Clinical Endocrinology and Metabolism,* 1995, *80*(12), 3567–3575.

Sampaio, E. P., and others. "Thalidomide selectively inhibits tumor necrosis factor alpha production by stimulated human monocytes." *Journal of Experimental Medicine,* 1991, *173,* 699–703.

Scevola, D., and others. "The imbalance of GH-IGF-I axis and adrenal axis in HIV-infected patients." *Nutrition and HIV Infection Second International Conference,* 1997, *13*(3), abstract no. P-0.

Strawford, A., and others. "The effects of combination megestrol acetate and testosterone replacement therapy in AIDS wasting syndrome." *Nutrition and HIV Infection Second International Conference,* 1997, *13*(3), abstract no. P-02.

Stuenkel, C. A., and others. "Sublingual administration of testosterone-hydroxypropyl-beta-cyclodextrin inclusion complex simulates episodic androgen release in hypogonadal men." *Journal of Clinical Endocrinology and Metabolism,* 1991, *72*(5), 1054–1059.

Subramanian, S., and others. "Clinical adrenal insufficiency in patients receiving megestrol therapy." *Archives of Internal Medicine,* 1997, *157,* 1008–1011.

Teruel, J. L. "Androgen therapy for anaemia of chronic renal failure: Indications in the erythropoietin era." *Scandinavian Journal of Urology and Nephrology,* 1996, *30*(5), 403–408.

Von Roenn, J. H. "Randomized trials of megestrol acetate for AIDS-associated anorexia and cachexia." *Oncology,* 1994, *51*(Supp 1), 19–24.

Von Roenn, J. H., and Knopf. "Anorexia/cachexia in patients with HIV: Lessons for the oncologist." *Oncology,* 1996, *10*(7), 1049–1056.

Wang, C., and others. "Testosterone replacement therapy improves mood in hypogonadal men: A clinical research center study." *Journal of Clinical Endocrinology and Metabolism,* 1996, *81*(10), 3578–3583.

Wolkewitz, O. M., and others. "Dehydroepiandrosterone (DHEA) treatment of depression." *Biological Psychiatry,* 1997, *41*(3), 311–318.

Zhang, L., and others. "Pentoxifylline enhances the antiviral activity of ddI against HIV-1 in cultured mononuclear cells." *International Conference on AIDS,* 1994, *10*(2), 103.

CHAPTER 13

•

Fighting the Virus

By now we've seen the importance of eating enough and eating right, of using vitamin and mineral supplements, and of fighting the process of wasting.

But we've also seen that those steps aren't enough. We also have to fight the *precipitants* of HIV wasting—those processes that initiate and magnify the changes that promote it.

We know that these processes start with HIV infection itself and are amplified by its increasing presence in our bodies. So we must also fight HIV progression directly. The more successful we are in our battle with the virus, the less it can cause us to waste.

This is the best argument I know for vigilant, uncompromising, early attention to anti-HIV treatment.

We've learned a great deal about HIV since this book was first published in 1995. We understand the virus better, can monitor it more closely, and have infinitely more powerful weapons against it. What was once characterized as bias in favor of early, aggressive, and comprehensive treatment has now become the standard of care.

What We've Learned About the Virus
•

We now know absolutely that the virus never sleeps.

Infection occurs in or through the lining of our sexual or gastrointestinal systems, or by veins or through breaks in the skin. Rapid, massive reproduction leads quickly to overwhelming infection. Over a short period of time, HIV enters different types of cells and tissues, called compartments, in the body. Cells in some of these compartments are short-lived. Others live longer.

As immune response kicks in, we mount our own massive effort, making fighter cells that recognize and attack HIV, suppressing but not wiping out the virus. Viral burden drops and is held at a new set point, a new equilibrium between the invader and our response. But this is a dynamic equilibrium. Enormous pressure from the virus is opposed by equal pressure from our defenses. It's a war. It's Armageddon.

So the lull that we experience between infection and HIV expression, often many years later, is not a lull at all. It is the eye of the hurricane, the center of the storm; the place where all seems still, while intense opposing forces hold one another in check.

This is not viral latency. There is no such thing as viral latency. The virus never sleeps.

As fast as HIV reproduces, our body makes immune cells, T cells and others, to fight it. That's how we keep it in check for the first few years, if we're not on treatment. Our body may hold the line for quite a while in this way, even without antiretroviral treatment. But we use up our resources in the effort. And unlike the virus, our ability to renew ourselves is finite. Sooner or later we seem to run out of parts. By the time we start to falter we have little left to work with. Without treatment, with very few exceptions, the virus always wins.

How We Monitor the Virus
•

Perhaps the most exciting development in the last two years—more even than the protease inhibitors—has been the introduction of viral load measurement and its validation as a marker for our success or failure in fighting HIV.

Viral Load

Before viral load was available, we could only judge our progress by T-cell, or CD4, counts, measuring damage after the fact. Viral load, on the other hand, warns us when the virus starts to get the jump on us, before damage occurs, so we can change our tactics. It can also tell us how a new approach is working, and whether an old one still has what it takes.

Viral load may be determined by two tests, PCR RNA or branched-chain DNA assay bDNA. This is because they measure different things. Thus, given the same blood sample, bDNA tends to be about half as much as PCR RNA would be. Either test is reliable, but you can't jump from one to the other. Commercially available tests can detect virus down to a count of 500 for bDNA, and as low as 20 in the case of PCR RMA. That's 20 free particles of virus in each fifth of a teaspoon of blood. More sensitive tests are available for research purposes and should become available clinically within the next year or two.

One final point: if your viral load is not detectable, you are still infected; *and you can still transmit HIV.* So can anyone who has sex or shares needles with you. That's because these tests measure only free virus in the blood; they don't measure your own infected cells that are still making virus. Nor do they reliably reflect the amount of free virus in secretions like semen or vaginal fluid, or in other compartments in the body. And the presence of a few viral particles—which can be all it takes to infect—will not be reported. *An undetectable viral load is not a license for unprotected sex or other risk behaviors.*

T-Cell Subsets

Until quite recently we've had no direct way to measure the amount of virus in our body, or the rate of its progression, outside the research laboratory. Instead we've relied on indirect markers that measure the changes resulting from progression.

Research trials take months and often years to run, and more time for collection and analysis of data. So most of what we've learned about treatment has been based on the use of these markers. T-cell subsets have historically been the most useful and are still of value today.

T cells are lymphocytes—some of the white cells that play a part in our immune response. While they are also present outside the bloodstream, they are most easily counted and differentiated in blood tests. A normal CD4 count will vary but is usually about a thousand cells.

There are several different populations of T cells, each with its own set of functions. CD4 cells, also called T-helper cells or T4 cells, stimulate the activation of other immune cells. They are infected by the virus, used by it to make more virus, and eventually destroyed. At a certain stage in HIV progression, their numbers in the blood begin to drop. This is why the CD4 count has been used as an indirect measure of progression.

We now know that the reservoir for most of our CD4 cells, as with most viral activity early in infection, is the lymph nodes. Once those lymph nodes are destroyed and the virus escapes, CD4 counts start to drop. Thus they help us measure progression, but only after it's happened. It's like having the burglar alarm on the silver cabinet instead of on the front door.

CD4 counts in the blood fluctuate widely, sometimes by as much as 20 percent on the same day. If you run up the stairs to the lab to have your blood drawn, they can go up; if you're sick, they can go down. Even the time of day your blood is drawn can make a difference. Thus readings that aren't part of a trend can be misleading. The percentage of T cells that are CD4s (called CD4 percent) is less subject to hour-to-hour fluctuation, and is thought to be a more reliable indicator.

T8 cells, or CD8 cells as they are now called, are suppressor cells. Their function is to mute the cascade of the immune response, balancing the action of the CD4 cells.

In HIV, CD8 cells are activated by the body in response to, and in defense against, the virus. A rising CD8 count tells you your body is hard at work fighting the virus. As HIV progresses, the number of helper cells falls as the number of suppressor cells increases. So the CD4-to-CD8 ratio (number of CD4s divided by number of CD8s) is another indirect marker of progression. A normal CD4-to-CD8 (or helper-to-suppressor) ratio ranges from 0.9 to 3.5.

Prior to 1996, most trials studying the effects of treatment against HIV used T-cell subsets to monitor viral activity. Now that viral load has been validated as a rapid and reliable measure of that activity, we can assess the power of drugs in the research setting and in your body much sooner—sometimes within a few days.

Antiretroviral Therapy
•

The explosion in our understanding of how the virus works, and how our bodies interact with the virus to promote or prevent infection and progression, has broadened the scope of HIV research throughout the world. We've learned how to assess who is most at risk for progression. We've opened new avenues for the development of drugs that can attack the virus at every stage in its cycle of growth and reproduction. We've proven that treatment can forestall the onset of illness in those who are asymptomatic; retard or reverse disease progression, even in those with massive immune compromise and advanced disease; reduce the risk of transmission to an unborn child; diminish the likelihood of infection from needle sticks for health care workers; lessen the chance of infection after exposure

Antiretroviral Strategy	
Hit early.	Start as soon as you know you're infected.
Hit hard.	Use three drugs at least, at full recommended doses.
Hit comprehensively.	Choose a regimen that covers all compartments; use drugs of more than one class to attack the virus from several sides at once.
Hit strategically.	Plan your antiretroviral strategy carefully, to preserve as many future options as possible.
	Take medicines on schedule and as directed.
	Try not to change regimens unless essential.
Shoot to kill.	Aim for viral suppression.

through unprotected sex or needle sharing; and perhaps even reverse infection itself, in a small group of those recently infected.

It takes drugs to do these things—lots of drugs, generally, and lots of commitment. But the results are much more promising than they once were. So learning how to fight the virus has become more critical than ever.

When to Start

There's an old story about two rabbits chased through the fields by a pack of dogs. They ran for miles; as they grew more and more weary, they found an old stone wall and wedged themselves into a hole between the stones. The dogs milled around, barking—still smelling rabbits, but unable to find them. "Well," said one rabbit to the other, "shall we go out and face them now, or wait till we outnumber them?"

The joke is charming, but the metaphor is ominous.

We now know that *there is no such thing as a period of viral latency*. The virus will not go away, or lie dormant, just because we don't attack it. Like the rabbits, it hides—but keeps on reproducing, out of sight, ready to emerge in more numbers than we can control.

That's been my bias for some time. But that bias has been increasingly validated by large-scale trials and studies. And while there is still controversy about holding back some weapons for later, I'm more concerned about *getting* us to later.

Just as there's a small group of people who are relatively resistant to infection, there are a few people who, through some miracle of genetics, can control or slow the progress of HIV infection themselves. As time goes on, we see eventual progression in this group as well, suggesting that they are in fact slow progressors rather than nonprogressors.

It's still a nice group to be in. If viral load is undetectable in these people, and infection doesn't progress, all they need to do is live right and keep watch—close watch.

A few other people have been infected with a viral strain that is too weak to take control. Again, the absence of detectable viral load makes it reasonable not to treat.

Most people and most viruses, though, are not like that. No matter how good you feel, the virus is hard at work; and it's not on your side. And if there's anything we should save for later when you need it, it's your immune system and your uninfected cells.

A detailed discussion of the stages of HIV infection is beyond the scope of this book. Briefly, though, we know that massive viral replication follows infection. This permits rapid entry into cells in different compartments in the body, committing them to turn out new generations of virus throughout their life span. Some of these cells last for more than ten years before they are replaced. Others may not be replaced at all. So the sooner we suppress virus, the sooner we may block infection of new generations of these cells.

We also know that every round of HIV replication, every couple of days, generates more mutations, more diversity, and more potential for resistance down the road.

We also know that not all CD4 cells are the same.

CD4 cells are able to respond to different foreign invaders. Until they find that invader, they have a long life span—perhaps ten or more years. In this stage they are called naive cells. Once they find their mark, they become memory cells. Memory cells divide and multiply rapidly, mounting a strong response against their particular enemy. But their life span is much shorter. And once memory cells that are specific for a given intruder die out, we can't make new ones. So if we wait to treat, some of those cells designed to fight specific infections will not come back, even when CD4 counts rise. Also, once we've lost our reserve of naive cells, we may not get new ones. Our vast repertoire of potential responses to new challenges may be lost.

These arguments for early treatment are convincing to me. But they're based on theory, not clinical results. And, now that we know that viral load predicts clinical outcome, we can each assess the consequences of our own strategy. If you don't share my bias for treatment, you can test your own bias, by following viral load.

When my son Corey was in high school, he bought tickets to a reggae concert the night before a calculus exam. I was furious; I told him he was incredibly irresponsible. "Well, Ma," he said, "I guess if I weren't getting straight A's, you might have a point there." Point well taken; he went to the reggae concert, he got his A in calculus, and I got off his back.

In other words, deciding whether or when to start treatment is no longer a theoretical or philosophical matter. It's an objective one; results talk. Like Corey and his mother and his A in calculus, it doesn't matter what any of us approve of or believe in. What matters is the outcome; and that can now be measured.

If you think you can fight this virus without drugs, get your viral load. If it's undetectable, you're right. If it's not, you're wrong. It's that simple.

That doesn't mean you have no choice as to how to deal with your infection. You're still free to choose not to treat. If you do so, though, you need to acknowledge the impact of that choice, and the price you may pay for that decision. Clearly, most of us will fight the virus better if we shoot to kill.

One final point: no responsible caregiver would advise against treatment once your lowest CD4 count has been 500 or less. At that point, even the most conservative, cost-conscious HIV doctor would urge you to get treatment.

How to Fight

We've learned that HIV infects T cells and other cells of the immune system, as well as other cell lines in our bodies. Infection has been documented in the brain, in the digestive and reproductive systems, and elsewhere. So we have to be sure that some of the medicines we use get into those places.

We also want to interrupt HIV reproduction at several places in the cycle, if we can. That way we maximize our impact and minimize side effects.

We've also learned that HIV is built to adapt and survive in changing environments. And since each free viral particle lives only a day or two, change can occur, be rewarded by survival, and rapidly express itself throughout the viral population. Thus the less we suppress reproduction, the greater the chance that a mutation will be successful, and the virus escape control. This property is called resistance, and we must account for it in our treatment strategies.

Resistance has less chance to develop when the virus is under massive and comprehensive attack. Thus the use of highly active antiretroviral therapy, or HAART, is essential to prevent or forestall resistance to the separate drugs we use. This explains the importance of using convergent therapy, hitting the virus from several sides at once. In addition, we have found that suppression is more durable, and resistance less likely, when we use antiretrovirals at the highest-tolerated effective doses.

Since resistance is less likely when the virus is suppressed, it makes sense to start treatment early. We also start early to avoid infection and recruitment of our own new cells for making HIV.

So by suppressing viral load we try to kill off new virus, made within our body, as soon as it hits the bloodstream. This may shut off reinfection cycles and promote lifetime suppression.

Because there will be times when the virus escapes control, we must conserve our options to fight back. So it's important to choose regimens with care, to use them properly, and to use them as long as we can. Any unnecessary change invites resistance and might cost us the protection of those drugs when we need them later. If resistance does occur, and the virus escapes control, we should change our regimen—preferably with all-new drugs.

Finally, because we still want to have a life, we should look for regimens that are as simple and tolerable as possible.

There are many drugs now, and several good combinations. If we choose them with care, plan ahead for the next move, and use them with respect, we should be able to hold the line until the next batch comes along.

In essence, then, we want to hit early, hit hard, hit comprehensively, hit strategically, and shoot to kill. If we have to change our mode of attack, we should change it as thoroughly as possible. And, when possible, we should settle for nothing less than complete suppression.

What to Use

There are currently eleven drugs, of three classes, licensed for fighting HIV. Many more drugs within these classes are in development or testing. Others licensed for other purposes may have activity against HIV. And new drugs of new classes, using entirely different mechanisms of action, are on the way as well.

Remember that while drugs were first tested alone, they should be prescribed in combination. *Two drugs are bad medicine, and monotherapy is malpractice,* in HIV management today.

Nucleoside Analogue Reverse Transcriptase Inhibitors. These drugs mimic the building blocks with which the virus copies its genetic material. They interfere with replication at the transcription phase. You need two of these for your regimen, and they all work well. Because the ones we have so far aren't as powerful as protease inhibitors, resistance tends to fade and they can be recycled if necessary. Five are currently approved.

Zidovudine (ZDV, AZT, Retrovir)

Dosage: typically 500 to 600 milligrams a day, in divided doses. Commonly prescribed at 200 milligrams three times a day. Used at 300 milligrams twice a day when twice-daily dosing is more convenient. In cases of HIV encephalopathy (or AIDS dementia complex), doses are larger and more frequent. Available in combination with 3TC as one pill combining zidovudine 300 mg and 3TC 150 for easy dosing at one pill twice a day (combivir).

Strong points: Good brain penetration; thus especially valuable for postexposure prophylaxis or HIV encephalopathy. Targets resting CD4 cells (not those preparing to divide). Treatment with zidovudine during pregnancy has been shown to reduce by two-thirds the risk of HIV transmission from a pregnant woman to her baby. Treatment has also been shown to reverse wasting. Can be taken with or without food.

Downside: Initial side effects can include nausea, headache, and fatigue. These normally subside after two or three weeks; those who can get through the first month of treatment are usually home free. Less-frequent side effects may include mild anemia (reduction in the number of red blood cells) and, rarely, muscle inflammation or myositis. Anemia usually responds to erythropoietin, when necessary, and should not be a reason to stop the drug.

Tips: Not to be used in combination with D4T. Resistance develops more rapidly in advanced HIV. 3TC appears to reverse or forestall resistance.

Didanosine (DDI, Videx)

Dosage: For people over 130 pounds, 200 milligrams twice a day. Reduce to 125 milligrams twice a day if under 130 pounds. Not to be taken with meals. Must be chewed. A 300-milligram daily dose is under study and shows good results for six months so far.

Strong points: Some brain penetration. In combination with D4T, no additive risk of peripheral neuropathy. Twice-a-day dosing; once-daily dosing is coming. Targets activated (dividing) T cells.

Downside: Side effects may include peripheral neuropathy, experienced as foot pain and less common at higher CD4 counts, and rare pancreatitis. Risk of pancreatitis is increased with alcohol use. Requires an alkaline environment for proper absorption, so can't be taken with food. Pills must be chewed. They taste, I'm told, like Alka-Seltzer. Also available in powdered form, which also tastes bad. Once resistant to DDI, anticipate reduced sensitivity to DDC.

Tips: In combination with D4T, no additional peripheral neuropathy. Especially well tolerated early in HIV, so this may be a good duo to start with.

Zalcitabine (DDC, Hivid)

Dosage: Generally .750 milligrams three times a day. Can be reduced to .375 milligrams twice a day if symptoms require reduction.

Strong points: Can be taken with or without food. Targets resting CD4 cells.

Downside: Side effects may include peripheral neuropathy or mouth ulcers (relatively common), and rare pancreatitis.

Tips: Don't use with DDI or D4T.

Stavudine (D4T, Zerit)

Dosage: Forty milligrams twice a day. If peripheral neuropathy is experienced, may reduce to 20 milligrams twice a day.

Strong points: Most "resistance-resistant" nucleoside analogue, thus offers increased chance of lasting effect; no overall change seen in DDI or D4T sensitivity after long-term therapy in combination. Good brain penetration. Twice-a-day dosing, with or without food. No increase in peripheral neuropathy when used in combination with DDI. Targets activated CD4 cells.

Downside: Side effects include peripheral neuropathy (but less than with DDI or DDC, and less at high CD4 counts). Resistance may result in reduced sensitivity to DDI and DDC.

Tips: Should not be used in combination with zidovudine (both mimic the same nucleoside).

Lamivudine (3TC, Epivir)

Dosage: 150 milligrams twice a day. Available in combination with zidovudine at 300 mg and 3TC 150 for easy dosing at one pill twice a day (combivir).

Strong points: Virtually no side effects, hence no impact on quality of life. Development of resistance is at the expense of zidovudine resistance and results in a weaker, less-fit virus. Treats or helps suppress chronic active hepatitis B while treating HIV. Targets resting CD4 cells. Good brain penetration.

Downside: Resistance develops quickly and appears to be lasting. Therefore, may want to try to hold it for use with an zidovudine-protease combination, since its first hit is the hardest—*and since true viral suppression may avoid the development of resistance and loss of effect.*

Tips: Should never be used alone or as only nucleoside analogue. Discontinuance in the presence of chronic active hepatitis B may lead to hepatitis flare. If resistance to HIV develops in such circumstances, don't count 3TC as one of your two nucleoside analogues for HIV therapy, but keep it on board to treat hepatitis B.

Nonnucleoside Reverse Transcriptase Inhibitors (NNRTIs). These drugs work at the same site as the nucleoside analogues to block transcription, but by a different mechanism. Two are approved to date.

Nevirapine (Viramune)

Dosage: Two hundred milligrams twice a day.

Strong points: Rapid, almost immediate absorption; good bioavailability (almost all of the dose taken gets into the bloodstream); excellent brain penetration. Thus a very interesting choice for postexposure prophylaxis (after needle sticks or unsafe sex), or for treatment of those recently infected who may not yet have seeded their brain with HIV. Also appears to have excellent performance in blocking mother-to-child transmission during childbirth.

Downside: Side effects include rash, which is fairly common. Rarely, a rash may be severe enough to require discontinuation. Dose titration reduces incidence (see "Tips"). Resistance develops rapidly as monotherapy. Induces rapid breakdown of some drugs, including protease inhibitors, by its effect on the CP450 system in the liver, and lowers the blood levels of those drugs.

Tips: As nevirapine induces or speeds up its own elimination, start with 200 milligrams only once a day, and increase to full dose after two weeks. Rash occurs less often with this approach and tends to be mild and temporary. Consider increasing the dose of protease inhibitors when used with nevirapine, as levels can be lowered by about 30 percent. Preliminary results of an HIV care trial suggest that nelfinavir levels do not appear to be lowered by nevirapine.

Delaverdine (Rescriptor)

Dosage: Four hundred milligrams three times a day.

Strong points: Increases protease inhibitor levels.

Downside: No increase in benefit over DDI alone when studied in combination. Some cases of congestive heart failure (CHF) reported.

Efavirenz (Sustiva, DMP 266)

Dosage: Two hundred milligrams a day.

Strong points: Powerful, well tolerated, penetrates CSF. Once a day dosing.

Downside: Side effects reported include malaise and dizziness, but are mild and generally resolve themselves. Reduces indinavir levels. FDA approval pending as of January 1998. Until approval, access restricted to lower CD4 counts.

Tips: Increases nelfinavir; don't change dose. Reduces indinavir; increase dose to 1000 milligrams every eight hours. Expanded access available pending approval.

Protease Inhibitors. These drugs are at the center of the current revolution in HIV care. They are exceptionally powerful at reducing viral load. Used alone, irreversible resistance is likely to develop and extend in some degree to other drugs in the class. Therefore, they are typically prescribed as the cornerstone of the "cocktail," their power protected and reinforced by other antiretrovirals, typically two nucleoside analogues. There is current interest in using two of these in combination, with nucleoside analogues and sometimes other drugs.

As a class, protease inhibitors can be complex to work with because of their potential for drug interactions. All are metabolized or broken down by one or more parts of the CP450 system in the liver. Since the body uses this system to break down many compounds, protease inhibitors may alter concentrations of other drugs to a significant degree (see Table 13.1). Other drugs may also change protease inhibitor concentrations.

These drug interactions can be quite intricate; a thorough dis-

TABLE 13.1.
•

Major Sources of Drug Interactions with Protease Inhibitors.

Type of Drug	Examples	Substitution
Antihistamines (allergy drugs)	*Seldane, Hismanal*	Benedryl
Seizure drugs	Dilantin, Phenobarbital, Tegretol	Depakote
Antibiotics	Erythromycin, Biaxin	Zithromax
Antimycobacterials	Rifampin, Mycobutin	a
Antifungals	Nizoral	a
Tranquilizers	Valium, Xanax, Halcyon, Restoril	Ativan
Antidepressants	*Welbutryn*	Paxil, tricyclics
Steroids	Decadron	a
	Birth-control pills	b
Antiretrovirals	NNRTIs, other protease inhibitors	Adjust doses

This is only a partial listing. Review all medications with your pharmacist. Drugs in italics are *very dangerous*; contraindicated with some or all protease inhibitors.

aComplex. Discuss with HIV specialist.

bDiscuss with gynecologist.

cussion is beyond the scope of this book. Readers are referred to the article by Evelyn Rose and Mary Romeyn in the September 1997 *Bulletin of Experimental Treatments for AIDS,* listed in the references at the end of this chapter. *Anyone taking protease inhibitors should review all current medications with her or his pharmacist, to rule out potentially dangerous combinations or the need for dosage adjustment. Any changes in medication thereafter should be reviewed as well.*

Saquinavir (Inverase)

Dosage: 1,200 milligrams of *soft-gel capsules* three times a day as of January 1998. Before then, FDA dose of 600 milligrams of hard-gel caps three times a day; in the community, had been dosed at double or quadruple that amount with high cost but better effect. *Bioavailability of soft-gel caps is four to nine times higher than that of hard-gel caps, with corresponding increase in blood levels.* Should be given within two hours after a full meal.

Strong points: Low side-effect profile at FDA-approved hard-gel doses. Side effects increase with higher dosage, but remain relatively low.

Downside: Very poor absorption in hard-gel formulation has led to low blood levels. Better efficacy at double or quadruple doses. Liver function tests may be elevated. Pancreatic or renal effects have been reported.

Tips: Take enough. Grapefruit juice with each dose has been shown to substantially increase blood levels. So does ketoconazole, ritonavir, or nelfinavir.

Indinavir (Crixivan)

Dosage: Eight hundred milligrams every eight hours, an hour before or two hours after meals (see "Tips"). A 1000-milligram, twice-a-day regimen is under study.

Strong points: Very potent in combination. Easily tolerated, with rare side effects. Response appears durable, reported out to sixty-eight weeks in combination with zidovudine and 3TC. One subject has made it to the four-year mark with continuing viral suppression—and he's just started law school! Good pill-takers have the most durable response.

Downside: Kidney stones reported in 4 percent. Bilirubin levels may be elevated. Mouth may be dry. May cause changes in fat deposition ("crix belly"). Dosage requirements are stringent. Durability of response is closely tied to compliance. Resistance to indinavir confers resistance to ritonavir.

Tips: Drink *a lot* of water. A low-fat, low-protein snack of 200 calories or less will not harm absorption. Don't use in combination with saquinavir; effect appears antagonistic.

Ritonavir (Norvir)

Dosage: Six hundred milligrams twice a day.

Strong points: Most potent protease inhibitor approved to date. Twice-daily dosing with food. Side effects may resolve after the first two to four weeks. Greatly increases saquinavir doses in combination.

Downside: Severe gastrointestinal side effects, especially at start of therapy. Tingling around the mouth and changes in taste perception reported. Side effects may be less if the dose is eased upward (see "Tips"). Broken down by many parts of the CP450 system, so it has the most significant drug interaction profile in its class. This makes it hard to work with when people are on multiple drugs. Formulation is 43 percent alcohol, so metronidazole (Flagyl) or disulfiram (Antabuse) must be avoided. Alcohol content may also pose a problem for those in recovery. Resistance to ritonavir confers resistance to indinavir.

Tips: Gradually increase dose at start-up, moving from 300 milligrams twice a day to the full 600-milligram, twice-a-day dose within two weeks. Because ritonavir induces or speeds up its own breakdown, a lower dose at the start of treatment should not result in lower blood levels. Ritonavir also appears to be powerful in combination with saquinavir at 400 milligrams each twice a day. Many of my patients report reduction of diarrhea with daily yogurt intake.

Nelfinavir (Viracept)

Dosage: Seven hundred fifty milligrams three times a day, with a meal or light snack.

Strong points: Well tolerated, with low side-effect profile for most. Taken with food, so easier to schedule. Twice-a-day dosing.

Downside: Most common side effect is diarrhea, which partially resolves over time. Most will continue to have two or three loosely formed stools a day; Lomotil or Imodium resolves. Not as strong as indinavir or ritonavir.

Tips: Early observation suggested that resistance, when it develops, may not confer resistance to other protease inhibitors. Thus, when suppression of viral load does not require one of the bigger guns, this may be a good place to start. Most studies, however, suggest some cross-resistance exists.

Because of their lifesaving, almost miraculous ability to suppress HIV replication, it's important to use protease inhibitors wisely. Taking them incorrectly, in lower doses or only some of the time, may give your virus the chance it needs to learn its way around them. If you haven't yet mastered the art of pill-taking, these may not be the pills to practice on.

If you *have* successfully developed the habit of taking your pills on schedule, the use of these medicines is worth the work it takes to learn about them, and well worth their price. To withhold them for the sake of cost control is not appropriate.

If you're currently using an antiretroviral regimen that does not include a protease inhibitor; if you're able to put up with the demands of staying on schedule; and if your viral load is not suppressed on your current regimen, you should discuss this with your doctor. Dollars that are saved at the cost of your right to life, and your chance to live out a full life span, are better left unsaved.

Other Drugs in Trials for HIV

Some exciting new drugs are in testing and should be released soon. Among them are:

Loviride, a nonnucleoside reverse transcriptase inhibitor.

Adepovir dipivoxil, a nucleoside analogue similar to cidofavir (Vistide). Acts against HIV and other viruses, including CMV, herpes simplex, and other herpes viruses. May offer once-a-day dosing, with low likelihood of resistance.

PMPA, a nucleotide analogue with powerful activity, excellent postexposure prophylaxis performance in animal studies, and less toxicity in lab studies.

GW1592-U89, Abacavir, a nucleoside analogue with the potency of a protease inhibitor, excellent CNS penetrance, and no CP450 drug interactions. A compassionate-use program has been announced as this book goes to press, but access has been gravely and arbitrarily limited despite widespread activist protests.

GW141W94 and *BMS-234475*, new protease inhibitors.

ABT-378, another new protease inhibitor that appears to be ten times as active as ritonavir, with activity against ritonavir-, indinavir- and saquinavir-resistant strains, and massively increased levels when given in combination with ritonavir.

Other experimental antiretroviral approaches include the use of *hydroxyurea (Hydrea)* in combination with nucleoside analogues. Hydroxyurea appears to increase the activity of nucleoside analogues, especially DDI. Some studies show increases in CD4 counts as well as viral load suppression. There is still some concern; as hydroxyurea's action results from its attack on cells infected with HIV, there is fear that it may suppress CD4 rebound. However, one report of viral suppression in hydroxyurea, indinavir, and DDI, with no return of detectable viral load after nine months off drugs, has caused great excitement. That combination is now in testing.

Immune-based therapies are also a focus of interest.

Tips for Success

Start by choosing a combination with enough power to suppress viral load. Look for one that's built to last. Resistance may be slower to develop, for example, with the combination of DDI and D4T.

Add an NNRTI or a protease inhibitor for your third drug. Base your choice on how much suppression you require, how organized and consistent you can be, and how you can fit a regimen into your lifestyle. For most of my patients, suppression—hence survival—is the first priority. Durability of response is the second. Lifestyle is the third, but quite important. If you can't remember to take your pills, practice makes perfect; but practice on something you can afford to lose.

Remember, for viral suppression in chronic infection, three may not be a magic number; combinations of four and five drugs are used in the community, when needed.

Where maximal suppression is needed, consider using two protease inhibitors in combination, backed by nucleoside analogues. Look for study results on combinations of nucleoside analogues, nonnucleoside reverse transcriptase inhibitors, and protease inhibitors, too. Regimens of four drugs, such as ritonavir, saquinavir, and two nucleoside analogues, already show promise, and studies may move to more than four. Recognize that today's news is paper for the cat tomorrow; we're learning something new every day.

Try to make it through initial side effects, if they don't damage critical functions. Often they subside, and you'll have saved the next regimen for a rainy day. Always let your doctor know about new side effects, though, so you don't miss something dangerous.

Monitor closely. Get a viral load before you start a new regimen and a month or so afterward, to see how you're doing. If your load is entirely suppressed, follow every three months or so. If not, follow more closely. Remember that at least threefold differences are needed to accurately reflect changes in viral load. If you're not suppressed, but differences are less than threefold, check again in a month or so to look for a trend.

When you must change, do so intelligently. Organize your options—holding zidovudine and 3TC, for example, to use in a truly suppressive regimen to avoid rapid resistance.

If you don't suppress at once, wait it out—as long as you're moving in the right direction. But keep checking.

Tables 13.2 and 13.3 offer some representative combinations and their relative power. Your prior antiretroviral experience will guide your choice, too. And news breaks every day about new options.

You and your doctor may want to work with the Antiretrovirogram—the form we use in my office to help make intelligent, individualized treatment decisions. You'll find it in Appendix XII.

Remember, these are pretty complicated concepts. Get yourself some crackerjack advice from your doctor or HIV expert. Use other information sources. Don't experiment on your own—and if you do, run your plan by someone who plays with this stuff day and night. As Joe Eron says, "we're professionals; do not try this at home." And always tell your doctor if you're doing something different on your own. Even if she or he doesn't approve, it will help the doctor to keep you safe.

TABLE 13.2.

•

Relative Potencies of Combinations in Patients with No Prior Treatment.

Drugs	Study	Duration (Weeks)	Decrease (Logs)
D4T/3TC	Katlama	24	1.7
DDI/D4T	Pollard	52	1.3
AZT/3TC	NUCB 3001	48	1.2
AZT/DD1	ACTG 175	104	0.5
AZT/DDI/NVP	Myers	28	2.3
AZT/3TC/NLF	Ho	16	3.9
DDI/D4T/RTV	Saimot	12	2.2
AZT/DDC/RTV	Mathez	60	1.9
AZT/3TC/RTV	Danner	8	3.0

Note: One log equals a tenfold change.

TABLE 13.3.

•

Relative Potencies of Combinations in Patients with Prior Treatment.

Drugs	Study	Duration (Weeks)	Decrease (Logs)
D4T/3TC	Katlama	24	0.7
DDI/D4T	Kalathoor	12	1.0
AZT/3TC	NUCB 3002	52	0.8
AZT/DDI	ACTG 175	104	0.5
RTV/SQV[a]	Murphy	48	3.2
D4T/3TC/IND	DeTruchis	24	1.4
DDI/D4T/NLF	Pednault	12	1.4
AZT/3TC/IND	Gulick	48	2.3

Note: One log equals a tenfold change.

[a]3TC added in some patients.

I'd like to follow Joe Eron's quote with three more that have helped to guide my course against the virus:

> Any regimen that includes only two drugs is doomed to failure. [Julio Montaner, program cochair, Eleventh International Conference on AIDS 1996, April 1997]

> I think we have regimens that are powerful enough that . . . they will work for a lifetime. [Calvin Cohen, research director, Community Research Initiative of New England, June 1997]

> I ain't goin' nowhere! [Mike Maron, patient, The Unquilt Celebration of Life, Andrew Ziegler Foundation, May 1997]

REFERENCES

Abrams, D. I. "Treatment options in zidovudine intolerance or failure." *AIDS*, 1994, *8*(Supp.), S3–S7.

Abrams, D. I., and others. "A comparative trial of didanosine or zalcitabine after treatment with zidovudine in patients with human immunodeficiency virus infection." *New England Journal of Medicine*, 1994, *330*(10), 657–662.

Baker, R. "AIDS treatment advocacy issues." *Bulletin of Experimental Treatments for AIDS*, December 1996, pp. 3–4.

Baker, R. "Three-drug therapy reduces deaths and new AIDS-related illnesses by 50 Percent." *Bulletin of Experimental Treatments for AIDS*, March 1997, pp. 3–4.

Bartlett, J. G. *Pocket Book of Infectious Disease Therapy.* Baltimore: Williams and Wilkins, 1996.

Bowers, M. "Hydroxurea." *Bulletin of Experimental Treatments for AIDS*, March 1997, pp. 9–11.

Carpenter, C.C.J., and others. "Antiretroviral therapy for HIV infection in 1996. Recommendations of an international panel." *Journal of the American Medical Association*, 1996, *276*, 146–164.

Cohen, C. "Maximizing treatment options: Starting, switching and sequencing in the new paradigm." Paper presented at the AMFAR Treatment Symposium: Rational Approaches to Antiretroviral Therapy in the Clinic, San Francisco, June 19, 1997.

Condra, J. H., and Emini. "Preventing HIV-1 drug resistance." *Science and Medicine*, 1997, *4*(1), 2–11.

Cooper, D. A. "Early antiretroviral therapy." *AIDS*, 1994, *8*, S9–S14.

Dormont, J. "Future treatment strategies in HIV infection." *AIDS*, 1994, *8*, S31–S33.

Henry, K. "Switching and combining antiretroviral therapies." *AIDS Clinical Care*, 1993, *5*(5), 33–38, 41.

Ho, D. D. "Quantitation of human immunodeficiency virus type 1 in the blood of infected persons." *New England Journal of Medicine*, 1989, *321*(24), 1621–1625.

Ho, D. "Can HIV be eradicated from an infected person?" Bernard Fields Memorial Lecture, Fourth Conference on Retroviruses and Opportunistic Infections, January 22–26, 1997, Washington, D.C. Abstract S1.

Jacobs, M., personal communication on nelfinavir/nevirapin pharmacokinetics.

Kempf, D., and others. "The duration of viral suppression is predicted by viral load during protease inhibitor therapy." Fourth Conference on Retroviruses and Opportunistic Infections, January 22–26, 1997, Washington, D.C. Abstract 603.

Kessler, H. A. "The next generation of antiretroviral agents." *HIV Newsline*, 1997, *3*(3) 73–79.

Lane, H. C. "HIV pathogenesis: Improving the management of HIV disease." *International AIDS Society–USA*, *5*(1), 4–7.

Leong, G. "Making sense of the data: Prescribing effective regimens that work in the real world." Paper presented at Amfar Treatment Symposium: Rational Approaches to Antiretroviral Therapy in the Clinic, San Francisco, June 19, 1997.

Man, K., and others. "Pancreatorenal syndrome associated with combination antiretroviral therapy in HIV infection." *Lancet*, 1997, *346*, 1745–1746.

Mayer, K. "Rationale for combination therapy: Available agents, viral load, and resistance." Paper presented at Amfar Treatment Symposium: Rational Approaches to Antiretroviral Therapy in the Clinic, San Francisco, June 19, 1997.

Mellors, J. W., and others. "Prognosis in HIV-1 infection predicted by the quantity of virus in plasma. *Science*, 1996, *272*, 1167–1170.

Mellors, J. W., and others. "Plasma viral load and CD4 lymphocytes as prognostic markers of HIV-1 infection." *Annals of Internal Medicine*, 1997, *126*(12), 946–954.

Mulder, J. W., and others. "Zidovudine twice daily in asymptomatic subjects with HIV infection and a high risk of progression to AIDS: A randomized, double-blind placebo-controlled study." *AIDS*, 1994, *8*, 313–321.

Panel on Clinical Practices for Treatment of HIV Infection. *Draft Guidelines for the Use of Antiretroviral Agents in HIV-Infected Adults and Adolescents*. Washington, D.C.: Federal Register, June 1997.

Perelson, A. S., and others. "HIV-1 dynamics *in vivo*: Virion clearance rate, infected cell life-span, and viral generation time." *Science,* 1996, *271,* 1582–1586.

Reynes, J. "Stadi study: Once daily administration of didanosine in combination with stavudine in antiretroviral-naive patients." Paper presented at European Zerit Symposium, Cannes, France, March 22, 1997.

Romeyn, M. "Report from the Third Conference on Retroviruses and Opportunistic Infections." *Bulletin of Experimental Treatments for AIDS,* March 1996, pp. 22–27.

Rose, E., and Romeyn, M. "Significant protease inhibitor interactions." *Bulletin of Experimental Treatments for AIDS,* September, 1997.

Sanford, J. P., and others. *Guide to Antimicrobial Therapy.* Dallas: Antimicrobial Therapy, Inc., 1997.

Sanford, J. P., and others. *Guide to HIV/AIDS Therapy, 1996.* Dallas: Antimicrobial Therapy, Inc., 1997.

International Association of Physicians in AIDS Care. "Three Drugs for Primary Infection, Four for Chronic Infection." *AIDScan,* Issue 2, Third International Congress on Drug Therapy in HIV Infection, Birmingham, England, November 8, 1996.

Valenti, W. M. "Antiretroviral therapy in the treatment-experienced patient." *HIV/AIDS Clinical Insight,* 1997, *7*(3), 1–6.

Volberding, P. A. "Initiation of antiretroviral therapy: Improving the management of HIV disease." *International AIDS Society–USA,* 1996, *4*(1), 4–6.

CHAPTER 14

•

Secondary Infections

As you start to learn about HIV, you'll find a great deal of information about opportunistic infections. These are infections that people normally fight off without help, but that can survive in the setting of immune suppression. Many are unique to HIV and other conditions that compromise immunity.

It's important to learn about opportunistic infections and to protect against them. But any secondary infection—any infection your body has to fight while it's fighting HIV—poses a greater threat than it did before.

We've seen that anything that triggers the immune response triggers the process of wasting.

We now know, also, that anything that triggers the immune response triggers HIV replication. Any activation of our immune system leads to release of new viral particles from our infected immune cells. So we have to be quick to recognize and help our bodies fight infection, to preserve lean body mass and viral suppression.

We have to avoid infection when possible. When we can't

avoid it we must diagnose early and treat vigorously. That's why you need to report symptoms quickly.

Never Trust a Fever
•

Before you had HIV, you could often shake off an infection. You wouldn't have run to your doctor with a fever, or a thick, wet cough, or diarrhea. You may still be able to cure such things yourself. But if you do so, it will be at the expense of lean body mass. Though you may have the immune power to fight off an illness, your protein stores will diminish as your body responds. And so will the force with which you and your medicines suppress the virus.

Years ago, we thought that fevers were a necessary part of HIV infection. "Oh well, that's AIDS," we used to say. We now know absolutely that this is not true. A fever of over 101 degrees, or a lesser fever that lasts several days, should always prompt a visit to your doctor. There will always be some other reason. And it is that very part of our immune response that causes a fever that also can cause us to waste.

In advanced stages of HIV, fevers can be common. But the cause can almost always be determined. It is rarely, if ever, attributable just to HIV.

Other Symptoms
•

Likewise, symptoms of infection can help guide us to the source of that infection. A cough, a facial ache, or crampy abdominal pain can be clues to the problem we seek.

Many of the secondary infections that promote wasting are not limited to people with HIV. Some of them are common to everyone. But in HIV they can be harsher. And they undercut your efforts to maintain nutritional competence. If you're early in the course of HIV, you owe it to your future to be vigilant. If you're further along, it's even more crucial.

Some causes of infection are more likely to present at different stages. Knowing where you stand on the continuum can help us know what to look for. We'll look at three stages separately below. But understand that they aren't exclusive: HIV disease is a continuum and doesn't fit precisely into boxes. Understand also that anything that can happen in one stage can happen in later stages too.

Early-Stage HIV (CD4 Nadir Above 500)
·

Any infection that could happen to anyone is more of a problem for you. Some, though, are more common, even early in the course of HIV.

Respiratory and Sinus Infections

Many of the germs that cause common respiratory infections—sore throats, bronchitis, even pneumonia—get a head start in people with HIV. These germs have a protective capsule, which surrounds them like a wall; we need our cell-mediated immunity, our T-cell immunity, to fight them effectively.

Thus we may not fight them as well—and if we do, it will be at the cost of immune activation in ways that help the virus.

These same germs are frequently the ones that cause sinusitis. Sinus infections are more common, more severe, and more lasting in people with HIV.

Just as our cellular immunity—the T-cell branch of our immune system—may be impaired, our humoral immunity—the B-cell branch, which makes antibodies—is more active. That's why people with HIV have heightened allergic responses. So in the case of sinusitis, we must balance that excess response. We treat the infection with antibiotics, and the allergic component with antihistamines, inhaled steroids, and decongestants. If we get in early, we can get out fast.

Routine sinus films aren't very sensitive; a limited CT (or CAT) scan is better. This study will show not only acute sinusitis, but also the localized thickening of chronic infection. Chronic sinusitis will not resolve without four to six weeks of treatment. That's four to six weeks of wasting, and of feeding the virus, if the diagnosis isn't made.

We treat HIV-associated sinusitis with the same drugs we use in noninfected people. People already on Bactrim for pneumocystis carinii pneumonia (PCP) prophylaxis are assumed to have a Bactrim-resistant infection, and a different drug is added. If there's no improvement, we refer to an ear, nose, and throat specialist for culturing. Fungal, microsporidial, and other unusual organisms have been seen.

Common Sexually and Injection-Transmitted Infections

Because HIV can be transmitted sexually or by the use of intravenous drugs, its presence may be associated with other, similarly transmitted infections.

Gonorrhea, Chlamydia, and Syphilis.   These infections are also concerns. Their presence tells us we've put ourselves and any partners more at risk. In the case of gonorrhea, resistance to the drugs that usually work is more frequent. And syphilis can be a special problem.

Normally we only see brain involvement, or neurosyphilis, in chronically infected people who've gone untreated for years. But people with HIV who contract syphilis can develop neurosyphilis early. It's more dangerous and harder to treat.

Some experts recommend a lumbar puncture, or spinal tap, in any HIV-positive person with syphilis to find out if the cerebrospinal fluid (CSF) that bathes the brain is infected. If it is, it will only be resolved with aggressive intravenous therapy. Even then it's hard to be sure of a cure. People with syphilis and HIV need close follow-up for at least six months, to watch for residual infection.

Human Papilloma Virus and Cervical and Anal Cancer.   This normally presents as genital or anal warts. The papilloma virus that causes these skin changes can also cause cancer at the site of infection. Progression to cancer appears to be faster in people with HIV. For that reason, women should be checked by pap smear at least every six months for changes in cervical cells; any changes must be more closely monitored.

Anal warts can likewise progress to anal cancer; therefore, annual anal pap smears are now recommended for women or men with any history of receptive anal intercourse or anal warts.

There appears to be a parallel between progression from anal papillomavirus infection to anal dysplasia and cancer and the same well-described progression to cervical cancer in women. Joel Palefsky at the University of California at San Francisco is doing landmark work in understanding what this means. A high proportion of the men with anal warts in his study do in fact show dysplasia, or abnormal cells at greater risk for progression to cancer, on anal pap smear. Our own office has seen dysplasia in a third to a half of patients with HIV and a history of anal receptive sex.

When high-grade dysplasia is found, it should be followed by serial examinations. A colposcope is used to provide magnification, and small biopsies are taken of suspicious-looking areas or at random. If there is no progression, we simply continue serial examinations and biopsies.

Any evidence of anal cancer with invasion should prompt aggressive evaluation, to avoid the risk of metastatic cancer.

Herpes Simplex (HSV). Outbreaks of herpes simplex in people with HIV are more likely to be reactivations of prior infection than new infection. People who test negative can acquire herpes and never know it; they may remain asymptomatic all their lives, or until another insult to their immune system allows symptoms to surface. Even those with recurrent outbreaks usually report only mild symptoms, after the initial episode. But herpes outbreaks in people with HIV can be more frequent, more persistent, and more severe.

It's essential to treat these events. Without treatment, herpes in the setting of HIV can progress to extensive, deep, and painful chronic ulceration. Other germs can infect the open sores. With anal or vaginal lesions, elimination can be excruciating. If lesions are in the mouth or throat, you may be unable to eat.

The presence of even one episode of herpes should prompt you to consider suppression. Viral shedding has been documented even in people without symptoms; it is suppressed with therapy. And the body's response to viruses other than HIV triggers many of the changes that favor HIV replication.

Treatment with acyclovir in late-stage HIV, even in people who test negative for herpes, has been shown to prolong life—reportedly by as much as 26 percent.

Acyclovir's effects on survival aren't clearly understood yet. Its suppression of other, less virulent or less apparent viruses may dampen the immune response that favors HIV replication.

In my office, we routinely prescribe acyclovir. We particularly urge treatment for people with any history of herpes simplex, shingles, or oral hairy leukoplakia, or with CD4 nadirs of less than 300.

Kaposi's Sarcoma–Associated Herpes-Like Virus (KSHV) and Kaposi's Sarcoma. Kaposi's sarcoma–associated herpes-like virus (KSHV) and Kaposi's sarcoma, or KS, is seen almost exclusively in gay men, and those who have acquired their HIV infection sexually. We now know it's caused by a herpes, or herpes-like, virus. About 25 percent of adults and 2–8 percent of children in our country are reported to possess KSHV antibodies, suggesting that infection is primarily, but not entirely, sexual. This virus appears to induce KS tumors in people with HIV. Researchers are working to characterize the virus and hope in time to treat it directly, to reduce the incidence of KS.

KS may present as one or more minor skin tumors, or it may involve the gastrointestinal and respiratory tracts as well. Treatment is local for minor lesions. If disease is widespread, chemotherapy may be used.

Hepatitis B and C. These are caused by viruses acquired through contact with blood and body fluids. HIV can significantly affect the development and course of these diseases.

Hepatitis B is highly infectious.

A much higher percentage of people will not resolve their hepatitis B in the setting of HIV. In one study, three times as many HIV-positive patients progressed to chronic infection as did those who were HIV-negative.

In those who develop chronic hepatitis the disease appears to be less severe, due to a compromised immune response. But viral replication, contagion, and resistance to therapy are greater.

Hepatitis C is most often transmitted by blood, via transfusions or IV drug use. While it is less contagious than hepatitis B, there is an even greater likelihood of chronic activity.

3TC, or Epivir, can help control chronic active hepatitis B. There is also a role for interferon alpha in some cases. Hepatitis B viral load by PCR, before and after treatment, can help assess results. Remember that people with chronic active hepatitis B are highly infectious to others through needle sharing or sex.

For people who have not been exposed to hepatitis B, a vaccine series may be protective. We try to do this early in the course of HIV, when the capacity to build an immune response is at its strongest. And we check hepatitis B surface antibody status periodically; if it's positive, immune protection persists.

There may also be a role for treating chronic active hepatitis C with interferon alpha. This should be discussed with a gastrointestinal specialist familiar with HIV care.

Tuberculosis (TB)

The alarming rise in cases of TB has been attributed in part to the HIV pandemic. In HIV-negative people, active TB is generally the result of reactivation, after the initial infection has been contained. About 5 percent of people who are exposed will reactivate within the first year, and another 5 percent each year thereafter throughout life. But people with HIV frequently move quickly from infection to active disease. There's also an increased risk of reactivation.

Because of changes in immune response, TB may not present in a typical fashion in a person who is HIV-infected. *Any HIV-positive person with an abnormal chest X ray should be presumed to have TB until proven otherwise.*

Treatment is with a multidrug regimen adapted to documented sensitivities of the organism. Compliance for the full term is essential. Isolation is necessary until smears of sputum show no organisms.

One of the gravest concerns facing our health system is the development of multidrug-resistant TB. This form of the bacillus has been reported to result in death in seven out of ten people infected, usually within one to four months. HIV-negative people are fully at risk. Health care workers are particularly endangered.

Multidrug-resistant TB has spread explosively throughout the HIV population in some parts of the country. Its frequency is enhanced by incomplete treatment, poor living conditions, and communal living settings. It poses a particular risk for patients who use HIV clinics. All the essentials are there: increased incidence, depressed immunity, and close quarters.

One especially disturbing study from San Francisco reported

the impact of homelessness on TB exposure. The likelihood of TB exposure was found to increase with the length of time a person remained homeless and also with residence in high-contact settings. *Of those who had lived in shelters or single-room welfare hotels for all of the year under study, 45 percent showed evidence of TB exposure.*

This is a terrifying glimpse into the future, at the public health nightmare that the epidemic of homelessness in America threatens to create. Given the rise in multidrug-resistant TB, it's a life-threatening crisis for all of us. It is especially frightening for those with HIV, who are least able to withstand such a threat.

Enteric Pathogens

This is a catchall term for parasites that infect the lower intestine. Some of them are known to cause diarrhea. Others may be innocuous in immunocompetent people but cause symptoms in people with HIV. Others remain clinically silent. *All* of them should be treated: any organism that must be contained and suppressed by our immune system will increase the burden of inflammatory stress on our bodies and accelerate wasting. An attempt should be made to eradicate the presence of any such organism found on routine stool evaluation.

Middle-Stage HIV (CD4 Nadir of 100 to 500)
•

This is the point at which we may see illnesses that are not found in people with intact immune response, except in conditions of stress.

Herpes Zoster (Shingles)

Herpes zoster is caused by reactivation of the chicken pox virus (varicella), which lives within nerve cells after infection. We see shingles in elderly people or people with extensive or chronic illness. Its symptoms and appearance are somewhat similar to those in herpes simplex outbreaks but appear in a localized area served by the affected nerve. Pain can be intense, especially when treatment is delayed. Rarely, it can involve the eye.

In people with HIV, herpes zoster often appears early, at CD4 counts of 500 or so. From 5 to 23 percent of cases will recur in the future. When immunosuppression is severe, recurrence can be chronic and can take different forms. Those forms are often resistant to first-line therapy.

Treatment is with high-dose acyclovir or famcyclovir. Rapid initiation of treatment can block or reduce residual pain. Acyclovir suppression therapy, at 400 milligrams twice a day, should be continued for life after such an episode.

Candida (Thrush)

Candida is a yeast, or fungus, that is universally present. Normally we can suppress it ourselves. When it is not suppressed, it first appears as a superficial infection in the mouth or vagina. Recurrence is common. With HIV progression, we may see it in the esophagus and other portions of the gastrointestinal tract. It's then classed as a deep fungal infection.

When immune suppression is not severe, oral or vaginal cases can usually be treated topically, with lozenges for the mouth or creams for the vagina. Deep or stubborn infections can be suppressed with systemic, or whole-body, treatment; fluconazole is effective for this. Fluconazole prophylaxis has also been shown to protect against oral and esophageal candidiasis, as well as cryptococcal meningitis and superficial fungal infections, especially at CD4 nadirs of fifty cells or less. Daily fluconazole in this group is more costly, but also more effective, than clotrimazole (Mycelex) troches. Resistance can develop. Resistance to fluconazole is much more common with once-a-week regimens, however.

The use of sensitivity studies to determine drug resistance is controversial, but a correlation between sensitivity and clinical resistance has been shown in recent work.

The new oral formulations of itraconazole (Sporonox) and amphotericin B (Fungizone) can be highly effective in suppressing previously resistant oral or pharyngeal thrush. We have found less need for IV amphotericin suppression since these have been available.

Because I want to avoid resistance, I don't use the common one-week-a-month-for-six-months regimen of itraconazole or other antifungals for fungal nails. We may need these drugs down the road for survival. We recommend nail polish, learning to love fungal nails (they go well with the new chunky shoes), or both. For severe cases, a podiatrist can remove them.

Pneumocystis Carinii Pneumonia (PCP)

PCP was once the most common initial opportunistic infection in HIV. It generally appears at a CD4 count of about 200 or less, although it can present sooner. With the advent of universal PCP prophylaxis, we see it much less often.

We have several good medicines for treating PCP, and people usually do well. But the best defense is a good offense. Prophylaxis is recommended if the CD4 count reaches 200, if there has been prior PCP infection, if oral thrush is present, or if there has been a fever of unknown origin for more than two weeks. Some doctors initiate prophylaxis earlier, as 18 percent of cases of PCP are said to occur at CD4 counts above 200.

Trimethoprim-sulfamethoxazole, also called Bactrim or Septra, is the medicine of choice. Patients take one double-strength tablet daily; three-day-a-week regimens are associated with more breakthrough infections. Tolerance is better if you start low and build up. We use pediatric Bactrim suspension, starting with a quarter teaspoon a day and doubling the dose weekly until two teaspoons a day are reached. Then we switch to a double-strength tablet. Many of the people who initially develop a rash—even a severe one—will tolerate full-strength Bactrim with gradual rechallenge. And once up to dose, breakthroughs are rare.

Try hard to use this drug. It offers the best protection against PCP, and also blocks routine bacterial infections and toxoplasmosis. And stay on it even if your counts go up.

Other medicines used for treatment or prophylaxis include dapsone, atovaquone (Mepron), and IV pentamidine. Aerosolized pentamidine is no longer recommended.

Toxoplasmosis ("Toxo")

This is another infection that was commonly seen in HIV before Bactrim prophylaxis. Toxoplasma gondi is a parasite that lives in the brain. Once CD4 cell counts fall to about 150, progression is possible. It presents as a change in brain function; the nature of that change depends on the site of infection within the brain.

Toxo is not only rare but also responds well to treatment.

Advanced-Stage HIV
(CD4 Nadir of 100 or Less)
•

There was a time when progression to a CD4 count of 100 was an ominous sign. It's a point at which many opportunistic infections — those that can be easily suppressed by a healthy immune system — have a chance to break through and emerge. It's largely because of our increasing sophistication, and in particular our use of prophylaxis, that people now do so well at counts of 100 and much less. Quality of life can often be good, even with counts down to zero. But we have to keep the doors locked and the lights on.

Here are the opportunistic infections to watch for at this stage.

Cryptococcal Meningitis ("Crypto")

Cryptococcus is another deep fungal infection. It generally presents as a neurologic infection, with headaches and changes in mental status. It can be treated, but once acquired it must be suppressed for life.

Prophylaxis is helpful, though costly, and has been discussed with candida, above. Treatment includes reducing excess intracranial pressure and using antifungals, typically amphotericin B (with or without flucytosine). High-dose fluconazole, or sometimes itraconazole, is used for suppression. Without suppression, relapse is common.

Cytomegalovirus (CMV)

This is another virus in the herpes family. It's present in virtually everyone. It's a true opportunistic infection, however, so we only see effects in immunosuppressed people.

CMV disease affects about 40 percent of people with advanced HIV disease, mostly below CD4 nadirs of 50. Highly active antiretroviral therapy, or HAART, has not been shown to reduce incidence. CMV presents most often as retinitis. Colitis is also common, and may be the cause of diarrhea, with negative stool studies. Neurologic infection, once a late and ominous finding, can now be detected earlier by PCR and responds to treatment. Treatment is followed by lifelong suppression therapy.

Eyes should be checked regularly to detect the development or progression of CMV retinitis.

Treatment options include:

- *Gancyclovir IV:* Good systemic activity; can cause low white count; resistance may develop.
- *Foscarnet IV:* Good systemic activity; potential for renal toxicity, generally easily managed. Also has anti-HIV activity. One study showed increased survival.
- *Gancyclovir eye implant or injection:* Excellent local activity but no effect on infection elsewhere. Immediate vision is blurry, and 10 percent develop eye inflammation or detached retinas.
- *Cidofavir IV:* Excellent, long-lasting activity, even against most gancyclovir-resistant strains. Dosage is weekly. Potential for severe, irreversible renal damage requires very careful use: cannot be used within two weeks of other drugs that stress renal function.
- *Combination gancyclovir and foscarnet IV:* Used for treatment failures, and as aggressive induction therapy.
- *Oral gancyclovir:* Less effective than IV, but may be good for suppression. Prophylaxis at CD4 counts less than 50 reduces cases by half. Clinical resistance appears rare.

Mycobacterium Avium Complex (MAC)

MAC is the most common systemic bacterial infection in people with HIV. As patients live longer, its incidence increases. It tends to appear at an average CD4 count of 50. Symptoms can include night sweats and fevers, enlargement of the liver and spleen, and abnormal liver tests. MAC infection is treated with a multiple-drug regimen.

Most doctors initiate prophylaxis at a CD4 count of 75; I'm a little old lady and I start at 100. Medicines used are azithromycin (Zithromax), clarithromycin (Biaxin), or rifabutin (Mycobutin). Clarithromycin requires some dose adjustment when used with protease inhibitors; rifabutin must not be used at all with some protease inhibitors.

Because azithromycin can be used with protease inhibitors, it has become the prophylaxis of choice. Once-a-week dosing of this drug (at 1,200 milligrams) doesn't seem to cause resistance.

Treatment requires two or three drugs, generally clarithromycin and ethambutol, with or without rifabutin.

Opportunistic Organisms That Cause Diarrhea

To discuss all the opportunistic infections that can cause diarrhea in AIDS would take another book. Two are of particular interest, though.

Cryptosporidium Parvum.   Infection with this organism is a particular risk for health care workers, day care kids and attendants, those who work with animals, and travelers, as well as the immunosuppressed. People who practice anal sex or oral-anal contact are also at high risk. It is estimated that 10 to 15 percent of people with HIV develop cryptosporidium. Drinking water is another common source that has generated much attention. See Appendix XI for tips on protection against water-borne infection.

In HIV-negative people, diarrhea and infection resolve. Eradication is much more difficult with immunosuppression.

Diagnosis is by stool tests for ova and parasites; cryptosporidium evaluation must be specifically requested. Treatment is difficult when counts are low. Paromomycin and azithromycin have been tried with some success. Other experimental drugs are in testing. Now that we have potent antiretroviral combinations, many cryptosporidial infections have resolved.

Microsporidium.   This is another persistent opportunistic pathogen. There are two main species: one appears to respond to albendazole, an investigational drug available for compassionate use, and one does not. Microsporidium is difficult to identify in stool samples unless the technician is highly skilled. Electron microscopy may be needed for diagnosis and differentiation of species.

Treatment may sometimes lead to resolution. When it doesn't, medications are needed to slow the diarrhea, and extra nutritional supplementation is required to prevent wasting. At present, the most effective treatment against microsporidiosis is aggressive antiretroviral therapy and living right.

Other Organisms That Cause Diarrhea.   The list of possible offenders is long, and will not be detailed here. But I want to emphasize again the importance of looking for a cause. Symptomatic and supportive care can help counteract the effects of wasting, but finding and treating the organism may resolve it.

Remember the basic premise of this book: CD4 counts can tell us what to watch for and what to suspect, and keeping your count up is important; but it's maintenance of lean body mass that will keep you alive and comfortable.

You'll find a recommended schedule for prophylaxis of opportunistic infections in Appendix VII.

JC Virus and Progressive Multifocal Leukoencephalopathy (PML)

JC virus is a slowly acting virus that is thought to reactivate with immune suppression, causing thought and motor changes by destroying the lining of cells in the brain. It is a rare illness and was considered incurable. Anecdotal reports of reversal and resolution with HAART, though, have given us hope for some with PML. Cidofavir and Ara-C have also been tried in isolated cases.

Keeping Well at Any Stage
•

We've talked about helping your immune system fight infections by diagnosing and treating them early and aggressively. There are a few other things you need to know as well.

The Virus Is the Primary Problem

HIV infection helps other infections to flourish, and vice versa. So one of the best ways you can keep from getting sick is to keep the virus sick. *Aggressive antiretroviral therapy helps suppress other infections.*

The Underlying Problems May Be Missed

Severe immune suppression reduces our ability to fight infection. Thus, when we begin to rebuild our immune systems, our bodies may recognize and react to invaders they were too weak to respond to before. MAC and CMV, for instance. are frequently diagnosed soon after we start a potent anti-HIV combination. It's not that we made ourselves sick; it's just that our bodies woke up, found a burglar in the bedroom, and started shooting.

If your CD4 count has been low, it's a good idea to screen for MAC and CMV as you start potent therapies.

Our Own Immune Responses Need Support

It takes a healthy body to mount an immune defense. Your white-blood-cell count, and especially your absolute neutrophil count, will help you and your doctor assess your ability to fight infection. Figure 14.1 shows you how to calculate this value.

Medicines and infections can lower this count. Filgrastim, or Neupogen, is a factor that stimulates your bone marrow to make more when you need it.

We used to think that an absolute neutrophil count of 700 was all you needed. But Mark Jacobson of San Francisco General Hospital has reported an exponential increase in serious secondary

---

FIGURE 14.1.
•
Calculating Absolute Neutrophil Count.

To find your absolute neutrophil count, look at the differential, a breakdown of your white cell count. Add together the poly-morphonucleocytes, or neutrophils, and the bands. Multiply your total white count by this number and divide by 100.

Example

Polys (or neutrophils)	44
Bands	+ 6
	50

White blood count 3,000

$$3{,}000 \times 50 = 150{,}000 \div 100 = 1{,}500$$

Absolute neutrophil count = 1,500

Greater than 1000? Yes
Safe level? Yes

---

infections and hospitalizations in people with HIV whose absolute neutrophil counts are 999 or less.

So you should keep an eye on your absolute neutrophil count. If it gets below 1,000, ask for treatment to get it back up. And watch it closely.

We Can't Forget TB and Pneumococcus

These infections put everyone, HIV-negative and HIV-positive alike, at risk. They can be deadly, and drug resistance is more and more common. Everyone with HIV should have a pneumovax as soon as possible after diagnosis. TB should be looked for annually with PPD and controls skin test (an anergy panel) or with an X ray if skin tests cause no reaction. Treatment should be aggressive, and attuned to drug interaction risks.

REFERENCES

Bartlett, J. G. *1996 Pocket Book of Infectious Disease Therapy.* Baltimore: Williams and Wilkins, 1996.

Benhamou, Y., and others. "Effects of lamivudine on replication of hepatitis B virus in HIV-infected men." *Annals of Internal Medicine,* 1996, *125*(9), 705–712.

Blackbourn, D. J., and others. "Infectious human herpesvirus 8 in a healthy North American blood donor." *Lancet,* 1997, *349,* 609–611.

Currier, J. "Recent advances in the prevention and treatment of mycobacterium avium complex disease." *Improving the Management of HIV Disease,* 1997, *4*(5), 15–18.

Fichtenbaum, C., and others. "Fluconazole resistant mucosal candidiasis in advanced HIV infection." Eleventh International Conference on AIDS, Vancouver, Canada, June 7–12, 1996.

Fischl, M. A., and others. "Clinical presentation and outcome of patients with HIV infection and tuberculosis caused by multiple drug-resistant bacilli." *Annals of Internal Medicine,* 1992, *117,* 257–259.

Framm, S. R., and Soave. "Agents of diarrhea: Management of the HIV-infected patient, Part II." *Medical Clinics of North America,* 1997, *81*(2), 427–447.

Haubricht, R. A., and Saag. "Management of HIV-associated fungal disease." *Improving the Management of HIV Disease,* 1997, *4*(5), 9–14.

Hoerr, R. "Colostrum based immunoglobulin as a natural biological agent." *Hyperalimentation: A Practical Approach,* Harvard Medical School Conference, 1994.

Jacobson, M. A. "Risk of hospitalization for serious bacterial infection (SBI) associated with neutropenia severity in patients with HIV." Eleventh International Conference on AIDS, Vancouver, Canada, June 7–12, 1996.

Jacobson, M. A., and others. "Failure of highly active antiretroviral therapy (HAART) to prevent CMV retinitis despite marked CD4 count increase." Fourth Conference on Retroviruses and Opportunistic Infections, January 22–26, 1997, Session 35, Abstract 353, p. 129.

Kaplan, J. E., and others. "USPHS/IDSA guidelines for the prevention of opportunistic infections in persons infected with human immunodeficiency virus: Introduction." *Clinical Infectious Diseases,* 1995, *21*(Supp.), S1–S11.

Lennette, E.T., and others. "Antibodies to human herpesvirus type 8 in the general population and in Kaposi's sarcoma patients." *Lancet,* 1996, *348*(9031), 858–861.

Lubeck, D. P., and others. "Quality of life and health service use among HIV-infected patients with chronic diarrhea." *Journal of Acquired Immune Deficiency Syndromes and Human Retrovirology,* 1993, *6,* 478–484.

MacGregor, R. R., and others. "Evidence of active cytomegalovirus infection in clinically stable HIV-infected individuals with CD4 lymphocyte counts below 100 microliters of blood: Features and risk of subsequent CMV retinitis." *Journal of Acquired Immune Deficiency Syndromes and Human Retrovirology,* 1995, *10,* 324–330.

Masur, H., and Public Service Task Force on Prophylaxis and Therapy for Mycobacterium Avium Complex. "Recommendations of prophylaxis and therapy for disseminated Mycobacterium avium complex disease in patients infected with the human immunodeficiency virus." *New England Journal of Medicine,* 1993, *329,* 898–904.

Mayer, K. H. "Epidemiology of HIV disease and associated opportunistic infections: Update 1996." In *HIV Treatment: New Options and New Hope* (pp. 24–30). Medford, Mass.: Tufts University, 1996.

Murphy, R. L. "Opportunistic infection prophylaxis." *Improving the Management of HIV Disease,* 1994, *2*(1), 1–2.

Nelson, M. R. "Foscarnet in the treatment of cytomegalovirus infection of the esophagus and colon in patients with the acquired immunodeficiency syndrome." *American Journal of Gastroenterology,* 1991, *86*(7), 876–881.

Northfelt, D. W., and others. "Anal neoplasia: Pathogenesis, diagnosis, and management." *Hematology/Oncology Clinics of North America,* 1996, *10*(5), 1177–1187.

Ocular Complications of AIDS Research Group. "Combination foscarnet and gancyclovir therapy vs. monotherapy for the treatment of relapsed cytomegalovirus retinitis in patients with AIDS." *Archives of Ophthalmology,* 1996, *114,* 23–33.

Palefsky, J. "Anal human papillomavirus infection and anal cancer in HIV-positive individuals: An emerging problem." *AIDS,* 1994, *8*(3), 283–295.

Para, M. F., and others. "ACTG 268 trial: Gradual initiation of trimethoprim/sulfamethoxazole as a primary prophylaxis for pneumocystis carinii pneumonia." Fourth Conference on Retroviruses and Opportunistic Infections, January 22–26, 1997, Abstract 2.

Powderly, W. G. "Recent advances in the management of cryptococcal meningitis in patients with AIDS." *Clinical Infectious Diseases,* 1996, *22*(S2), S119–S123.

Powderly, W. G., and others. "A randomized trial comparing fluconazole with clotrimazole troches for the prevention of fungal infections in patients with advanced human immunodeficiency virus." *New England Journal of Medicine,* 1995, *332*(11), 700–705.

Sanford, J.P., and others. *The Sanford Guide to Antimicrobial Therapy, 1996.* Dallas: Antimicrobial Therapy, Inc., 1997.

Sanford, J. P., and others. *The Sanford Guide to HIV/AIDS Therapy, 1996.* Dallas: Antimicrobial Therapy, Inc., 1997.

Smith, G. H. "Treatment of infections in the patient with acquired immunodeficiency syndrome." *Archives of Internal Medicine,* 1994, *154,* 949–973.

Spector, S. A., and others. "Oral gancyclovir for the prevention of cytomegalovirus disease in persons with AIDS." *New England Journal of Medicine,* 1996, *334,* 1491–1497.

CHAPTER 15

•

Special Problems

This chapter addresses specific symptoms that commonly arise in the course of HIV infection and interfere with our ability to nourish ourselves. We've addressed some of them in great detail already. But a brief and directed approach to their management can serve as a working model.

Problems Directly Related to Nutrition

•

Some of these problems have already been discussed in earlier chapters of this book. This chapter will offer further suggestions to help you work around them.

Anorexia

We've already said a great deal about anorexia in HIV—how it happens and how it affects our ability to maintain nutritional competence, in Chapters One and Two; how to assess it, in Chapter

Three; and how to fight it, in Chapters Six and Twelve. The amount of time we've spent addressing anorexia is a direct reflection of its importance.

Our most important task is to see it, accept the challenge it provides, and recognize that, in most cases, we can reduce its degree and its effects.

Anorexia has its roots in HIV itself. But it is the presence of a secondary process, beyond HIV, that greatly increases its effect. And it is the *absence* of other sources of joy and pleasure that reduces our will to overcome it. So the most important way to combat anorexia is to do *everything*—to address all aspects of fighting HIV, and of living a healthy and satisfying life, with the same careful attention.

Problems with Eating and Swallowing

In order to take in food, you have to be able to eat. Problems that interfere with the mechanical process of eating require special attention.

Mouth Sores or Ulcers. These develop from a variety of causes and can make the act of eating and swallowing painful. Treatment of the underlying cause is the most effective approach. Offenders to consider are fungal infections (like thrush), viral infections (especially herpes simplex; consider also CMV), and medications (DDC in particular). A gentle scraping of the spot for microscopic examination may show fungal forms; a viral culture may grow herpes viruses. If another cause isn't found, and you're on DDC, you and your doctor may need to consider a change of nucleoside analogues. If that's not possible, you may have to reduce the DDC dose. If mouth pain persists, however, we must also treat the symptoms.

Topical applications of soothing substances can often provide relief, permitting us to eat. We suggest triamcinolone 0.1 percent dental paste, applied by cotton swab directly to the painful spot about three times a day. Hurricane Spray, an aerosolized lidocaine product, can be used as needed for temporary numbing before eating or when pain is not controlled. We also use the swish-and-spit method with soothing liquids like Kaopectate or Mylanta. Swallowing one to two tablespoons of the first two, after swishing in the mouth, may help esophageal ulcer pain as well; Kaopectate will also firm up stools, and Mylanta may ease stomach pain. Another product, called Mouth Kote, is specifically designed for soothing the pain of mouth ulcers; it can also be found at pharmacies.

For severe pain, your doctor can prescribe viscous lidocaine, a topical anesthetic for the mouth and throat. Its effects are more complete and last longer.

Xerostomia.   Also called dry mouth, xerostomia responds to the same soothing measures described above. In addition, the pain of xerostomia can be avoided by frequent use of artificial saliva products. Oralube is one; your pharmacist may recommend others as well. Some patients prefer the feel of Mouth-Kote and use it in preference to artificial saliva.

Dental Disease.   The pain of deep tooth decay, dental abscesses, or gum disease can also impair eating. These conditions must be treated. Until these conditions resolve, however, pain medicine should be prescribed as needed.

If you no longer have teeth, a mechanical, soft diet is required. I urge you, though, to get false teeth made. Food will taste better, with greater variety and texture. You're likely to eat more.

Trouble Swallowing.   With severe weakness or neurologic dysfunction, the ability to swallow may be impaired. This can increase the risk of inadvertent aspiration, or passage of food into the lungs. Pneumonia can result.

When your swallowing capacity is impaired, it must be evaluated closely. This is done by speech or occupational therapists, who can then recommend a safe diet. Thick liquids are usually easier to swallow than thin ones. A product is available, called Thikit, to thicken liquids and make them safe to swallow. You can thus have your favorite tastes in a texture you can handle. The therapist who evaluates you can tell you where to purchase Thikit, if it's indicated.

Pureed foods, ground foods, or soft but intact foods, such as well-cooked stews, are sometimes recommended. Keeping the head of your bed elevated at about thirty degrees at all times can reduce the risk of aspiration.

Malabsorption

Malabsorption is integral to the process of wasting in HIV. We've discussed its causes, investigation, and treatment earlier in this book. This section addresses the symptoms, other than wasting, that can result from malabsorption.

The most frequent symptoms of malabsorption result from lactose intolerance and fat malabsorption in the large intestine. Pancreatic insufficiency can also cause discomfort.

Lactose Intolerance. As we saw earlier, alterations in the intestinal wall can cause a deficiency of lactase, an enzyme needed to break down milk sugars, even early in the course of HIV. The unabsorbed sugars remain in the gut. They provide food for bacteria naturally present in the gut, resulting in their overpopulation. As these bacteria digest the milk sugars you can't digest, they liberate gas. Bloating, cramping, and excess burping or passing wind are the primary manifestations; they tend to increase within an hour or two after eating milk products.

You can avoid this by avoiding those foods. Still, milk products offer good nutritional value other than lactose, and are often a source of comfort and pleasure.

One way to ameliorate these symptoms is to use special products made for the many other people with lactase deficiency. Sweet acidophilus milk has been treated with cultures of *Lactobacillus acidophilus*. These bacteria convert lactose to sugars your body can digest. Acidophilus milk, therefore, is 80 percent to 90 percent reduced in its lactose content, and is well tolerated by most people who are lactase deficient.

Another approach is to use Lactaid, milk treated with lactase enzyme. It's said that 80 percent of people with lactose intolerance will be able to tolerate this product. Lactaid milk can be purchased at health food stores, pharmacies, and some supermarkets. Lactaid tablets are also available.

Malabsorption of Fats. You'll notice the effects of fat malabsorption during periods of active secondary infection and late in the course of HIV. In particular, damage to the large intestine by organisms causing diarrhea impairs fat uptake. Again, undigested remnants in the gut allow for overgrowth of natural bacteria, extra gas, and a feeling of fullness or bloating. In addition, caloric value is wasted.

Keeping the fat content in your diet low will help your symptoms; since fats aren't digested well anyway, you won't lose net caloric value by such restriction. If you do need those calories, though, some fats are more easily absorbed than others. These are called medium-chain triglycerides, or MCTs. They are found naturally in palm kernel and coconut oils.

MCTs offer another advantage, too. They cannot be combined into larger fat molecules, so they are more likely to be used as fuel for instant energy.

MCTs are a component of medical foods designed specifically for people with fat malabsorption. If you're using medical foods as supplements, you may want to choose the ones that incorporate MCTs. Table 12.1 includes a list of representative medical food supplements to point you in the right direction.

In cases of severe malabsorption, there may be a role for more directed supplements. Lipisorb, for instance, which is not marketed publicly, contains a large proportion of MCTs (85 percent). This can be recommended by a dietician if need is shown. Studies at Harvard University's Deaconess Hospital in 1994 showed that Lipisorb significantly improved fat absorption, compared to a similar formula without MCTs, in patients with microsporidial or nonspecific diarrhea. Treatment with either supplement also reduced daily bowel movements by almost half.

As fatty acids are irritating to the gut, avoidance or careful choice of fat sources can help break the vicious cycle of injury, malabsorption, and increased transit time.

Pancreatic Insufficiency. This condition can result in indigestion. Pancreatic enzymes needed for efficient digestion may not be present when there is injury to the pancreas. In these cases, enzymes can be supplemented before meals.

Diarrhea

Diarrhea holds a critical position in the spectrum of HIV care. It is commonly the first gastrointestinal symptom to appear. Estimates of its presence in the HIV population range from 30 to 90 percent.

The list of possible causes is broad and often hard to differentiate. Nonetheless, with rigorous evaluation, a cause can be determined in almost all cases; up to 10 percent of cases have multiple causes. And frequently, organisms that are easily eradicated or suppressed in HIV-negative healthy people can persist and cause chronic diarrhea in the presence of HIV.

Because it represents an assault on the very system that must absorb nutrients, infectious diarrhea poses a triple threat to maintenance of lean body mass. An injured gut wall cannot absorb well; an irritated gut moves nutrients through too fast for optimal absorption; and the presence of pervasive secondary infection activates the inflammatory response that leads to wasting, even in the absence of other stressors.

We'll focus on four aspects of diarrhea—prevention, evaluation and treatment, symptom control, and nutritional support.

Prevention. Diarrhea in the setting of advanced immunosuppression frequently results from organisms that can be controlled, or eradicated with treatment, with a more intact immune system. That's why, ideally, we want to know what you've got *before* it can hurt you—while you're still fully able to defeat it.

From the moment you know you are HIV-infected, you should look for the presence of infection in the gut. Even in the absence of symptoms, the search for gastrointestinal infestation should begin at once.

For any HIV patient who has ever practiced receptive anal intercourse, I send three separate stool samples, from different days, for examination for ova and parasites. I repeat these studies routinely once a year.

Prevention can also involve not exposing yourself to new infection; we've looked at that in Chapters Seven and Eight. Thoughtful attention to the risk of infection from drinking water or ice; careful attention to hygiene in the preparation of food; avoidance of unprotected anal sex, or contact between mouth and rectum; particular care about hand washing in the presence of others with diarrhea—these steps may help to protect or defend against infection that can cause great harm down the road.

Evaluation and Treatment. The evaluation of HIV-related diarrhea should be thorough. Frequently, it is caused by the presence of intestinal parasites called protozoa. These will be found on examination for ova and parasites ("stool for O and P"), as mentioned above. When sending these samples, your doctor must specifically request evaluation for cryptosporidium and microsporidium, as these require special techniques. Microsporidium, for example, can sometimes only be detected and identified with electron microscopy.

In addition, a stool sample for white cells and routine culture should be sent. People with HIV can get normal kinds of diarrhea, too. Stool should be studied for the presence of *Clostridium difficile* (C diff), which can flourish when normal gut bacteria are destroyed by antibiotics. If your CD4 cells are low, your doctor should also request evaluation for fungal and viral organisms. *Anything found should be treated with appropriate medicines.*

If nothing is found, a gastroenterologist can look inside with a soft flexible tube, called a colonoscope, and take biopsies. Cytomegalovirus (CMV) and mycobacterium (MAC, MTB, tuberculosis, and others) will be sought in this way. It's estimated that 30 percent of people living with AIDS have CMV disease in the intestine. Multiple biopsies, throughout the colon, may be needed to find it.

Fungal infection and herpes should also be considered. Also, your gastroenterologist will look for noninfectious causes of diarrhea, such as Kaposi's sarcoma.

Flexible sigmoidoscopy, an abbreviated look at the lower colon that can be done in the office, is likely to miss CMV, because of its tendency to infect the more remote segments.

A colonoscopy doesn't hurt; they give you pain and anxiety medicine, before and throughout the procedure. They won't knock you out completely, but you won't care what happens. I watched mine cheerfully from start to finish—reportedly with running commentary.

The evaluation and management of diarrhea in HIV have been the focus of close scrutiny and intense controversy. In 1990, a hotly debated paper recommended minimal evaluation and largely symptomatic treatment as the most "efficient" approach to the management of HIV-associated diarrhea. A rash of papers was published in rebuttal, showing the possibility of at least one detectable cause in 50 to 80 percent of all such patients; even those researchers who were not focused on the metabolic changes caused by secondary infection stressed the importance of knowing what people had, and trying to fix it, rather than masking the results with symptomatic treatment.

The original paper is often quoted, in the interest of "efficiency," by those whose primary concern is cost control in HIV management. But its conclusions are misleading. First, no attention was paid to clinical end points—measures of overall health, hospitalizations required, and length of life. There was also no consideration of diarrhea's effects on wasting. Even in terms of cost, no assessment was made of the long-term implications of limited evaluation.

Cost control is best achieved by the practice of early and thorough evaluation and care. In any given month, caring for healthier people costs less than caring for sick people. And costs saved by reducing length of life are unethical and unconscionable. In an era of managed care, where cost-effectiveness is often sought at the expense of excellence, it is important for everyone with HIV to know what is possible, what can and should be done, to evaluate and treat the causes of diarrhea.

Symptom Control. When a cause cannot be found or does not respond to treatment, we must find ways to change the result. Agents that slow down the gut, such as Lomotil and Imodium, are a good start. If they fail, tincture of opium may help. The use of medical foods has been shown to reduce the number of stools in chronic, HIV-associated diarrhea by about 50 percent. And one medical food, Optimune, may be particularly effective in this regard.

When diarrhea is chronic and severe, more aggressive methods may be necessary. Somatostatin-A, or Sandostatin, is a long-acting version of our body's own hormone for slowing gut movement. It must be given by injection, usually three times a day. If a patient is receiving TPN, or total parenteral nutrition, some doctors add it to the bag. Somatostatin-A is costly, and should be reserved for cases that don't respond to simpler measures. Its results can be dramatic, though. As a last-ditch effort, it has much to offer.

You must also maintain high fluid intake, as diarrhea wastes a lot of water. Because electrolytes—elements that must be present in your blood in precise amounts to maintain homeostasis—are selectively lost with diarrhea, Gatorade or other electrolyte-balanced sports drinks can make it easier to maintain their regulation. Fig-

FIGURE 15.1.
•
**Hydration Formula for Dehydration
Due to Diarrhea.**

Mix together:
  1 liter boiled or cryptosporidium-safe bottled water
  1 tablespoon sugar
  1 teaspoon salt

Flavor with:
  Frozen orange juice concentrate to taste, or
  any other nonalcoholic flavoring. (If this option is used,
    eat a banana for each two liters of fluid consumed.)

Drink as much as tolerated.

ure 15.1 offers a simple, inexpensive replacement approach for hydration in diarrhea, if cost is an issue.

Nutritional Support.   Diarrhea reflects injury to the gut wall, reducing its capacity to take in nutrients. It speeds up bowel contractions, increasing transit time and allowing briefer contact with the gut wall for absorption. It can be triggered by intake, causing people to limit or avoid eating. It is essential to evaluate a person with diarrhea of more than a few days' duration for wasting. Some of the studies reported above have shown the value of early supplementation with appropriate medical foods. The presence of documented wasting is grounds for such supplementation, but you can get a head start by demonstrating the process of wasting, rather than its effects.

Increasingly, aggressive early oral or enteral supplementation has been found to avoid the need for TPN. Where such supplementation is not successful, and where there is still an opportunity for good quality of life, TPN is appropriate and should be considered. This is discussed more fully in Chapter Twelve.

Even if you need TPN, it's still important to eat *something*. A gut not used will atrophy. Supplements containing some substances actually help the gut repair itself. Glutamine is one of these; it is a component of some medical foods.

Physical Problems
Indirectly Affecting Nutrition
•

Fever and pain, both symptoms of physical illness, also have an impact on nutritional status.

Fever

Fever is almost always accompanied by anorexia. The inflammatory factors that alter temperature control are the same ones that impair appetite. These are also the factors that disturb our metabolic regulation, changing its pathways and causing us to use what we eat less efficiently. So a fever is always a sign that something important is happening. It should never be disregarded. Also, fever makes you feel sick. Under such circumstances exercise and play are no more appealing than food. So fever needs to be treated for comfort.

We've talked at length, in Chapter Fourteen, about seeking out and eliminating the infections that lead to fever. But since the cytokines that cause fever promote wasting, it makes sense to also treat the fever itself. Many of the medicines we use for this purpose act by blocking those cytokines and their actions.

Fever can be attacked either centrally, by changing the brain's response to inflammation, or peripherally, by reducing the inflammation itself. Acetaminophen, or Tylenol, is an example of a drug that acts centrally; aspirin, ibuprofen, and certain other compounds typify peripherally acting drugs. These latter medicines are part of a large class of nonsteroidal anti-inflammatory drugs, or NSAIDs, which have a long history of use, chiefly for the treatment of arthritis or muscle inflammation.

Early animal research explored the effects of NSAIDs on cytokine levels and wasting. Mice were given an infusion of IL-2, an important cytokine in wasting. Food intake dropped dramatically with administration. Giving the mice ibuprofen blocked this effect; giving them acetaminophen did not.

The point of this research was to learn where this cytokine action takes place—either centrally, by changing brain response, or peripherally, by contributing to inflammation.

This is how we learned that cytokine effects occur throughout the body. But it raises another question: if NSAIDs reduce the inflammatory response associated with anorexia and wasting, might they have a role in helping to block wasting?

I've been waiting since 1991 to see some studies on this concept, but have found none so far. So at this point there's no firm scientific basis for recommending chronic use of ibuprofen or aspirin—particularly since constant use can cause stomach upset. Clearly, though, there must be some benefit to using them during periods of cytokine activation, as evidenced by fever. If ibuprofen restores appetite in mice with high cytokine levels, it may do the same thing for people.

So a fever should be treated to make you feel better. And if you can tolerate NSAIDS, it should ideally be treated not with acetaminophen, but with aspirin, ibuprofen, or another drug in the same class. In addition, new data on low levels of intracellular glutathione in people with HIV make the use of acetaminophen less attractive, as it also reduces intracellular glutathione concentrations.

My patients generally find ibuprofen gentler on their stomach than aspirin, and take one or two 200-milligram pills, with food, every eight hours when their temperature's up. It's available over the counter as Advil or as a generic drug (the same drug, but made by a different company and sold under a different brand name). If fevers are high, your doctor may want to prescribe a higher dose. Acetaminophen and ibuprofen can be taken together, if ibuprofen alone isn't enough.

If you have a history of ulcers or gastritis, you should not take ibuprofen or aspirin without your doctor's approval. You should not take ibuprofen or *any* NSAID if you've had a true allergic reaction to aspirin. If you're not sure, ask your doctor. Check with your doctor before taking acetaminophen, also, if there's a problem with your liver.

A cool, damp washcloth can be placed on your forehead, or under your armpits, to help make a fever less distressing. Very high fevers can also be helped by immersing yourself in a tepid, or barely lukewarm, bath. Don't use cold water for this, because it may cause chilling; a temperature below your own is good enough.

Fevers can also cause dehydration, so be sure to drink enough liquids. Avoid overexertion and abrupt climate changes. And especially avoid chilling. Wear your rubbers in the rain and a hat in the cold. Your mother was right about that.

Abdominal Pain

As with fever, it's important to look for the cause of abdominal pain. Paying close attention to your symptoms will help your doctor narrow down the possibilities and respond more effectively. Here are some questions to ask yourself, before your appointment:

- *Where's the pain?* High up, just below the rib cage? In the middle, or to one side? Down low above the groin? Try to point to the spot that feels the worst.
- *How did it start?* Did it come on gradually, over days or weeks, or abruptly? Is it getting progressively worse?
- *What does it feel like?* Is it constant or spasmodic? Sharp or dull, burning or aching? Does it feel as though it's close to the surface, or down deep?
- *When does it come?* After eating, or after a period of not eating? After eating specific foods—fatty foods or highly spiced ones or milk products? After a big meal? After you lie down? During or after diarrhea? How long does it last?
- *What symptoms are associated with it?* Is there gas or bloating? Fever? Diarrhea or constipation? Nausea? Pain somewhere else too?
- *What makes it worse?* Does it change when you move or change position?
- *What makes it better?* You'll find that your body makes adjustments, in the way you move, eat, or even breathe, to relieve it. What are these adjustments? Do you self-medicate with over-the-counter remedies? Which ones? Do they help?

If you pay close attention, you'll find you're already doing things to make it better; other things you can do will occur to you based on your observations. And the information you bring to your doctor will help pin down the cause.

Often pain relieved by eating, especially when it is high in the abdomen or under the rib cage, will respond to drugs called H2 blockers, which reduce the acid content of your stomach juices. Avoiding eating before going to bed may help, too. Not using cigarettes and alcohol is also recommended.

Pain that comes after eating fatty foods may suggest fat malabsorption, gall bladder inflammation, or other processes your doctor will consider. You can help by avoiding those foods.

Crampy abdominal pain may respond to antispasmodics, like Donnatal. Ask your doctor if these may be helpful.

Pain that results from pressure when the liver or spleen are enlarged can be reduced or avoided by eating several small meals.

Other Pain

Pain can accompany many of the conditions encountered in people living with HIV. More than a quarter of asymptomatic people report pain; more than half of those hospitalized for HIV-related causes, and four-fifths of those with an AIDS diagnosis, require treatment for pain. The impact is particularly noticeable on our emotional state: new or severe pain is frightening, and chronic pain exhausting. If we are to give our best efforts to getting or staying well, we need to address this distraction.

Studies show that pain is adequately controlled in only about 60 percent of cancer patients. That's bad enough; but William Breitbart estimates that pain control is satisfactory in only about 15 percent of people who live with HIV.

Pain control is most likely to fall apart in periods of transition—from home to hospital, or vice versa; when changing doctors or health care systems; when traveling.

The medical management of pain is best accomplished when it respects every complaint from every patient, seeks and treats the underlying cause, treats adequately, and addresses emotional as well as physical pain and distress. And the most important thing a doctor or caregiver can do to address pain is to ask if it's there. If we're not assessing it, we miss untreated pain, with its multiple direct and indirect costs.

Here are some helpful hints for controlling pain:

- *Treat early.* Pain is easier to suppress than to overcome. Take steps to block it when it first appears.
- *Treat consistently.* Don't wait for recurrence of pain to take the next pill. A regular schedule of pain control will require less medication and provide greater relief.
- *Treat appropriately.* Start with nonopioid (nonnarcotic) drugs such as aspirin or ibuprofen. If your stomach can't tolerate these medicines, acetaminophen is appropriate; consider NAC also, if you're taking acetaminophen. Use them consistently; if they don't work, consider with your doctor a change to opioids. Start with a weak one, progressing to stronger drugs only as needed. But *do* progress if needed. Start with a short-acting drug, while you assess its effects and your response. When relief stabilizes, or when pain breaks through repeatedly, consider long-acting forms. Sustained-release morphine products can avoid pain escalation, or the excessive attention to symptoms that can result from the need to rely exclusively or heavily on short-acting narcotics for treatment or breakthrough. I also like to use a fentanyl, or Duragesic, patch. It's initially placed on the body every three days, providing for sustained release through the skin. This gives us a stable level of pain control without focusing attention on achieving that control. People can concentrate on life again, taking extra medicine only if or when pain breaks through. My patients report they are less drowsy, and more involved in living their lives, with this approach.
- *Treat specifically.* Treat direct pain, the pain of tissue damage, by addressing its cause. Fight infections; reduce inflammation when there is swelling or injury. NSAIDs are especially helpful here. Use creams, where indicated, to heal or relieve skin conditions. Treat neuropathic pain, the pain of nerve damage, with agents that quiet nerves, like amitriptyline (Elavil), or agents that numb them, like lidocaine and mexiletine.
- *Treat holistically.* There is more relief available than that from pills alone. Massage can do wonders for musculo-

skeletal pain. Exercise, *when it doesn't increase symptoms,* releases your own natural opioids. Cuddling does, too. Eating may help a migraine. A regular program of meditation can increase your pain threshold. Hot baths relieve muscle pain and abdominal cramping. And sleep can be especially restorative.

- *Treat sturdily.* Try not to give in to despair. Acceptance is hard, sometimes; but if you refuse to be a victim of your pain, it will interfere less in your life.

Doctors are sometimes afraid to prescribe habit-forming drugs to those who have a history of drug abuse. And it is better to avoid them, *if pain can still be adequately controlled.* But if not, relieving pain is more important. A prior or current history of opiate use may require a higher dose now, for pain control. And control of pain is the greater priority.

Emotional and Cognitive Disturbance
•

The suffering of depression and anxiety directly affects appetite; we have talked about that already in Chapter Seven. So does confusion, which interferes with our ability to obtain and prepare food.

Depression

There's a lot to be unhappy about if you have HIV. It's hard to face your own vulnerability. Young people, especially, are not prepared for this. Money is frequently an issue, at a time you need it most. Old sources of pleasure and entertainment must often be avoided to protect your health. Old sources of validation—success in work, pride in physique, and others—may be lacking. Gay people often face prejudice from others around them; intravenous drug users may face even more. Pain and other symptoms can wear you down as well.

Physical problems affect how we feel. But just as our body can act on our moods, our moods also act on our body. The result can be a vicious cycle, a downward spiral into clinical depression. One effect of this depression is a weakened immune system, with lowered resistance to attack. Another may be immobilization—entrapment in our misery, without the tools to dig ourselves out.

Our body regulates emotions through the use of chemicals. Among these are neurotransmitters, chemicals used by brain cells to talk to one another. Just as pain is our body's way of telling us we're in danger, sorrow is a survival signal too. It is neurologically directed and chemically transmitted to alert us to conditions we should avoid.

The trouble is, it's not a perfect system. It's soft-wired when we are children, so early experiences are formative. Neurologic pathways formed in childhood become neurologic highways of the future—wider, deeper, more easily traveled, even when they take us somewhere we don't want to go.

Those things that trigger hidden memories of early experiences engender an intense response, and we often don't understand why in a way that allows us to change it.

So our emotions, as adults, are often not proportional to the events that trigger them. And because our neural pathways are more or less hard-wired by now, we can have feelings that are not appropriate to the events that cause them. When we were children we didn't reason analytically. We may do so now, but our emotions often follow their old tracks.

So often, the first thing to do is to remember that what we feel is real, *but it may not be true.* We have every right to our emotions and should not be apologetic for them. But the perception of our circumstances, colored by those emotions, may be inaccurate.

Another task can be to bring those hidden maps to light, so we know when we're taking a wrong turn and can choose to redirect our course.

Contrary to popular opinion, brain cells can rebuild connections; pathways of response can be changed; amounts of neurotransmitters, and the receptors that recognize them, are in constant flux. There is real value to bringing old experience to light, where you can evaluate it with the analytical skills you've built by now. There's also value to be gained from confirming your experience in the eyes of others.

So there are several ways we can address depression, breaking a cycle that could otherwise entrap us.

Know When You're Depressed. Often, we're so cut off from our emotions that we don't even know we're sad. We just feel tired. Or we hurt all over. Or our appetite is gone. We may sleep poorly, or too much. We may lose interest in things that used to please us. We may stop seeing friends or family. Eventually, we may just stay in bed, not even bathing, getting dressed, or going out.

Any of these changes should alert you to look hard at your feelings and consider the possibility of depression.

Get Help. It doesn't even matter much where you start—*as long as you do start.* If you've really slowed down, that first step may be a hard one. Talk to your doctor or to friends. See if they share your concern. Ask them to help you find more specific help.

Try a Support Group. Studies of women with breast cancer have shown a significant survival advantage—a longer life—when people meet regularly with others who face the same fight. For you, the practical benefits are obvious: someone else may have a better remedy for mouth sores or know where to get cheaper vitamins. Others will have tackled the maze of social service supports and can help you chart your own way to money, better food and housing, household help. Apart from the practical benefits, you'll find you're not alone: others share the feelings you're ashamed of, and they may not feel ashamed; others have surmounted what seems to you insurmountable. You'll even find that you help them—your practical experiences in dealing with HIV can be shared too, saving time and effort for all of you.

When we meet in groups together, we see the extraordinary power of the human spirit and its incredible will to survive. We find the humor hidden in our pain and use it to sustain us. Together, we are each much stronger.

Even strangers won't be strangers if they share your problems and concerns.

Seek Counseling. Even where there's no money, counseling is often available for people living with HIV. The Ryan White Act has allocated funds to serve the needs of people with HIV infection. These funds are available to AIDS service organizations and other nonprofit agencies. In many cases they are used to provide counseling. Many health care providers who fight HIV privately will also adjust their fees on a sliding scale, tailoring the costs of care or counseling to the income of people with HIV.

If you can get counseling, you'll be able to address, safely, those issues that are too painful to look at alone. You'll be able to grieve when you need to, and not be overwhelmed. You'll seek out your own values and see them reinforced. You may start to recognize unproductive sorrow and reject it. You'll begin to see and value your own heroism.

We pay a high price for keeping our feelings suppressed. The relief that comes from letting them go can be immeasurable. It can free up new energy for improving our comfort and pleasure.

Consider Medications. The feelings we have, triggered along familiar pathways formed by old experience, are often inappropriate to our survival now—and are often incorrect.

Our body's preprogrammed responses are carried out by the use of chemical messengers. People self-medicate for pain, using alcohol or drugs to alter the effects of those messengers. Those are imprecise treatments, though—dirty drugs, as I call them—and their use carries with it a high price.

We now have cleaner drugs—medicines that act precisely on our neurochemical responses and hence improve their actions. The best among them don't replace the chemicals we're low on; rather, they improve our brain's efficiency at using what we have.

These drugs are called antidepressants. The very name scares many people off. But if you understand that they simply give your brain cells a little longer to use each molecule in your own store of natural chemicals, they won't sound so dangerous. And they have other beneficial effects, too. Those that improve the action of serotonin or norepinephrine, for instance, may also reduce the experience of headache or other pain. We use them to protect against migraine, or to reduce the symptoms of peripheral neuropathy.

Antidepressants won't take your problems away, I promise you. You'll still be sad when you should be. But they can keep you from sliding into the destructive downward spiral that characterizes clinical depression. You'll still have your problems; but you'll have more strength to address them.

I tend to recommend selective serotonin reuptake inhibitors, or SSRIs, for people with HIV. In particular, I like the newer ones. They last only a short time in the body, and can be stopped quickly if need be. There's less danger of overdose. I use paroxetine, or Paxil, which can sometimes make you sleepy, for people with insomnia. For others I recommend sertraline, or Zoloft, which has the least chance of drug interactions. Prozac, or fluoxetine, stays in the body a long time, so I try to avoid its use in HIV. It's very important to use these drugs with respect for your other medications; protease inhibitors in particular may raise their levels and delay their clearance.

There are other classes of antidepressants that may be helpful, too. Welbutryn is low in side effects, but *must not be taken with ritonavir, which greatly increases its levels.* Other protease inhibitors may also raise its levels, although to a lesser extent. Other new antidepressants include nefazodone (Serzone) and venlafaxine (Effexor).

When prescribing these or other drugs, your doctor should always check with her or his pharmacy adviser on drug interactions that might result, given your current drug regimen. You should do this too.

If patients have peripheral neuropathy, amitriptyline, or Elavil—or another drug of its class—is a good choice. Elavil is cheap, and it's indicated for treatment of neuropathic pain.

If depression is not severe, I start at half the recommended starting dose of each drug and raise it after two weeks. And I continue it, if tolerated, for at least six months. I want those new highways well paved.

Many of us who practice primary care are comfortable prescribing these medicines in cases of mild to moderate depression, referring more severely affected patients to psychiatrists. Others routinely seek the expert help of psychiatrists. Certainly, any suicidal patient should be so referred. If your doctor wants to refer you to a psychiatrist, that's fine. They work with these medicines more than we do, and can often tailor a regimen to closely suit your needs. In our office, we don't prescribe Welbutryn together with protease inhibitors without a psychiatric consult.

• • •

You don't have to buy the values or emotions that were instilled in you in your childhood. You may be right, even when you *think* you're wrong, to have these current feelings or desires. But you may need a little extra muscle to help you redirect. With the right help, you can build and strengthen your own hard-wiring, creating pathways of positive response that need not lead to pain.

Anxiety

Like depression, anxiety is common in people with HIV, for many of the same reasons. Support and counseling are equally important. Regular exercise can provide emotional, as well as physical, conditioning, reducing the symptoms of chronic anxiety.

I also tend to use medications for anxiety fairly often in people with HIV. We've seen studies that show that the immune system is temporarily affected by acute episodes of anxiety. We know that a body dealing with emotional stressors has less strength left to deal with physical ones. And we know that you don't have time to suffer.

The management of anxiety medication, though, should be in the hands of your doctor. Because diazepam, or Valium, and other drugs of its class are abusable drugs, people can buy them on the street. Because they are addictive, withdrawal can be deadly. Unintentional withdrawal when you can't eat, for instance, can kill you. In addition, careful dosing is needed. Too much can cause confusion and loss of balance—symptoms we associate with other serious problems in the setting of HIV. And many antianxiety drugs must not be used with some or all of the protease inhibitors, or may need dosage adjustment. Self-medication for anxiety in HIV can get you in a lot of trouble.

If you're anxious, don't be ashamed to ask your doctor if medication will help you. Properly managed, it can make a big difference. But don't use it lightly. And don't treat yourself.

Confusion

In most cases we care even more about maintaining the integrity of our mind than that of our body. And the specter of dementia—or HIV encephalopathy, as it's properly called—is ominous. So if we lose track of time or our thoughts, forget to eat or miss appointments, or can't keep up with medicines, it can be frightening.

In most cases, however, there's another explanation for confusion. Depression is a frequent cause and can be hard to differentiate from dementia. Delirium—a temporary disturbance of brain function due to illness, fever, or medications—is also common. Both of these problems resolve with treatment.

Medications may contribute to confusion in a person with HIV. In particular, the use of antianxiety medicines, drugs for peripheral neuropathy, and pain prescriptions should be considered as potential causes when confusion presents.

Infections and other disease in the brain and its linings should also be ruled out.

In those rare cases where the diagnosis of HIV encephalopathy is made, there still is room for hope. With the advent of zidovudine, we began to see a marked reduction in the incidence and progression of HIV encephalopathy. AZT penetrates the brain, blocking injury by suppressing the virus. Encephalopathy is less likely in people who take zidovudine. We now know that nevirapine (Viramune), DMP 266 (sustiva), and some nucleoside analogues (D4T, 3TC, and DDI) also penetrate the central nervous system and can be helpful in treatment or prevention of encephalopathy.

Elyse Singer of UCLA reports that education appears to help protect against impairment in dementia—but the best defense is a good offense. *Properly and aggressively treated HIV infection should block development of dementia.*

Risk factors for dementia include youth, old age, advanced disease, wasting, increased cytokine release, MAC infection, anemia, and cigarette smoking. Risks are increased by delay in diagnosis and treatment, limited education, and poverty affecting access to care. No surprises there.

When present, its effects often respond to high-dose zidovudine therapy. This is the one remaining set of circumstances where high-dose treatment—200 milligrams, five times a day—is indicated.

If you are experiencing confusion, *the critical step is to see your doctor early.* Depression can be treated; medications can be adjusted; a workup can be begun, if necessary, to evaluate the brain for other causes. If encephalopathy is present, zidovudine can be instituted or increased. If you truly can't take zidovudine, DDI has been shown to penetrate the brain as well. And unpublished studies suggest that D4T may do so also.

What If I Get Well?
•

Up until the last couple of years, getting well was hardly considered a problem. But with the revolution in HIV management, with better drugs, better understanding, more proof to force provision of proper care, and the increasing power of HIV advocacy, we've seen a drastic change. Hospices are shut down, hospitals underfilled. Viatical companies are dying like flies. (Don't you love it? You bet your life *and won!*) People all over the developed world have taken up their beds to walk.

The problem is, there isn't a guidebook for how to get well. What's to be done about work, after years of disability? Can we in fact support ourselves? How do we square ourselves with credit card companies and tax collectors? How do we reconcile our new health and natural aggressive drive with the spiritual values we had begun to live by? What about sex, and love? How strong a fabric of acceptance did we really weave with our families when we thought it was time to say good-bye? A whole generation of women and men who had made their peace with death must now face life again.

For those who were permanently damaged before the revolution, the return to health brings an even more basic challenge. How do I learn to walk again? To think again? To leave my parents, after I went home to die? What medicines must I now be withdrawn from? Where will I find the strength to walk and dress myself? How can I take back my life at the most elemental level?

I don't think we have solutions for this delicious problem yet, but we're trying to address them. Some of the approaches people are putting together are provocative and hopeful, such as the following:

- *Jumpstart!* This is an intensive ten-day rehabilitation effort aimed at those who have been weak, confused, in pain, or handicapped and want help to find their way back. This program includes a comprehensive physical examination and evaluation of HIV management; planning and initial supervision of an individualized rehabilitation program; movement and body-patterning assessment and treatment; evaluation of neurological, cognitive, and emotional status, with treatment initiation as needed; a comprehensive nutritional assessment; and counseling to help set goals for a new life, in accordance with each participant's values. After completion, members of the Jumpstart! faculty will be available to work with participants' own local doctors, therapists, and rehabilitation specialists, with direct follow-up in San

Francisco if needed. Contact: Paul Nemrow, M.D., Director, Jumpstart! 415–750–5762.

- *The Lazarus Program.* In this project, people meet in small groups to explore their emotional and spiritual response to coming back to life from HIV, and to find a spiritual context within which to live their new life. We currently seek funding for this project from multidenominational religious sources. Contact: Jeremy Hollinger, Lazarus Program Coordinator, Andrew Ziegler Foundation, 415–566–0130.

- *PLUS-II.* This is described by its creator, Alfredo Armendiarez, as "spring training camp for activists." An outgrowth of the popular PLUS seminars, funded through the National Task Force on AIDS Prevention, it expands on the "HIV 101" holistic education and intense emotional bonding of that weekend training session, to offer those recovering from HIV a way to give back to their community. The original PLUS seminar will go on the road to other communities when requested, as well. Contact: Alfredo Armendiarez, Director, PLUS Seminars, 415–356–8100, ext. 129.

We at the Andrew Ziegler Foundation would love to learn about other innovations and programs that address coming back to life from HIV. Write us at:

The Andrew Ziegler Foundation
2350 Irving Street
San Francisco, CA 94122

• • •

By focusing your attention on those aspects of HIV infection that manifest in your body, you can find ways to change them. An individualized approach targeting the problems that affect you will greatly improve your care.

REFERENCES

Bowers, M. "Diarrhea in AIDS." *Bulletin of Experimental Treatments for AIDS*, June 1997.

Breitbart, W. "Beyond the AHCPR cancer pain guidelines: Management of pain in AIDS." *Pain Management Refined: New Approaches.* 1997 Program Development Meeting, Santa Monica, Calif., March 14–16, 1997.

Breitbart, W., and Lefkowitz. "Pain management in AIDS: BETA Live transcript." *Bulletin of Experimental Treatments for AIDS,* June 1995, pp. 68–77.

Cello, J. P., and others. "Effect of octreotide on refractory AIDS-associated diarrhea. A prospective, multicenter clinical trial." *Annals of Internal Medicine,* 1991, *115*(9), 705–710.

Connolly, G. M., and others. "Non-cryptosporidial diarrhoea in human immunodeficiency virus (HIV) infected patients." *Gut,* 1989, *30,* 195–200.

Connolly, G. M., and others. "Investigation of seemingly pathogen-negative diarrhoea in patients infected with HIV-1." *Gut,* 1990, *31,* 886–889.

Eeftinck Schattenkerk, J. K., and others. "Clinical significance of small-intestinal microsporidiosis in HIV-1-infected individuals." *Lancet,* 1991, *338*(8762), 323.

Framm, S. R., and Soave. "Agents of diarrhea: Management of the HIV-infected patient, Part II." *Medical Clinics of North America,* 1997, *81*(2), 427–447.

Greenson, J. K., and others. "AIDS enteropathy: Occult enteric infections and duodenal mucosal alterations in chronic diarrhea." *Annals of Internal Medicine,* 1991, *114,* 366–372.

Greenspan, D., and others. "Association between oral lesions and smoking in a clinic population." *International Conference on AIDS,* 1992, *8*(2), B147.

Grossman, I., and others. "Blastocystis hominis in hospital employees." *American Journal of Gastroenterology,* 1992, *87*(6), 729–732.

Gunzler, V. "Thalidomide in human immunodeficiency virus (HIV) patients." *Drug Safety,* 1992, *7*(2), 116–134.

Hecht, F. M. "Diarrhea and AIDS." *Annals of Internal Medicine,* 1990, *113*(10), 804–805.

Kaljot, K. T., and others. "Prevalence of acute enteric viral pathogens in acquired immunodeficiency syndrome patients with diarrhea." *Gastroenterology,* 1989, *97,* 1031–1032.

Kantor, T. G. (ed.). "Evolving trends in the management of chronic pain." *American Journal of Medicine,* 1996, *101*(1A), 1S–62S.

Kotler, D. P., and others. "Small intestinal injury and parasitic diseases in AIDS." *Annals of Internal Medicine,* 1990, *11,* 444–449.

Miaskowski, C. A. "Beyond the AHCPR guidelines: Home care issues." Pain Management Refined: New Approaches. 1997 Program Development Meeting, Santa Monica, Calif., March 14–16, 1997.

Muzyka, B. C., and Glick. "Major aphthous ulcers in patients with HIV disease." *Oral Surgery, Oral Medicine and Oral Pathology,* 1994, 77(2), 116–120.

Passik, S. D. "Transdermal fentanyl in HIV/AIDS substance abusers." Pain Management Refined: New Approaches. 1997 Program Development Meeting, Santa Monica, Calif., March 14–16, 1997.

Payne, R. "Beyond the AHCPR guidelines: 1994 to 1997, What's Next?" Pain Management Refined: New Approaches. 1997 Program Development Meeting, Santa Monica, Calif., March 14–16, 1997.

Power, C., and others. "HIV dementia scale: A rapid screening test." *Journal of Acquired Immune Deficiency Syndromes and Human Retrovirology,* 1995, 8(3), 273–278.

Silverman Jr., S., and others. "Prednisone management of HIV-associated recurrent oral ulcerations." *International Conference on AIDS,* 1992, 8(2), B148.

Simon, D., and others. "Treatment options for AIDS-related esophageal and diarrheal disorders." *American Journal of Gastroenterology,* 1992, 87(3), 274–279.

Singer, E. "Central nervous system disease." Paper presented at National Conference on Women and HIV, Pasadena, Calif., May 4–7, 1997, Session 112.

Smith, P. D. "Intestinal infections in patients with the acquired immunodeficiency syndrome (AIDS)." *Annals of Internal Medicine,* 1988, *108,* 328–333.

CHAPTER 16

•

Joining Studies

Hiv is more complex and pervasive than we ever dreamed possible when it first appeared. I suspect we'll be surprised again a few times at the extent of its impact on our civilization. But every year, we've seen our understanding of its life cycle and behavior grow. Every year we learn to fight it more effectively.

As researchers in laboratories work to understand the nature of HIV from a molecular or genetic standpoint, doctors in the trenches work to fight it. Some of the best of them are also researchers; every time we find something that might work, we need to test our hypotheses on people.

Those tests, when they prove beneficial and safe, result in new drug approvals, or in changes in the way the medical community understands and responds to HIV.

Traditionally, the process of new-drug approval by the Food and Drug Administration (FDA) has been agonizingly slow. We often watched a drug's performance for years in other countries before we could use it here. But because of the strong voices of AIDS advocates, that process has speeded up. A drug that shows promise can be placed on a fast track for approval, sometimes making it to market within two or three years of its first tests in humans.

We don't have time to wait with HIV. Saving years of waiting has prolonged many lives. So our treatment of this illness reinvents itself, over and over, every year.

If you're working with a doctor who keeps abreast of changes, your care is already immeasurably better than it was, for instance, in 1996. But even state-of-the-art AIDS treatment lags behind the newest developments from studies.

Joining trials to test new drugs or treatment protocols propels your care into the future. The results aren't certain; but it offers you a chance to get twenty-first-century care in the twentieth century. It's a hard gamble to pass up, if you're committed to the best.

Studies are often not restricted to a given area. Community trials, linked together for pooling of data, make new approaches available to people all over the country. What it takes is to seek them out, to understand the risks and benefits, and to choose carefully the trial that's best for you.

Types of Trials
•

After a new drug has shown potential activity in the laboratory setting, it's tested on animals for safety. It then goes to human trials. These trials are performed in phases.

Phase I Trials

These are trials to assess the safety of a drug in humans and determine the appropriate dosage range. Their advantage lies in the early access they offer to the newest treatments. They also pose the greatest risks. A medicine may have unexpected toxicity or side effects that were not seen prior to testing in humans. Known or unknown toxicities may present or escalate at higher doses. Lower doses may not be effective.

Data gathered from a Phase I trial will be used to evaluate the safety of a drug and its optimal dose—the dose that is expected to offer the least toxicity for the most effect.

Phase II Trials

Once we've determined, in a successful Phase I trial, that a drug is safe, we begin a Phase II trial to determine if it works. These trials enroll more people and are more likely to be widely offered at sites around the country. Subjects may be assigned to an active-drug arm of the trial or to a placebo arm. Those in the placebo arm will receive an inactive substitute. If the study is "blinded," subjects won't know which one they're getting. If it's "double-blinded," their doctors won't either.

Because people join these drug studies for benefit, arrangements are generally made to provide active drug to all participants after the period of study is complete, or at another given end point. This is called an intent-to-treat design. If early data are spectacular, the trial may be halted or changed to permit all participants to be treated while awaiting drug approval.

Some Phase II trials use currently approved types of therapy in one arm of the study, instead of placebo. The new, experimental treatment will make up the other arm. Again, people won't know what they're getting.

Another approach may be to do a crossover trial, treating you with one treatment for a period and then switching you over to the other—comparing you to yourself, so to speak.

People who take part in Phase II trials often receive free drugs for a period of time after the study has ended.

During the period of testing in a Phase II trial, there may also be parallel-track testing, which makes the drug available to those who don't qualify for the formal trial. The compound may also be available under a compassionate-use protocol for people who have failed all currently approved methods of treatment.

If a drug is successful in Phase II trials, the FDA will consider its rapid, tentative approval, so that all people can have access to treatment while the Phase III trials go forward.

Phase III Trials

These are large studies, conducted all around the country, monitoring and quantifying response to treatment and answering questions left unanswered in the Phase II trials before approval. They provide us with information at the level that used to be required before a drug could be released.

Choosing a Trial

Many studies are available, in various phases. Some look at new drugs, as we've discussed above. Others compare new treatments to those already in use, seeking to improve our skills with the tools we already have. Others compare new approaches—the use of new antiretroviral combinations, for example, or the effects of acupuncture on peripheral neuropathy. There are studies addressing Kaposi's sarcoma, or pneumocystis prophylaxis, or the symptomatic treatment of diarrhea. There are very exciting studies exploring the treatment of wasting and the maintenance of nutritional competence. Now that the urgency of opposing HIV-related wasting has become common knowledge, we see an exponential increase in nutritionally related research.

Because trials are designed to assess results, there's not room for too many other variables; therefore, joining a trial may exclude you from another treatment. The manifestations of HIV in your individual case will help you determine what's most important.

You can't choose frivolously. If your antiretroviral recipe is working, for instance, you don't want to give it up for an unproven treatment—even a treatment that's unproven only in you. If you've arrested CMV retinitis with one drug, you shouldn't risk your vision on a new approach. The best way to use trials, then, is to start with the things that aren't working for you, the parts of your illness that don't respond to current conventional treatment, and try to find new ways to treat them.

You also need to look at what a trial will cost you. A trial with a placebo arm, for instance, may leave you less treated for a problem than you are right now. Risking placement in the placebo arm of a trial only becomes worthwhile when nothing else works anyway.

Be sure to consider the side-effect profile of any new drug offered for trial, and what those effects mean for you. If your white cell count is low already, for instance, you'll want to think twice about trying a drug that might lower it still further.

If your care is working, you need to find trials that enhance it, either by increasing your options for fighting the virus itself or by protecting against future assaults. Remember, more may be better than less; early may be better than late; adding may be better than switching.

So the best trial for you is a trial that

- Addresses a problem you can't otherwise fix
- Does not take from you any protection that you already have
- Stresses your body only in ways it can handle
- Increases your preparedness for the future
- Propels your care into the future

Talk to your doctor about the trials that interest you, or ask her or him to review the options with you. You will need to coordinate any treatment received in a study with the treatment your doctor provides.

Access to Trials

•

There are so many treatment approaches under study that it's hard to keep up with them all. Even if you stay up to date with the literature or with activist sources of information, you need to plug in to the places that offer the treatments you want.

There are several sources to point you in the right direction. Some of them are national, others regional.

National Directories

The National Clinical Trials Database keeps a record of all open studies for HIV care in the country. You can access this by computer yourself (see Figure 19.1). There are other sources of this information that are easily accessible by phone. They can help you find the study you want and put you in touch with the people you need to talk to in order to enroll.

- AIDS Clinical Trials Information Service
  800-TRIALS-A
  English and Spanish; offers customized searches of
  the National Clinical Trials Database

- American Foundation for AIDS Research
  212–682–7440
- Project Inform Hotline
  800–822–7422
- People With AIDS Coalition of New York Hotline
  800–828–3280

Regional Directories

- *Connecticut, New York, New Jersey, and Philadelphia*
  AIDS Treatment Data Network
  212–260–8868
- *Gulf Coast*
  Tulane University, Infectious Disease Section
  504–584–3605
- *Missouri*
  AIDS Project of the Ozarks
  800–743–5767
  417–881–1900
- *New England*
  Community Research Initiative
  617–566–4004
- *New York*
  AIDS Institute Experimental Treatment Infoline
  212–239–5523 (outside New York State)
  800-MEDS-4HIV (within New York State)
- *Northern California*
  Community Consortium
  415–476–9554
- *Northern Georgia and Alabama*
  AIDS Survival Project
  404–874–7926
- *Pacific Northwest*
  Seattle Treatment Educational Program (STEP)
  206–329–4857
- *Wisconsin*
  Directory of Wisconsin HIV/AIDS Clinical Trials
  800–359–9272
  414–225–1600

- *Canada*
    Canadian HIV Trial Network
    604–631–5327

Contacting a national or regional directory of trials will help you add the best and newest treatments to your regimen and maximize your options for health. And when you do this for yourself, the information you and others provide will help others in the future.

CHAPTER 17

•

Women and HIV

In 1996, more than three million people in the world became infected with HIV; half of them were women.

In the United States, the first six months of 1996 showed a 15 percent decrease in death rates for men. Death rates for women, however, increased by 3 percent.

Women currently represent 42 percent of people living with HIV and AIDS. In Zimbabwe and Botswana, 40 percent of the women presenting for pregnancy care are HIV-infected.

And every twenty seconds, a woman in the world is infected with HIV. That's three women a minute. Four thousand women every day. So the first lesson we must learn is that in this crucial aspect we are not different; women are not immune to HIV infection.

Most of these women are infected by injection drug use, or by sex with an infected male partner. Many of those infected sexually have had only one partner in their lifetime. Many are unaware of the risks to which that partner has exposed them. Martina Clark of the United Nations, herself infected, calls this "the monogamous housewife syndrome." It's possible to contract this disease while living a life even Jesse Helms would approve of.

There are many ways in which women and men infected with HIV do not differ. We seem to respond equally to antiretroviral treatment. Our prognosis, the prediction of how well we will do given the same care, tends to be about the same. How we get there, however, can be different. This has only been a focus of major research interest in the last few years.

Early research into HIV and women tended to focus on our reproductive role: women as breeders, we called it. Our own health needs were overlooked, except for our role in transmission to our children. By early 1995, interest had expanded to the health of our genital organs. This was a step in the right direction, but we still had far to go. Women are more than uteruses and vaginas.

In the intervening years, activists have helped ensure inclusion in trials formerly closed to those capable of pregnancy. The requirement that trials include women has changed the face of research. Now, our care and progress are subjects of intense scrutiny; studies and trials work hard to recruit us.

As science awakens to our presence, we are waking up too. We're starting to assert ourselves: to require that we understand the rationale for decisions affecting our care; to take an active part in making those decisions; to join other activists in pushing for social change; to demand access to treatment for our children.

At the Pasadena, California, conference on women and HIV in spring 1997, I was enormously moved by the numbers and the nature of the women who came. Advocates from migrant worker camps in Florida; Philadelphia inner-city activists who sought to help others get started; intense, exquisitely expressive artists; newly infected women just getting their feet wet; and, everywhere, mothers of children—moved to education and activism by protectiveness and passion for their kids. Presenters spoke not only as scientists and administrators, but as advocates and sisters. Speakers struggled to explain complex research in understandable terms. Participants demanded no less. Women of all backgrounds volunteered as mentors for those who sought their help. I was witnessing the beginning of a great and mighty movement.

And out of that meeting came a wealth of new information about the ways in which we *are* different. Much of this does in fact relate to our sexual anatomy. Much relates also to the cultural roles of women—our commitment to our children, our heightened vulnerability to violence and to sex without permission, our reduced earning power and authority because of gender bias, and the subtler manifestations of growing up in a male-dominated culture. We looked at our concern about our beauty, about being loved and cared for, about seeing one another as competition, about playing dumb. And remembering that we could put all that down if it didn't work for us, we tried on other behaviors. Confronting authority and demanding explanations was a favorite one. Some presenters were threatened, others outraged, others gentle and respectful. I loved it.

There is so much to hope for, when we put down the things that separate us and support one another. And no one will fight to give us the best care possible until we will accept no less. So we have to learn about ourselves, to learn what the best care is.

What's Not Different About HIV in Women
•

Women infected with HIV are every bit as likely as men to progress to illness and death without treatment. They respond to antiretroviral therapy just as well, require monitoring just as closely, and are as subject to wasting, vitamin deficiencies, hormonal alterations, and secondary infections as men. Their primary infection is characterized by the same large rapid increases in viral load we see in men. Just as in men, that initial increase is followed by establishment of a viral set point, the point of impasse between invader and immune response. That set point helps predict the tendency for progression, as it does in men. Studies of women who are long-term nonprogressors also parallel similar studies in men. So if you are a woman, the rest of this book is about you too.

What's Different About HIV in Women
•

To begin with, women's anatomy is different. Our chief receptive sex organ, the vagina, is designed to maintain a healthy environment that can resist infection. Changes in that environment make us more susceptible to HIV infection, as well as to other infections that may promote its progression.

HIV Prevention

Those changes can result from the presence of another sexually transmitted disease, or STD. Treatment of STDs has been shown to drastically reduce the rate of HIV infection. And STDs have been found to be prevalent in young women, even those with a history of only one or two partners. It's a jungle out there.

What to do: Avoid and/or treat all STDs.

Antibiotic treatment for unrelated illness can alter the balance of healthy vaginal bacteria; imbalances can result that favor infection. Wasting also alters the vaginal environment, making it more susceptible to infection. So do new sex partners (sorry) and vaginal sex more than eight times a week (sorry again).

What to do: Avoid unnecessary antibiotic treatment. Studies are currently under way in Pittsburgh to replace healthy bacteria, called lactobacillus, by suppository. Be sure you want that new partner. Address nutritional status.

Change also results from our own interventions. There are probably factors in vaginal secretions that inactivate the virus. Douching destroys the natural balance of healthy bacteria and the factors that help protect against infection, putting us at greater risk for HIV. Artificial scents can alter that balance also. And spermicidal gels and foams may cause irritation, increasing the risk of infection.

What to do: Don't douche, don't perfume.

Oral contraceptives may thin the vaginal wall. Just beneath that wall lie the cells that provide HIV with a point of entry into the body. Sex itself may cause abrasions, exposing those cells to the virus. Nonoxynol-9 can irritate the vaginal lining, increasing exposure.

What to do: Rubbers, rubbers, rubbers. There is also a new female condom, discussed in Chapter Eight. A 1996 National Institutes of Health consensus panel recommends that you stay on oral contraceptives if you're on them (they appear to reduce gonorrhea and chlamydia), until we know more. There are new contraceptives under study that work to restore a healthy vaginal environment.

In young women or in pregnancy, cells from within the cervix, which are more susceptible to HIV, can also be found on the outside. Infected white blood cells from semen can pass into the bloodstream between these cells.

What to do: Rubbers, rubbers, rubbers.

Anal sex heightens the risk of HIV transmission; this can be especially concerning when anal sex is practiced to avoid pregnancy.

What to do: Reconsider this type of sexual activity. If you continue, insist on rubbers.

In other countries, genital mutilation increases transmission risk. The sale of children for sex work leads to infection, abandonment, and death. Both here and abroad, sexual abuse and incest leave little girls not only damaged but also infected. And early sexual abuse and violence appear to strongly influence, if not predict, increased sexual risk-taking in later years.

What to do: We all need to share in political activism to expose and abolish such intrusions on the bodies of young women. Those of us who have been abused should consider seeking counseling, to minimize the effects of such treatment on our control over our own lives.

HIV Infection

Unlike men, women show variations in their viral population early. This is especially marked in women using oral contraception. It may be that more virus gets through, so that more than one population of virus is transmitted from the same partner. Or it may be because of the transmission of HIV-infected cells, rather than free virus. We do not yet know whether such diversity makes a clinical, or practical, difference.

Unlike their mothers, infected infants appear to display less HIV variety.

Julia Overbaugh, who reported these findings in Pasadena in 1997, summed them up as follows. In patterns of viral transmission:

- Women are different from men.
- Women are more complicated than men.
- Men are more like babies.

Secondary Infections

Women have more candida (oral, vaginal, or esophageal yeast infections), more pneumococcal pneumonia, and more chronic herpes simplex virus infections than men.

What to do: Pneumococcal vaccination is critical, and should be done early; acyclovir suppression can be prescribed at 400 milligrams twice a day. Fungal suppression with fluconazole should be considered where clinically appropriate.

Pelvic inflammatory disease, or PID, represents the spread of sexually transmitted diseases (gonorrhea and chlamydia in particular) that ascend from vagina to cervix and uterus and upward to fallopian tubes and ovaries. People with HIV tend to have more severe disease and more need for surgery. The bacteria causing PID may be different in HIV, also.

What to do: Monitor closely for fever and pelvic pain, as well as for increased discharge seen earlier in the disease. See your doctor right away if you have these symptoms.

Infection of the cervix by human papillomavirus (HPV) can lead to cervical dysplasia and eventually to cancer. Dysplasia is much more common and can be more severe, but rates of cervical cancer do not seem to be higher. According to Joel Palefsky, treatment may not be as successful. In addition, those with cervical HPV infection or dysplasia are likely to also have similar changes on anal pap smear.

The rate of progression to anal cancer increases with falling CD4 count. HIV cells may make factors that turn on HPV viral replication, and vice versa.

What to do: Get cervical pap smears every six months. If they are abnormal, repeat paps or colposcopy (microscopic evaluation) of the cervix. We should consider screening for anal dysplasia or cancer in women with cervical dysplasia, whether or not they report a history of anal receptive intercourse.

Women have CMV less often than men. It's seen less often in intravenous drug users. But if the CD4 count has been less than 25, 25 percent of women (compared to 31 percent of men) will show infection. And CMV colitis is actually more common in women than in men.

What to do: Monitor and treat for CMV infection. Consider prophylaxis when appropriate.

Twenty percent of HIV-positive people with tuberculosis in New York are women. They tend to be younger, with higher CD4 counts and fewer AIDS-defining conditions than men. Of women who had both TB and HIV infection, 81 percent had CD4 counts less than 200.

What to do: Test for TB annually. Dawn Smith of the HERS study recommends anergy testing; patients sometimes react. If they are anergic, monitor TB by annual chest X ray. If fever and cough are present, always evaluate sputum for AFB (acid-fast bacillus) as well as pneumocystis and bacterial pneumonia.

Pregnancy

Pregnancy causes a reduction in immune response. This makes sense; we don't want to reject and attack our babies while they grow inside us. But that immune suppression, which reverses after delivery in HIV-negative women, does not reverse in women who are infected. Rather, it progresses. So pregnancy, and especially multiple pregnancies, are not without cost.

What to do: Consider carefully the risks of becoming pregnant, and of carrying a child to term. If you do choose to have a baby, be sure to get adequate antiretroviral therapy for yourself and your baby. One in four babies born to HIV-positive mothers were once born infected. By 1995, zidovudine treatment had reduced that number to one in twelve; we now have less than one in twenty. If your water breaks or you develop a reproductive-tract infection, delivery should be quickly accomplished, to increase the baby's chances for a safe and uninfected birth.

Nutrition

Women with HIV appear to lose more fat than men do when they waste. There is currently controversy over whether they regain what has been lost as fat or lean body mass. And androgenic therapies like testosterone can masculinize appearance.

What to do: Exercise will help protect lean body mass. And there are nonandrogenic therapies that will help build more mass, sometimes with an associated loss of fat. Oxandrolone and growth hormone have both been used safely in women. Next to come will be trials of physiologic replacement of testosterone in those whose levels are low even for women.

New data on loss of bone density in men raise important new questions for women, especially now that we have a chance to live out our whole life. Do we have early loss of bone density too, if we're infected? If so, when does it start? What triggers it? Should we be taking estrogen? Are our estrogen and testosterone levels low? What about calcium and vitamin D supplementation? Will exercise help? If we do lose bone mass, should we try to replace it using current osteoporosis medications?

What to do: I don't know yet. We'll be asking these and other questions over the next couple of years. For now, I recommend following bone density and not dieting. If you have to get that perfect body, do it with exercise.

Neurologic Aspects

Women have more cognitive loss (poorer intellectual function) and more demyelination, or loss of the normal nerve coating, than men.

What to do: Aggressive antiretroviral therapy, targeted to ensure brain penetration, is urgent. Education can help protect against dementia, as can estrogen replacement therapy.

One study has shown that women with HIV and pain report no greater frequency or duration of their pain, but do report greater intensity and are more likely to have their pain undermedicated than men with HIV. Another paper reports that women experience pain more intensely but cope with it better.

What to do: Insist on adequate pain control, according to the guidelines set forth in Chapter Fifteen.

The Role of Gender Expectations
•

Women are classically caregivers, taught and expected to attend to the needs of others before we attend to our own. Most single-parent families, in particular, are headed by women. Many of these women must work as well as care for their children. Those who do not must manage on very little money. The needs of the children are bound to come first.

Consequently, women work more hours, stretch fewer dollars, enjoy less rest and privacy, and are hard-pressed to satisfy the demands of everyday life. The addition of illness, and the need for special care to stay well, can make the burden overwhelming. It's even hard to go to the clinic when you have to take three kids along.

One of the most difficult parts of parenting is the setting of proper priorities. Especially when kids are infected too, our instincts are to care for them first, at the expense of our own health, if necessary. I spoke to a man at one conference who told me how he took the protease inhibitors prescribed for him, reduced the dosage size, and gave them to his infected daughter instead. Women are often faced with similar choices. This story has been repeated over and over to me since then.

Now we have access to powerful drugs for kids. But the conflict remains between care for our children and care for ourselves. If a mother is due for a follow-up visit and her child is sick, chances are that the mother will cancel her own appointment. If her child's appointment conflicts with her own, the child's appointment will win out. And if a parent's vitamins or food supplements—even, sometimes, medicines—take money from a budget that must feed and shelter the children, they may well take a back seat.

Young mothers especially need support. It's hard enough to be a child and raise a child. If one or both of you are sick, it's even harder. You need a little help from your friends.

What to do: There are two ways to approach this problem. First, and most helpful, we can try to make it simple for a mother to care for herself and her children—by scheduling appointments together, by providing enough money and services so that critical needs are met for all of the family, and by maintaining hope. If a mother sees that care of herself and her family is not an impossible task, she's less likely to give up.

Second, we have to remember that the best way to care for a

child may be to ensure that the child *has* a mother. I'm always struck by the safety video on airplanes. The oxygen masks drop down, and parents are instructed to put theirs on first—so that they'll be physically able to get their child's on.

You can't give your children any better gift than the gift of a mother who loves them. So you have to make room for your own needs, too. Not just medicines, but warmth and sleep and food and love and play and vitamins. Keep some of that for yourself, to help keep you here for your child.

Other gender expectations involve our body image. We are acculturated to the aesthetics of slenderness. But our survival depends on maintaining our bank of nutritional stores.

What to do: Exercise. Eat well. Don't diet; and if you must diet, do so with care and monitoring, to assess the effects on lean body mass.

The Role of Power
•

Despite the strides we've made, women are unequal participants in many aspects of life. We make less money, get fewer promotions, and do more work than our male counterparts. We are also likely to be unequal partners in relationships.

Women are more vulnerable to physical abuse, and to sex without permission, than are men. If we have experienced these as children, we may not resist them later. If we don't know we can choose whom to sleep with and when, what work to do and for whom, how we will look and dress and act, we won't choose. In particular, if we are in dependent relationships, we lack the reinforcement from others that might make us expect and demand our fair share.

Sandra Thurmond, a national AIDS policy director, offers these priorities for women with HIV:

1. Access to comprehensive drug HIV-positive treatment programs
2. Needle exchange programs, to halt the spread of infection for women with HIV
3. An end to domestic violence—"a broader meaning for safe sex"
4. Access to excellent care, with proper drugs and monitoring

Martina Clark of the United Nations adds:

5. Placing women with HIV on trial committees, on ethical review boards, and as paid workers at trial sites

My own priorities, especially after Pasadena, would include also:

6. Providing women with a way to talk to one another, share what they have in common, and use their abilities to help each other up the rock

Barrier Protection
•

If you're infected, it's critical that you not infect others. Condoms are a good step toward safer sex. You are also more infective while you are menstruating; sex at that time, even with a condom, should be avoided.

It isn't only your partner you have to worry about. As we saw in Chapter Eight, you remain at risk for contracting sexually transmitted diseases. Other infections are more likely and will be more severe in their effects.

There is a new condom, tested in six countries and now marketed here, made for women. While there is concern that it may not provide as much protection as a male condom, it has been shown to be fairly effective in reducing HIV transmission. Instructions for use can be found in Chapter Eight. Nonoxynol-9, a spermicide that also acts against viruses, is also reported to reduce the risk. Again, it's not as safe as condoms; but you control its application, and your partner need not know.

You need to use a condom, if you can. If not, nonoxynol-9 is better than nothing.

• • •

If you're a woman living with HIV, you must care for yourself, even while you are caring for others. You should do what you can to avoid or resist any actions of others that harm you. You should take control of decisions on whether or not to bear children. If you're pregnant, you should be on aggressive antiretroviral therapy, aiming to suppress your viral load.

You need close routine follow-up for gynecological care. You need to maintain good nutrition. You should consider entering studies, for your sake and for the sake of other women.

You should strengthen your own role in healing, and in the direction of your care. You should learn all you can about your body and the virus. And you should find a doctor you can trust.

REFERENCES

Anastos, K., and Greenblatt. "Epidemiology and natural history of HIV infection among women." *HIV Advances in Research and Therapy,* 1994, *4*(2), 11–19.

Bearden, E. M. "Multicultural outreach project." National Conference on Women and HIV, Pasadena, Calif., May 4–7, 1997.

Breitbart, W. "Gender differences in the pain experience of AIDS patients." National Conference on Women and HIV, Pasadena, Calif., May 4–7, 1997.

Centers for Disease Control. "Change in AIDS deaths in first six months of 1996, by gender," February 28, 1997.

Connor, E. M., and others. "Reduction of maternal-infant transmission of HIV-1 with zidovudine treatment." *New England Journal of Medicine,* 1994, *331*(18), 1173–1180.

Cotton, D. J. "Planning antiretroviral therapy for HIV-infected women." *HIV Advances in Research and Therapy,* 1994, *4*(2), 21–27.

Davids, J., and others. "Demanding quality treatment for HIV: The Act Up Philadelphia women's standard of care." National Conference on Women and HIV, Pasadena, Calif., May 4–7, 1997.

Duerr, A. "Gynecologic infections: Challenges and response." National Conference on Women and HIV, Pasadena, Calif., May 4–7, 1997.

Grossman, C. J. "Interactions between the gonadal steroids and the immune system." *Science,* 1985, *227,* 257–260.

Hankins, C. A., and Handley. "HIV disease and AIDS in women: Current knowledge and a research agenda." *Journal of Acquired Immune Deficiency Syndromes and Human Retrovirology,* 1992, *5*(10), 957–971.

Hankins, C. A., and others. "Cervicovaginal screening in women with HIV infection: A need for increased vigilance?" *Canadian Medical Association Journal,* 1994, *150*(5), 681–686.

Hillier, S. "Effects of the genital tract ecosystem on transmission of HIV to women." National Conference on Women and HIV, Pasadena, Calif., May 4–7, 1997.

Hitchcock, P. "The vaginal ecosystem: Nature's gate-keeper for reproductive health of women." National Conference on Women and HIV, Pasadena, Calif., May 4–7, 1997.

Kirkman, R., and Chantler. "Contraception and the prevention of sexually transmitted diseases." *British Medical Bulletin,* 1993, *49*(1), 171–181.

Legg, J. J. "Women and HIV." *Journal of the American Board of Family
Practice,* 1993, *6*(4), 367–377.

Levine, J. "Androgyny, creativity and locus of control as predictors of
depression in HIV positive women." Unpublished doctoral dissertation, California Institute of Integral Studies, San Francisco, 1993.

Mayer, K. "Phase 1 study of a new vaginal microbicide, Buffergel: Rationale and clinical data." National Conference on Women and HIV,
Pasadena, Calif., May 4–7, 1997.

Overbaugh, J. "HIV in the genital tract." National Conference on
Women and HIV, Pasadena, Calif., May 4–7, 1997.

Palefsky, J. "Human papillomavirus infection among HIV-infected individuals: Implications for development of malignant tumors." *Hematol-
ogy and Oncology Clinics of North America,* 1991, *5*(2), 357–370.

Palefsky, J. "Cervicovaginal human papillomavirus in HIV+ and high-
risk HIV– women." National Conference on Women and HIV,
Pasadena, Calif., May 4–7, 1997.

Seidman, S. N., and Rieder. "A review of sexual behavior in the United
States." *American Journal of Psychiatry,* 1994, *151*(3), 330–341.

Shah, P. N., and others. "Menstrual symptoms in women infected by
human immunodeficiency virus." *Obstetrics and Gynecology,* 1994,
83(3), 397–400.

Singer, E. "Analgesia and pain management in HIV infected women."
National Conference on Women and HIV, Pasadena, Calif., May
4–7, 1997.

Sobo, E. J. "Inner-city women and AIDS: The psycho-social benefits of
unsafe sex." *Cultural and Medical Psychiatry,* 1993, *17*(4), 455–485.

U.S. Department of Health and Human Services. "Recommendations of
the U.S. Public Health Task Force in the use of zidovudine to reduce
perinatal transmission of human immunodeficiency virus." *Morbidity
and Mortality Weekly Report,* 1994, *43*, RR-11.

Voeller, B. "AIDS and heterosexual anal intercourse." *Archives of Sexual
Behavior,* 1991, *20*(3), 233–276.

Warren, D. L., and Duerr. "HIV infection in non-pregnant women: A review of current knowledge." *Current Opinions in Obstetrics and Gynecology,* 1993, *5*(4), 527–533.

Weiser, B. "The biology of HIV-1 infection in women and men." National
Conference on Women and HIV, Pasadena, Calif., May 4–7, 1997.

Wyatt, G. "Redefining the balance of power in relationships." National
Conference on Women and HIV, Pasadena, Calif., May 4–7, 1997.

CHAPTER 18

•

What to Do
Algorithms for Care

By now, you pretty much know what there is to know about wasting in HIV. You've learned why lean body mass is lost, and how. You've learned how to watch for it, and how to address it when it occurs. You've looked at the things you can do on your own, and have a basic grasp of what you and your doctor can do together—monitoring, investigating factors that contribute, and counteracting those factors.

This chapter, then, is a review of what you've already learned. Here you will find suggested approaches, relative to each stage of HIV progression. By focusing attention directly on *you*, and on where you stand right now in the continuum of HIV infection, you can direct your efforts most efficiently and individualize the suggestions made in this book.

Algorithms are cheat sheets—recipes, normally made for and by doctors, that tell us where and how to direct our efforts most efficiently. They may be set up as flow charts, or as short lists of recommended actions or things to look for. You'll find them frequently as you begin to read the scientific literature. In this chapter we'll offer them as lists, with comment as needed to help it all make sense.

Start Early
•

This is a fight that is best begun early. Prevention is key. Close monitoring, right from the start, will pay off for years to come. Aggressive intervention and treatment of *all* aspects of HIV-associated illness will help fight the wasting process.

If you're ill or symptomatic at this point, you'll need to address those issues that are relative to your stage first. Even so, suggestions made for earlier stages will still have relevance for you. But wherever you are in the course of HIV, now is the time to start.

Right Now, Whatever Your Stage of HIV
•

HIV

- Assess CD4 status, to estimate stage of progression.
- Assess viral load, to document current viral activity (use branched-chain DNA (bDNA) or PCR RNA).
- Consider highly active antiretroviral therapy, or HAART. Use at least three drugs, and aim for viral suppression.
- Consider antioxidants, to lower rate of viral replication.

Secondary Infections

- Search for them, and treat if found. Check stools for ova and parasites, including cryptosporidium and microsporidium. Also test for tuberculosis if no history of exposure (PPD and controls still advocated if no prior PPD positive history; chest X ray if no response to skin tests). *Evaluate any diarrhea aggressively.*
- Obtain cervical pap smear if female; regardless of gender, obtain anal pap if any history of cervical dysplasic, genital warts, or receptive anal sex.
- Present quickly to your doctor for *any* sign of infection, especially fever, night sweats, respiratory complaints, facial pain, herpes, or female pelvic symptoms.

Nutrition

- Complete your nutritional assessment (from Appendix II).
- Monitor calorie and protein consumption; adjust your eating patterns to improve intake.
- Obtain measurement of body cell mass or lean body mass, by bioimpedance analysis (BIA) or by DEXA.
- Obtain bone densitometry to assess for osteopenia or osteoporosis.
- Begin progressive resistance exercise if energy permits.
- Address anorexia.

- Check B_{12}, folate or RBC folate, and magnesium levels.
- Begin vitamin supplementation.
- Check testosterone level.

Maintenance

- Start learning all you can about HIV infection and the weapons we have to fight it.
- Address any discomfort or pain; treat the symptom as well as the cause.
- Evaluate support systems, especially friends and family. Consider a support group. Consider counseling, if depressed or overwhelmed. Seek out social programs for help with money, food, and housing.
- Evaluate life stressors. Change those that are easily changed; consider ways to change others over time.
- Evaluate recreational habits—sleep, sex, cigarettes, alcohol, drugs. Change those you can change, to promote a healthier lifestyle. Prioritize; don't try to change them all at once.
- Evaluate work habits. Make time for sleep and recreation.

ALGORITHM TWO

HIV-Positive, Asymptomatic, at Diagnosis

CD4 Count 500–1,000,
No AIDS-Defining Illness, Weight Stable

•

HIV

- Assess viral load (with bDNA or PCR RNA) and T-cell subsets.
- Consider early highly active antiretroviral therapy (HAART). Follow T-cell subsets and viral load every three months, to monitor for progression. If progression is seen, recheck viral load before changing therapy. If therapy is changed, recheck viral load in two to four weeks to assess effects.

Secondary Infections

- Screen yearly for
    Enteric, or gut, infections (three stools for ova and parasites, including cryptosporidium and microsporidium).
    Tuberculosis (PPD and controls).
    Condyloma (genital or rectal warts) by physical exam; rectal pap smear if *any* history of receptive anal intercourse.
- Screen every six months for
    Cervical changes due to condyloma; screen more often if abnormal (by pap smear).
    Vaginal infections (wet mount for bacterial vaginosis; potassium hydroxide (KOH) prep for yeast; chlamydia and gonorrhea tests if *any* sexual activity; vaginal culture if any discharge not resolved by treatment for the above causes).
- See your doctor at once for symptoms of infection, as well as other symptoms of discomfort or pain.

Nutrition

- Redo nutritional assessment every three months; adjust eating patterns to improve intake.
- Monitor weight monthly, and lean body mass every three months. Set goals for weight gain if needed.
- Follow albumin at each doctor visit or lab draw (at minimum, every three months).
- Begin progressive resistance exercise—ideally, at least three times a week (free weights; machine weight training; Theraband). Set goals for increase in body cell mass. Skip sessions if deeply fatigued.
- Address anorexia if present.
- Consider food supplements if needed.
- Supplement vitamin intake.

Maintenance

- Keep learning, from objective learning sources and from others.
- Consider volunteering to help others with HIV.
- Consider HIV political activism.
- Consider counseling to address issues raised by diagnosis.

ALGORITHM THREE

HIV-Positive, Asymptomatic

CD4 Count 500 or Less, No Active Wasting
•

HIV

- Follow T-cell subsets and viral load every three months, to monitor for progression.
- Initiate HAART, if not already begun.
- Consider joining trials for new regimens of combination therapy.
- Consider antioxidants.

Secondary Infections

- Screen yearly for
    Enteric (gut) infections.
    Tuberculosis (by PPD and controls). If anergic, obtain yearly X ray.
    Condyloma, genital or rectal warts, or rectal dysplasia (by physical exam; rectal pap smear if *any* history of receptive anal intercourse).
- Screen every six months for
    Cervical changes due to condyloma; more often if abnormal (by pap smear).
    Vaginal infections (by pelvic exam, wet mount, KOH prep, vaginal culture if discharge present, chlamydia and gonorrhea if *any* sexual activity).
- Consider acyclovir for herpes suppression if any episodes.
- Look for occult infections if triglycerides rise substantially.

Nutrition

- Redo nutritional assessment every three months; adjust eating patterns to improve intake.

- Monitor weight monthly, and body cell mass every three months. Respond aggressively to any loss.
  - Address anorexia.
  - Consider food supplements.
  - Follow albumin levels at each doctor visit or lab draw (at minimum, every three months).
- Monitor bone densitometry every other year at least; consider yearly evaluation if osteopenia reported, or any signs of wasting or disease progression, or in the presence of long-term or high-dose prednisone treatment.
- Supplement vitamins.
- Begin or continue progressive resistance exercise—ideally, at least three times a week. Skip or reduce intensity of sessions if deeply fatigued.

Maintenance

- Keep learning all you can about HIV and its control.
- Consider volunteer activities; activism.
- Maintain support networks. Consider an HIV support group. Consider counseling if indicated.
- Make time for sleep and recreation.

Fight Aggressively
•

If you're farther along in the course of HIV, it's increasingly important to leave no stone unturned—to do everything you can to fight wasting. As we've seen, this involves more than just food. A complete approach to prevention or treatment of the wasting syndrome requires a high level of vigilance on the part of you and your doctor: opposing any increase in replication of the virus itself; protecting against, monitoring for, and treating secondary infections decisively; and addressing wasting, when it appears, with an early and vigorous program.

I can't emphasize enough the increased value we can gain, from all the interventions available to fight wasting, when we reach for them right at the start of the process. It's just like gravity. It's easier not to fall down the mountain than it is to climb back up.

The algorithms that follow, then, offer an aggressive approach. If you are opposed to some of these methods, or find they require more of your will and attention than you are willing to dedicate, that's fine. Just take and use what feels right. If you aren't ideologically opposed to these treatments, though, and you want to fight the fight with all you have, you have a right to do so.

You also have a right to take part in decisions about your health care that affect you so critically. Understanding the basis for these recommendations, from your readings here and elsewhere, will help you to argue for such a program.

ALGORITHM FOUR

AIDS, No Active Intercurrent Infections
•

HIV

- Follow T-cell subsets and viral load every three months, to monitor for progression.
- Continue HAART; consider a change of regimens according to the principles discussed in Chapter Thirteen, if viral load rises more than half a log (by more than three times) or if CD4 count drops. Recheck load at once if levels are rising significantly. If currently available antiretroviral therapies have failed, reevaluate the options carefully. Seek a trial or a compassionate-use program that offers new therapy.
- Consider antioxidants.

Secondary Infections

- Screen yearly for enteric infections, tuberculosis, condyloma, or anal dysplasia.
- Screen every six months for cervical changes due to condyloma—more often if abnormal—and vaginal infections.
- Screen every six months, or sooner if instructed, for CMV retinitis (ophthalmology consult).
- Consider acyclovir for herpes suppression if any episodes. *Once CD4 cells are below 100, survival benefit has been shown with addition of acyclovir to antiretroviral therapy;* start acyclovir suppression therapy at that point, at least, and consider using it sooner.
- Initiate prophylaxis for pneumocystis, toxoplasmosis, and MAC as indicated by CD4 counts (see Chapter Fourteen).
- Consider prophylaxis for deep fungal infections.
- Consider CMV prophylaxis.
- Use systemic, not local, therapy for esophageal and other deep fungal infections. Try to avoid ketoconazole (Nizoral), as it lowers testosterone levels.

- Look for occult infections.
- Report fevers or any change in symptoms promptly.

Nutrition

- Begin or continue progressive resistance exercise—ideally, at least three times a week. Choose a level that challenges but doesn't tire you. Skip or reduce intensity of sessions if deeply fatigued.
- Continue nutritional assessment every three months; adjust eating patterns to improve intake.
- Monitor weight monthly. If at all possible, begin lean body mass measurement. Respond aggressively to any loss: address anorexia, consider food supplements, consider malabsorption as a contributing factor.
- Consider annual bone densitometry if CD4s less than 100 or prior episode of wasting.
- Consider anabolic therapies for documented loss of body cell mass or loss of 5 percent or more from documented baseline weight—testosterone for men, oxandrolone and/or growth hormone for men or women, nandrolone decanoate if approved. Consider convergent therapy with anabolic treatment if required.
- Follow albumin levels at each doctor visit or lab draw (every month or two, if possible).
- Supplement vitamin intake.
- Monitor for B_{12}, folate, and magnesium deficiency.

Maintenance

- Limit your workload, and your volunteer and activist activities, as needed, to avoid fatigue or burnout. But do all you want to do if it feels good.
- Consider application for disability, if work is too tiring.
- Align yourself with social service programs for money, food, or shelter assistance.
- Maintain support networks; consider an HIV support group; seek counseling if indicated.

ALGORITHM FIVE
AIDS, Active Wasting

Acute Onset, Loss of Weight or Lean Body Mass,
Anorexia, Fevers or Night Sweats, Deep Fatigue,
Marked Increase in Triglyceride Levels
•

HIV

- Recheck viral load to assess for escape from control.
- Continue HAART; consider a change of regimens according to the principles discussed in Chapter Thirteen, if viral load rises more than half a log (by more than three times) or if CD4 count drops. Recheck load at once if levels are rising significantly. If currently available antiretroviral therapies have failed, reevaluate the options carefully. Seek a trial or a compassionate-use program that offers new therapies. Repeat viral load before changing, to make sure it isn't just a blip.
- Consider antioxidants.

Secondary Infections

- Maintain prophylaxis according to schedule. If one drug can't be used, change to another.
- Seek underlying intercurrent infections aggressively: monitor closely for symptoms and investigate them.
- Consider possible presence of opportunistic infections according to CD4 counts, as listed in Chapter Fourteen.
- Consider presence of nonopportunistic infections.
- Rigorously evaluate diarrhea, abdominal pain, abnormal tests of liver function; also shortness of breath, cough (even if chronic), or chest pain; also difficulty swallowing or throat pain, *or any focal symptom.*
- Use systemic, not local, therapy for esophageal and other deep fungal infections. Avoid ketoconazole (Nizoral) if possible.
- If wasting signs and symptoms persist in the absence of

any proven infection, consider referral to an infectious disease (I.D.) specialist for consultation.

Nutrition

- Closely monitor weight and body cell mass.
- Monitor bone densitometry if not done within the past year. Consider anabolics or other therapies if osteopenia or osteoporosis is reported.
- Follow albumin. Consider testing prealbumin, transferrin, or total iron binding capacity (TIBC), to monitor immediate status during periods of active wasting.
- Address anorexia aggressively, using appetite stimulants, medical foods as supplements, and practical tricks discussed earlier. Get help if food or money's not available.
- Use symptom medicines to help control mouth, throat, or abdominal pain, and to combat diarrhea.
- Consider malabsorption as a contributing factor. Evaluate according to the tests listed in Chapter Twelve. If malabsorption is present, attempt to counter it with special medical foods designed for such cases. *Start early; don't wait for wasting to progress.*
- Fight metabolic dysregulation leading to wasting, in response to other stressors.
- Consider cytokine blockers.
- Treat fevers with nonsteroidal anti-inflammatory drugs, unless contraindicated.
- Initiate anabolic therapy: testosterone in men, if total level is not above 600 nanograms per deciliter; oxandrolone or growth hormone, depending on clinical picture. If wasting has not been reversed with diagnosis and treatment of the underlying infection and with first-step anabolics, consider convergent therapy with more than one. Monitor body cell mass closely during this period, to assess your nutritional status and your response to treatment. Even if you have not yet shown loss of body cell mass or a weight loss of more than 5 percent, you should strongly consider anabolic approaches dur-

ing a period of active secondary infection and its associated wasting. It's easier to stop falling down the hill than
it is to climb back up.

- Suspend exercise.
- If wasting does not respond to oral supplements, consider a course of total parenteral nutrition (TPN) until the
underlying cause of your wasting can be found and fully
treated.
- Do your best to keep up some oral intake whenever possible, even if TPN is provided, to help preserve gut wall
integrity.
- Supplement vitamin intake.
- Monitor for B_{12}, folate, and magnesium deficiency. Supplement these as needed.
- Withdraw special supports, such as TPN, as wasting resolves with treatment of underlying infection.
- Continue medical food supplements as long as possible,
to help you regain what you've lost and to consolidate
that gain.
- Continue TPN in the face of unresolved diarrhea or
untreatable infection, at least until you can maintain
lean body mass with medical foods and other interventions.

Maintenance

- Reduce activities as needed to limit fatigue.
- Put volunteer and activist activities on hold. *Let others
take care of you while you are ill.*
- Consider application for disability, temporary or permanent as your case indicates, if work is too tiring.
- Align yourself with social service programs for money,
food, or shelter assistance. *Ask for more help when you
need it.*
- Maintain support networks and support group participation. *Ask for and accept help when you need it.*
- Address depression aggressively, with medication as well
as with counseling and social supports.

Stay in Charge: Choosing When to Stop
•

We've spent almost the whole book, so far, talking about and reaching for empowerment.

If you're reading this book—especially if you've read this far—you care about what happens to your body and want to understand it. And you *have* to understand it to argue for and contribute to the best, most thorough, and most uncompromising care you can have. Your doctor, unless her or his time is unlimited, must have your help to stay on top of details. The more you understand, the better your care will be.

Some of us, though—some doctors—are as caught up in this effort as you are. We want to pull out all the stops, offer everything we can to fight this fight. And the more we see the virus as the enemy, and the challenge as our life's work, the less we're willing to stop fighting.

If you have a doctor who is personally invested in the war on HIV, you have a strong ally for the battle. But you must remember that *you* are the one in charge. Just as you have the right to insist on the best, most comprehensive, and most careful HIV treatment, you also have the right to refuse it, or to modify it in ways that allow you the degree of quality of life you determine to be necessary.

This becomes especially important if you are very ill.

The struggle against AIDS is a marathon. We train for it; we set aside other matters to attend to it; we try to pace ourselves throughout it and be good to ourselves along the way. At every point, there are decisions to be made about how fully we'll commit, and how much we'll hold back, to maintain a life of quality.

When you're sick, it's hard to eat if you don't want to. It's hard to submit to testing, and to intravenous lines and spinal taps and CT scans. If you do so, it's because the quality of life you expect to gain is greater than the quality you surrender.

Sometimes, that quality doesn't seem to be there. Chronic pain, while controllable, can play a part. Weakness, or loss of the ability to do the things we love the most, can erode our expectation of a happy outcome, and with it our commitment. Fatigue or confusion can make the act of taking pills all day, forcing ourselves to eat, even performing the activities of daily living, seem like a mountainous chore.

If our perspective results from depression, we're probably wrong. With appropriate treatment, things may look much brighter. We may have a lot to keep struggling for.

If our life's work isn't done—if we haven't come to terms with ourselves and those we've loved, with the lives we've led and what we'll leave behind—it's often worthwhile to fight on until we find completion, no matter how many pills we have to take, or symptoms we must accept.

But if the time comes when fighting the virus feels like all work, with no reward in sight; if you've used every miracle that science has to offer, and the virus is still winning; if you're not depressed and have tried the care and medicines that help depression; if you've given your perspective a good while to sort itself out; if you are at peace with how you've lived your life; *and if you are peaceful about letting go*—you have the right to do so.

I am surprised and humbled by the grace and acceptance I've seen in people with HIV who have come through my office and have died. It's not always so, but it's common. And those who are happiest, most peaceful, most curious, most entirely unafraid are often those who, earlier on, fought the hardest.

So if you are living with serious illness, and your options have narrowed severely—only you can decide when to fight and when to let it go.

There is no reason for anyone with HIV to die in pain and suffering. The struggle and effort you go through is *for you*—to buy you the most time, the most pleasure, and the best shot at being here when and if we beat this thing.

This is your game. If you decide you're not in it anymore, your doctor will still be there. Any quality remaining to you can be maximized. And your doctor can see to it that the time remaining to you will be comfortable and pleasant, naturally and without effort. As my friend and teacher Kevin Schram, who's been a nurse forever, says,

"This is the nineties, Baby. Nobody has to hurt."

This section is for those who have fought the good fight, and don't want to fight anymore.

AIDS, End Stage

for Patients and Caregivers
•

HIV

- Stop antiretroviral therapy, unless HIV encephalopathy is present or suspected.
- Stop antioxidants.
- Stop all labs and testing.

Secondary Infections

- Treat any that are symptomatic and reduce quality of life, as long as consciousness is present.
- Treat painful or distressing symptoms aggressively.
- Treat fevers.

Nutrition

- Offer food and drink only as wished.
- Offer comfort foods and favorite dishes.
- Whenever possible, provide companionship at mealtimes.
- Stop vitamin supplements and appetite enhancers. Consider continuing Marinol (if marijuana is not available), for effects on mood, appetite, and disposition.

Maintenance

- Support autonomy as fully as possible. Offer, and defer to, choices.
- Ensure that maximal social supports are in place: money, food, and housing, as available. Consider hospice benefit, providing higher levels of care at home or in residential hospice.
- Provide home help for housework and personal care.
- Encourage visits from friends and family as tolerated. Provide quiet, loving companionship.

- Support full discussion of any topic initiated: support memories when recalled; assist with any necessary settling of affairs; support spiritual introspection only when invited to do so.
- Take time to say good-bye.
- Maintain a pleasant environment: sunlight, fresh air, outdoor time as tolerated; music, good kitchen smells, fragrant flowers, laughter; clean, dry sheets and clothes.
- Continue activity out of bed as wished. Assist where needed. Consider hospital bed, where appropriate, for comfort and ease of care.
- *Treat all symptoms:*
  Use long-acting narcotics in as high a dose as needed to control chronic pain. Consider a fentanyl patch, which doesn't need to be swallowed. Don't undertreat.

  Consider short-acting morphine, or Percocet or other narcotics of choice, for breakthrough pain.

  Use laxatives to avoid constipation from narcotics. Treat anxiety, depression, nausea, and shortness of breath aggressively.

REFERENCES

Bartlett, J. G. *The Johns Hopkins Guide to Medical Care of Patients with HIV Infection.* (6th ed.) Baltimore: Williams and Wilkins, 1996.

Bayle, K. E. "The role of the primary care physician in end-stage AIDS." *AIDSfile,* 1993, *7*(2), 7–9.

Jewett, J. F., and Hecht. "Preventive health care for adults with HIV infection." *Journal of the American Medical Association,* 1993, *269*(9), 1144–1253.

Kantor, T. G. (ed.). "Evolving trends in the management of chronic pain." *American Journal of Medicine,* 1996, *101*(1A), 1S–62S.

Miaskowski, C. A. "Beyond the AHCPR guidelines: Home care issues." *Pain Management Refined: New Approaches.* 1997 Program Development Meeting, Santa Monica, Calif., March 14–16, 1997.

Passik, S. D. "Transdermal fentanyl in HIV/AIDS substance abusers." Pain Management Refined: New Approaches. 1997 Program Development Meeting, Santa Monica, Calif., March 14–16, 1997.

Payne, R. "Beyond the AHCPR guidelines: 1994 to 1997, What's Next?"

Pain Management Refined: New Approaches. 1997 Program Development Meeting, Santa Monica, Calif., March 14–16, 1997.

Sanford, J. P., and others. *The Sanford Guide to Antimicrobial Therapy, 1996.* Dallas: Antimicrobial Therapy, Inc., 1997.

Sanford, J. P., and others. *The Sanford Guide to HIV/AIDS Therapy, 1996.* Dallas: Antimicrobial Therapy, Inc., 1997.

PART IV

•

Taking Charge: How to Direct Your Own Healing

•

CHAPTER 19

•

Taking Charge
of Your Medical Care

The one person most intensely concerned with your health is yourself. It's important to have a doctor you can trust. But if you just turn the job over, you lose the most important part of a critical partnership.

I'd like to suggest that you think of your doctor as a resource: a scientific adviser; a skilled technician, available to help you determine, and then serve, your needs; a gateway to testing and treatment. With luck, he or she can also be your cheerleader and will become your friend. With great luck, teaching will flow in both directions. But it's you who bears final responsibility for guiding the direction of your care.

You are the one who will choose how much effort to make. Only you know what you are capable of, *can* be capable of, when you set your mind to it. You need to understand *why* you make sacrifices if you are to make them with a willing heart. If you're not convinced of the value of treatment, it simply will not work as well. And in the final analysis, only you reap the rewards.

In fact, it's the very people who stay in charge—who listen to their advisers and stay current with medical knowledge, but reserve the right to make decisions based on that knowledge—who seem to do the best, for the longest time.

Integrating Other Disciplines
•

You can design a plan of care that incorporates alternative methods. You may refuse some of the treatments Western medicine has to offer, if they conflict deeply with your values. Just as we don't have to share your bias, you don't have to share ours. In some cases you will teach us, by following your own program and doing well.

Remember: you're not locked into any decision. There's always room for change if things go poorly, as long as you keep up your monitoring, so you'll know in advance if they do.

Just as your trust in your doctor is a good placebo, your trust in the path you choose is an excellent medicine, too. And there's nothing wrong with placebos, traditional or alternative—as long as they work.

Be Curious

We've listed some resources, in Chapter Five, for learning about alternative treatments for HIV. They're often complementary to traditional Western medicine: you needn't choose one or the other. And in many cases, they rest on a whole different philosophical approach to the body and its care. Because of this, there may be aspects of health we ignore, in traditional medicine, that they can address more profoundly.

Doctors, on the whole, won't have time to learn other disciplines. You will, and you may wish to.

Be Careful

Be sure that what you learn is based in fact, and not in someone else's prejudice. Look at the sources of information. Watch out for misleading claims, for anger or unacknowledged bias on the part of the proponent, or for arguments that sound like sloppy science. You may find reports of some treatments in the activist literature cited below. This is particularly helpful for avoiding things that can hurt you.

In particular, be wary of claims about ozone therapy, or taking hydrogen peroxide. I've researched this, both in the underground press and in the medical literature. The claims sound scientific, if you don't know your science. But if you understand the workings of your body, and of HIV, as explained in this book, you'll see how conflicting they are.

Ozone *is* used for purification of blood—but it's used on blood *outside* the body, to prepare it for transfusion to someone else. Ozone's value in that application lies in the fact that *it creates an environment that is unhealthy for living things.* Red blood cells can tolerate a lot of free radicals and a temporary atmosphere of oxidative stress. Germs can't. Some viruses can't. Your body can't.

Recognize also that peroxide ingestion and ozone treatment are touted *for* their oxidizing properties—the very opposite of what we're trying to achieve with our use of antioxidants. Peroxide and ozone do provide you with more oxygen atoms on breakdown, as claimed, but it's the wrong kind of oxygen, the kind that can hurt you.

Oxygen—molecular oxygen, two atoms bonded stably together without free radicals—is a fine thing. Breathe a little extra, if you want to; a little more can't hurt you. But oxygen molecules or atoms in their free radical form are just what the virus needs for replication. And they damage your structures and cells.

This is a perfect example of a fashionable, but dangerous and potentially damaging, alternative treatment.

If you're using herbs, don't experiment; look to an herbalist for advice before you start making up recipes.

If you're trying some new drug from a buyers' club, read up on it first. And always let your doctor know you're trying something new. Other medicines or treatments may need to be adjusted.

Do your homework. This stuff is real. Don't be any less thoughtful about alternative therapies than you'd be about traditional medical approaches.

A partial list of buyer's clubs can be found in Appendix IX.

Being Prepared
•

The better prepared you are for your doctor visit, the more you'll get done.

Keep Records

Get copies of your lab reports at doctor visits, so you can work on your flow charts at home. Keep them up to date. Know when weight or lean body mass changes, when albumin slips on repeated occasions.

Know when you're due for T-cell subsets, or a test for viral load. Consider your next step before you see your doctor, whether it's upgrading to combination therapy, applying for a new trial, or evaluating for viral suppression. Keep your antiretrovirogram up to date, and stay a step or two ahead of current treatment. Do this piece of homework with your doctor—well before it's time to change—if she'll take the time.

Keep track of your symptoms—where they are, when they appear, what brings them on, and what helps them.

Do an emotional inventory before every visit. Report depression, anxiety, uncontrolled anger. Be prepared to ask for specific assistance. In managed care, especially, few doctors can offer referrals for counseling, or address your emotional status, unless you ask for it. Medicines can be helpful. And if you also need someone to talk to, speak up.

Use Appointment Time Efficiently

In my residency training I was taught to address no more than two problems per outpatient visit. That's ridiculous, even for perfectly healthy people. It's entirely unresponsive to the needs of people with HIV who are trying to stay healthy.

The trick, I think, is to first prioritize your issues. Put the urgent ones first, in case you don't get to everything. Then present all your issues up front. "I have four problems I want to discuss, and I'm due for my bDNA and my second hepatitis B shot. And I want to address my depression."

The first time your doctor hears this, she may experience a little depression of her own! But the fact is, it works. It helps doctors to apportion their time most effectively, saves them time spent figuring out what you're due for, and lets them know right where you stand. If they're used to being totally in charge, they may be startled at first, but you need to be gently assertive if you want to be part of the game.

In time your doctor will come to love you for this approach. It helps us to do a good job—and it beats getting sandbagged with one problem at a time. Once we've spent fifteen minutes discussing somebody's fungal toenail, we and our day can be ruined when we hear about fevers, diarrhea, and thoughts of suicide as we're on our way out the door.

Keeping Informed
•

If you're going to help drive the car, you'll need to know the terrain. You've made a good start, but you have to continue to keep up with new developments in HIV treatment—ideally, almost as fast as they happen. There are manageable ways to ensure this.

Written Sources

Perhaps the best source for clear, up-to-date information is *BETA, Bulletin of Experimental Treatments for AIDS.* Published by the San Francisco AIDS Foundation, it's written by experts and intended for people without a scientific background. Before publication, it's reviewed for accuracy by physicians and activists together. The information offered is current and presented in a form that's easy to read. Any major scientific findings about HIV will be covered in *BETA* before they are published in medical journals.

AIDS Treatment News, written by John S. James, is a newsletter particularly respected by the HIV community.

A lighter approach, looking at the lifestyles and attitudes of people with HIV, is offered by *POZ,* published bimonthly in New York. It's a magazine, and a classy one.

You'll find a list of information sources, meaty but intelligible, in Appendix IX. Some of these offer scholarship programs if you can't afford a subscription. Where they don't, they may be able to tell you where in your area you can look at a copy.

If you *can* afford subscriptions, consider paying double, extending a scholarship to someone who can't.

Telephone Sources

BETA, funded by the San Francisco Aids Foundation, offers periodic national teleconferences. People in the forefront of HIV care—researchers, professors, clinicians, and those from other disciplines whose work has had a major impact on HIV management—are engaged to speak and answer questions from the telephone audience. Attendance at these teleconferences is easy (all it takes is a phone) and free. Normally each program is offered three times, to allow for more questions from a larger audience.

You can sign up for a session of *BETA* Live, as it's called, by phoning 800–707–BETA. Program content is advertised in each issue of *BETA* magazine, and transcriptions of prior teleconferences may be printed in the next issue.

Computer Sources
•

There's an amazing amount of information available by computer, if you have the access and skills. Some of it's free, once you get on the computer. Some of it's interactive, letting you discuss HIV-related issues with others like yourself.

Every issue of *BETA* is presented on computer in its entirety and made available to interactive networks.

Perhaps the most exciting benefit of computer access is that you can get a summary of anything in the current medical literature by plugging into the National Library of Medicine through Grateful Med (800–423–9255 for more information or to start service).

Grateful Med enables you to search all published studies in peer-reviewed (respected) journals, written by and for doctors. Titles, authors, and sources are cited, so you can look up any article in a medical library; but even better, this service will provide you with abstracts—brief summaries of findings for each paper.

For MEDLINE, the journal database that covers all aspects of medicine, there is usually a per-minute charge. One free site is http://www.ncbi.nlm.nih.gov/pubmed. But if you're searching on AIDSLINE—a separate database dealing only with medical publications that relate to HIV—your search will be free. In 1994, Congress felt that HIV was so critical, and its understanding so essential, that the public good would best be served by providing government support for this service. AIDSLINE can also be searched via the World Wide Web. (Figure 19.1 offers a list of computer sources for HIV-related information.)

FIGURE 19.1.

•

Internet Information Sources.

HIV InSite

This is an excellent website for basic and detailed information about HIV. Features include **AIDSLINE,** a fully searchable collection of medical articles about HIV/AIDS and an easy-to-use, complete database of **Clinical Trials** that can be searched by medical condition, treatment, medication, and state.

http://hivinsite.ucsf.edu

Immunet

A professional, easy-to-use site that features **AIDS Treatment News,** community forums, an exhaustive, searchable Global AIDS Resource Directory, and information on new treatments and trials.

http://www.immunet.org

AEGIS

The AIDS Education Global Information System lives up to its imposing name. This is the website with the **largest indexed, searchable knowledge base** out there, which means you can learn about almost anything from the same sources your doctor would use. This is a good place to access *BETA* and the National Library of Medicine's **AIDSLINE, AIDSDRUGS,** and **AIDSTRIALS.**

http://www.aegis.com

CDC AIDS Clinical Trials Information

This is the Centers for Disease Control's listing of AIDS clinical trials. They call it a partial listing, but it is still a good source of information.

http://www.actis.org

(continued next page)

The Body

This user friendly website is a good source for basic information about the HIV virus, treatment, and quality of life. Transcripts of the major national HIV conferences are also available here.

http://www.thebody.com/learning.html

Project Inform

Focusing on **upbeat advocacy** and getting current information in a concise form to people with HIV, this is a very useful site. In addition to a searchable list of excellent Project Inform publications, there are listings of town meetings, hotline numbers, and much more.

http://projinf.org

International Association of Physicians in AIDS Care

IAPAC's stated goal is to optimize the survival and quality of life of people with HIV globally. This translates into a focus on big-picture issues and an international perspective that differentiates it from most other websites.

http://www.iapac.org

Critical Path AIDS Project

This Philadelphia-based site has national links to HIV resources and is a great place to keep abreast of **what's new in HIV treatment.**

http://www.critpath.org

San Francisco AIDS Foundation

The SFAF site features excellent local and national content, HIV policy watch, needle-exchange information, and much more. This site is available in **Spanish.**

http://www.sfaf.org

AIDS New York City

The place to go for links to many community-based New York City organizations.

http://www.aidsnyc.org

This is a tremendous boon for those of us doing HIV research. It means we can afford to stay right up to date; all it takes is our time. But these benefits aren't just for doctors. They're for anyone who has access to equipment, knows enough to get value from scientific papers, and signs up. It's that simple.

This means that you, given a computer and a modem, can search on AIDSLINE for hours—printing out abstracts, as well as their sources; following controversies; getting the newest published information; knowing where to go, if you want, for more details. You can learn new ways to care for yourself, and make and defend your decisions.

I want to suggest strongly that, if you've made it this far through the book, there is value in AIDSLINE for you. Much of the basic science literature will be unintelligible—it is for a lot of doctors, too! But there are reviews and reports of new clinical research—reports you are now ready to understand—on almost all facets of HIV and AIDS. With AIDSLINE, you can look at every current paper that's been published on any topic, however obscure, that pertains to your particular case. The Grateful Med software even helps you learn how to search.

With the explosive growth of the World Wide Web, vast amounts of information are becoming available via the Internet. Information on clinical trials, new treatments, community resources, HIV/AIDS conferences, AIDSLINE, and much more has been placed on the web and is available to you. *While Internet access is not free, it may represent a good value for people with HIV.* If you can use a computer, you can build intellectual muscle and use it to help you stay well, in a way that has never before been possible.

• • •

Whatever you do, keep on learning. Look at many approaches. Look critically. Know your own case like you know your own face in the mirror. Keep talking to others. Share information, as well as support. Take part in your health care; but do so in a way that is informed, knowledgeable, and thoughtful.

Knowledge truly is power. This is personal activism at its best.

CHAPTER 20

•

Feeding the Soul

Most of what we've talked about so far has dealt with the physical aspects of HIV infection. There's so much to understand about the physiology, the body workings, of HIV in order to play a substantive role in your care. I could write a book about it.

But you're not just a body. If you're to make the most of your life, there's other healing, other work to be done.

The Connection Between Mind and Body
•

A lot of attention has been devoted over the past twenty years to the inseparability of body and spirit. That's not a new concept, but the body of scientific knowledge that addresses it is in fact fairly new.

Psychoneuroimmunology

Psychoneuroimmunology is the scientific term for something we have all suspected, if not built our lives on—the concept that those who feel better, do better. Research not only confirms this, but attempts to unravel the physiologic mechanisms through which it occurs.

Josie Levine, a San Francisco psychologist who has studied women living with HIV, defines psychoneuroimmunology as "the concept of interconnecting biological pathways through which emotions can affect the physiological body and the immune system." Put more simply, it defines the study of how your attitudes, your personal responses, and your emotions can affect your health.

It's been shown that feelings, attitudes, and coping strategies can directly affect resistance and response to disease. Essentially, your brain releases substances that initiate, and respond to, emotions. These substances trigger other changes in your endocrine or glandular system. Those changes act in turn on your immune system. That's especially important in a process like HIV infection, which acts principally through the immune system.

This is how placebo effects kick in. Your attitude of belief in a treatment creates certain emotions, such as hope—an expectation of success. These emotions are experienced, or felt, through the release of chemicals in your brain. These chemicals in turn affect endocrine and immune function, with the result that your expectation of success enhances your body's ability to bring about that success.

It has been estimated that *about 55 percent of the success of any medical treatment is due to placebo effect.* That's a powerful reason to be fully committed to any treatment you undergo.

But this system works both ways. Acute distress or depression can impair immune response. It's possible that grave internal conflict may thus be as bad for you as alcohol or cigarettes. And just as regular exercise can stimulate endorphin release, strengthening the immune response, distress or depression inhibits the release of certain other neurotransmitters. Not only are fewer of them made, but receptors—the paths by which other cells receive their signals—are also reduced. The spiral turns downward. The more depressed someone becomes, the harder it is to get out.

Fifty percent of people with HIV will experience a reactive depression within six months of diagnosis. Many of these are severe enough to be classed as clinical depression. Studies suggest that the result can affect not only your life, but your resistance to HIV.

That's one of the reasons it's critical to get help when distress becomes chronic or deep. It's hard to get out by yourself, and it's hard to stay well if you don't.

Let's look at some other things we've learned from the study of psychoneuroimmunology.

Just as type-A people—highly stressed, time-pressured, hostile—are at more risk for heart disease, people classed as Type C are more at risk for immune dysfunction. The characteristic that researchers use to define Type C is *compliance with external authority.* One's own feelings and needs are repressed in order to comply with another's. Eventually, numbing occurs; feelings and needs aren't heard when they're consistently denied. So people end up feeling helpless, not believing that anything they do can affect what will happen to them, and numb, not knowing why they are sad. The effects of learned helplessness on the immune system have been shown to be drastic.

Dr. Levine suggests that this is of special concern for women, whose conditioning and life circumstances more often support surrender to the will of others, and therefore to such feelings of helplessness.

Type-C behavior is a learned behavior. The brain is not hardwired. If you're there now, you don't have to stay there.

Traits that appear to *improve* immune function include:

- *Instrumentality.* The tendency to act when faced with a problem. This trait also seems to be associated with increased self-esteem and reduced anxiety about death.
- *Sense of personal responsibility.* The belief that one is accountable for one's actions and their results.
- *An internal locus of control.* A determination to make personal choices, to control a situation and its outcome. This trait is associated with decisive action in situations involving personal risk.
- *Flexibility.* The potential for moving from action, once defined as a masculine behavior, to expressiveness, once considered a feminine behavior, as the situation requires. The presence of both traits, or *androgyny,* appears to be most successful and confers the most flexibility.
- *Creativity.* The potential for seeing options where none

were seen before, for entertaining and communicating possibilities.

- *Commitment.* The ability to find meaning in work, relationships, and personal values.
- *Challenge.* The capacity to respond well to stressors, with less anxiety and greater expectation of success, viewing change as challenging and liking it.

No one has all of these traits. But this list gives us an idea of what to look for, what to reinforce in ourselves. And while change can be frightening at first, a step in these directions is likely to pay off in a renewed sense of power and personal integrity. These are good goals to work toward.

So the study of psychoneuroimmunology tells us that we should get help for depression; we should question our feelings of helplessness; we should look hard to learn how we feel; and we should cultivate those qualities that impel our commitment, put us in charge, and help us to handle our lives well. And, it suggests, to do so will help us stay well.

Lessons from Survivors

In his book *The Healing Path,* Mark Barasch reports on interviews with people who, once diagnosed with serious illness, lengthened their expected life span or reversed their disease. We call these people "medical miracles"; in the HIV community we might call them "long-term nonprogressors."

Certain traits were found to be common to many of Barasch's subjects. Some greeted their diagnosis with outrage, if not frank disbelief. They refused to accept their prognosis. Sometimes they refused or postponed treatments that were said to be critical to life.

Others accepted that they were going to die, but claimed for themselves the right to spend what time was left as they wished. And some of them didn't die.

Most informed themselves fully about their condition, seeking knowledge not only from doctors but from other sources of healing. They considered and often practiced alternative and spiritual approaches. When faced with great internal conflict, they listened, only accepting invasive or frightening treatment when they could make peace with it. Most of all, they insisted on being in charge.

They were willing to risk death, if need be, rather than surrender to a course they were wholly opposed to.

They looked deeply into their lives—not blaming themselves for their illness, but seeking roots of conflict—of "dis-ease"—within their own lives. They faced up to pain that they'd buried. They listened to symptoms; stopped working themselves, sometimes literally, to death; became less concerned with prestige; began to live life according to personal values, rather than those imposed from outside.

They looked at the ways they had cost themselves love in the name of protection. Once they weren't safe anymore, they could choose to take risks: exploring new levels of openness; becoming more creative, more tender, more playful.

They decided to do what they wanted with the time that was left. Sometimes that involved first *finding out* what they wanted; some of us are so used to caring for others, we don't even hear our own voice. Often, they had to deny the wishes of others. And many times, they risked ridicule. But when you know you're not immortal, ridicule loses its sting.

Psychoneuroimmunologists call this "adopting an internal locus of control"; I call it raising yourself.

Barasch also tells us that these people didn't try to travel alone. They found helpers—therapists, alternative healers, wise and close friends, often their doctors. They formed close alliances, choosing to learn and understand their helpers' approach to healing. The helpers were said to be empathetic, and not arrogant; to relate to them as individuals; to offer sanctuary; and to touch them. The qualities describing such a relationship sound a lot like qualities honored in psychoneuroimmunology: empowerment, control, commitment, creativity, and challenge.

Of course, the author interviewed only those who did well. Many of the others were dead. Many of *them* had been resistant to treatment, too, and might have done better with submission to conventional care.

The point is not that you should refuse care. It's rather that you should consider, investigate, and take part in every major step in treatment that you make—coming to peace with it and supporting it, rather than simply submitting. And you should address healing in every facet of your life. We have to bring healing to *all* of our being—not only our bodies, but our souls as well.

The Connection with Others
•

One of the important lessons we learn from Mark Barasch's subjects is to not try to do it alone.

Support Groups

Studies have shown that people who work in support groups live longer than people who don't. Judging by my own participation in groups at the Center for Attitudinal Healing, they probably have more fun, too. It's a huge relief to talk openly with others who face the same journey you do. It's thrilling to see how much you can offer to others. It's humbling to see how much love is available, and how easy it is to accept it.

People with chronic or life-threatening illness just don't have time to be petty. They talk about what matters: life, sex, relationships, secret fears, and pleasures. Thoughts that wake you at night and overwhelm you lose their fear when they're not held in secret — and when you find that others have laid them to rest.

These people talk in more practical terms, too. Some of the best tricks for comfort I've learned have come from the groups I attended.

And they're *funny*. There's so much absurdity, so much that's frankly ridiculous about dealing with chronic disease. Somehow laughter takes all the power from the pain. I don't think I've ever laughed harder than I have in support groups.

I have patients who won't go — they don't want to see sicker people or acknowledge that they're infected. But HIV is a trip to be shared. These groups are a haven, a place where you needn't pretend, needn't be what you're not. Acceptance from others — warts and all, so to speak — is often the first step toward accepting yourself as you are.

You'll also find critical information. HIV knowledge is building so rapidly that none of us can truly keep up with it; that's why the partnership between you and your doctor is so crucial. You'll have much to contribute if you catch up with other HIV warriors every week.

Friends and Family

It's important to maintain those relationships that have fed you. You'll find they will change: some will strengthen, others lose significance. Still others will appear and deepen. That's because *you* are changing, as you grow in response to your challenge. But family and old friends maintain a context and a depth of loyalty that comes from years of care. Supporting your attachments to the circle around you will stand you in good stead, now and later.

In particular, relationships with family may be easier than they used to be. Your family's on notice now: they know it's your turn, and they don't want to add to your stress. If they do, you can educate them. Tell them what you need. When one of their members is threatened, families often grow in ways never thought possible.

Your family needs your love and acceptance. It's okay to tell them how to make that possible.

Keep in contact. Pick up the phone. If you're starting to withdraw, let people know that. Let it be their turn to call you.

Try especially to share meals with people you love, when you can.

Social Service Networks

If you're ill, you may already have someone helping you. This kind of companionship is especially valuable, because it's undemanding. You can have company without even talking. And if you're open to it, an AIDS volunteer, chore worker, or companion may actually become a close friend.

Nurses and home care workers are in it because they love it, too. Even though the work is hard, and the loss is often painful, people who choose these professions do so because of the personal fulfillment they find in service. The comfort they offer to others fills genuine needs of their own. And again, in this case it's your turn.

The Importance of Touch

One of the greatest costs illness exacts is the loss of being touched. Older people experience this also, when the family's gone and they're on their own.

We need touch to know where our edges are. We need it to feel connected. That's why sleeping with someone, even without sex, leaves you so full in the morning. And touch can reduce pain, help us to find where we're causing our pain and let go, and take away sorrow even better than sleep. And it feels good.

If you have a partner, keep up sexual contact. Be careful about safety, but don't let it go. If sex isn't working, see your doctor. It may be your medicines, or low testosterone.

If sex doesn't interest you — or if it's not happening in your life — look for other sources of touching. Sleep with your partner, if you have one. Sleep with your pet, if you don't. Some people get a sense of being held from sleeping with a full-length pillow. If you don't have a partner, or a pet, or a pillow, you *really* need to be touched.

Are you being hugged? Are you hugging people? If not, can you change?

Massage is a wonderful way to be touched. It fills the basic need we all have; and it also relieves tension, gives sensory input to our whole body, touches and awakens our feelings, offers true communication. I can't believe we don't *all* get a massage every week.

Some massage therapists donate time to people with HIV. Others work on a sliding scale. If you're strong enough, you may find someone to trade with.

Music and Laughter

Music speaks directly to us, with no need for others to share it. But there are aspects of music that offer a lot to communication, and aspects of sharing that enrich us immeasurably.

If you have a religious tradition, you know the power of music. You know the reverence it elicits, and how much greater this is when your church or synagogue or temple is full of other people. Without a word spoken, music supports common values, reminds you of community. The pain of the world falls away.

I'm a Jew, but I go, almost every week, to a church in San Francisco called Glide Memorial. People pack the house — all types, all backgrounds, all beliefs. Clothes, money, religions may vary, but everyone wants to get in. And what do we do there? We sing. Loud, rocking gospel, song after song. In between, we hold hands. Or we all hug each other. There's even a sermon stuck in there somewhere. And we're so primed, we listen. Nobody even gets bored.

Cecil Williams, the man who heads this church, is famous. Not for the music of the Glide Ensemble, but for the incredible array of social service programs his church offers; for his outspoken support of people who are homeless, drug-addicted, ill, of different colors and sexual persuasions; for the people Glide feeds every day and those it's preparing to house; for Williams's ability to bring people together for social action, reaching beyond themselves to help their neighbors.

And he does it, to start with, with music. When you're hearing such sound—dancing to it, clapping to it, singing, letting go—you join that community unreservedly and are fed by it. You get happy. You find your best self. You feel strong again and let go of the pretense, the disillusionment, the belief that what you do makes no difference, the fear that you're in this alone.

You get honest, because you are safe. And you'll do anything you can, give money or time or your presence, to help others in that community or the community of the world. For me, I am brought to that innocence by the power of the music in the company of others.

Most of us have other musical traditions, as well. Playing certain music brings back the same feelings. Sharing it with others breaks down barriers, reminds us of our commonality.

You can use music for comfort, for energy, to honor or alter a mood, to lift a relationship closer to trust. And it's always there.

Laughter also speaks to the heart. It's contagious—a delicious form of communication, more physical than verbal in effect.

Norman Cousins was the first to let us know the power of laughter; he swore that he laughed himself well. In his case, he deliberately sought it—with movies, books, comedic settings—as therapy for immunologic illness. The benefits to his soul were secondary.

And he may have been right. Just *try* to stay stuck in your anger or misery, if someone can get you to laugh.

Laughter's a great example of the mind-body connection. It doesn't just reflect your mood—it changes it. You're different before it than after. I bet you can't laugh for one full minute, right now, over nothing, without feeling better when you're done.

The Connection with the World
•

The soul is also fed by helping others. In the case of people with HIV, it's especially important.

We need to fight this disease fully. We can do so not only through caring for our own bodies, but by caring for others with HIV.

It's a good survival mechanism, first of all: the people who survived the concentration camps, for instance, were those especially concerned with others. It made them determined to stay alive.

It strengthens our fighting stance. If we are uncompromisingly committed to fighting HIV, I think the body will hear that and respond. But more than this, it feels good. We know we're part of a larger community. We know we can help make a difference.

I believe this kind of empowerment will help keep you well. And regardless of that, it will feed your soul.

Volunteering

Many AIDS organizations have a volunteer corps. In most cases volunteers provide support to a person with AIDS—helping with housework or errands, walking the dog, assisting with bills, or just visiting. Volunteers may also be needed to help deliver meals to people who are ill. If you have a special skill—like massage or haircutting, lawyering or counseling—you may choose to offer that service instead.

This is a good thing to do when you're well. There's often a fair amount of physical effort required. It's good to help others, but you must guard your own body, too.

Activism

Much of the change that has come about in this country in support of people with HIV has occurred due to the work of activists. Political organizations like Act Up strike fear into the hearts of businesspeople and bureaucrats alike. Their work has resulted in important gains—early access to new treatments, for example, and lower prices for some drugs.

Organizations that provide programs and information help to educate those who would learn, enabling them to take part in and understand decisions about their care. This is true activism also.

If you choose to take part at this level, you'll know you are helping the cause for people for years to come. You may find it's a constructive outlet for your undifferentiated anger, too.

The Connection to Self: The Value of Solitude
•

Because many people living with chronic illness are lonely, we tend to focus more on maintaining contact with others than we do on going within. But this internal quest is also crucial.

Loneliness means needing contact and not being able to get it. But solitude can also be a pleasure. Developing an appetite for the pleasure it provides can help us get closer to ourselves.

Introspection

We looked at the importance of introspection when we considered lessons from survivors. The people discussed there all chose to look closely at themselves. They worked to strip away the false fronts they'd put on for others, in order to find their own voice. Along the way, there were surprises. Hidden memories, particularly of childhood, were often quite painful to face. Their own anger and ugliness—traits present in everyone—also took work to accept. The work wasn't easy, and the course was often slow, as it is for most of us. But they found, as they made their way through, that recalling their pain would release or soften it. By truly experiencing long-repressed pain, they were freed of its power.

The energy they saved by allowing those parts of themselves to surface was now free. They had more strength in the present, to live and to make themselves whole.

Internal work of this depth is best served if it's done with another. The intensity of suffering is diminished when shared. This is the value of therapy or counseling.

But the bulk of the work is internal. It takes time, time alone to reflect on these matters. It takes listening. To listen, there has to be quiet.

This, I think, marks the difference between productive and unproductive sorrow. Depression, or pain you can't handle, gets stuck. It should not be allowed to drag on or become too severe to be borne. But the secrets we find when we listen alone often free us. Even when we cry, we cry old tears. Letting them flow lets them go.

This is often the first step toward raising ourselves, toward learning what we really want and what our needs and values really are. There's an important role for solitude, I think, to permit time for self-exploration.

Solitude is also needed for the full expression of our creativity. When you're still, and not distracted, new ideas arise. You can follow them up, write them down, act on them. You cannot create and respond simultaneously.

Meditation

We need solitude, like sleep, for our healing. We need time to be only ourselves, entirely at rest. Meditation offers us this time. When directed, it may bring us to some spiritual realization we are reaching for. But even mindless meditation—perhaps most of all mindless meditation—allows our body to reorganize itself and address its own healing beneath the cognitive level.

Mindless meditation, actually, is not likely to result without years of practice. There's too much lined up waiting for attention. But to simply *be*, without direction, for a part of every day, can offer peace and healing to your body.

Music

Music heightens our relationship to others and to the community at large. That's much of its extraordinary value. But it also has a value just for us.

It deepens the experience of our moods. It comforts us, perhaps especially when we're alone. There's a gentle healing to it. Nothing is required in response. It helps us find our spiritual core—that inner strength that's not reactive to the world around us.

• • •

Cultivate your appetite for solitude. Let it be a balance to your appetite for companionship and your drive to help others.

Cultivate your soul. In the spare time remaining, between learning and eating and exercising and treating, be sure to have a nice time.

• • •

Last May we had a celebration at my office, to express together our gratitude for coming back to life from HIV. I looked around at maybe sixty people. Many of them had been written off and left for dead by someone, some time within the last three years. And with our support and agreement, they had decided not to die. And they didn't. We played kick-the-can with them long enough to get them to the next place, where they are firmly planted now. They wanted it, they asked for it, they earned it. And they have taken back their right to life.

That victory and sense of gratitude is not peculiar to our office. Clinics and offices and buyers' clubs and activist organizations all over the country have had the same experience.

A lot of these people made it to this moment because they had access to costly therapies, nutritional and medical—used judiciously and appropriately, and sometimes in combination—when they were needed. They refused to roll over and die on schedule and looked for another way. Others—their doctors, their friends, the advocates and activists who have made this fight their life—heard their call and joined their battle. And now they are here, and starting over.

You can make that decision, too. Whether you, like Ignacio, are learning and teaching from a prison cell in Florida; or dancing in the Castro or in Chelsea; or fighting for your own rights in Montgomery—whatever you have done with your life before this moment, wherever you stand in the continuum of HIV infection, you can choose, at this moment, to take charge.

Be hungry; learn everything you can. Be generous and open, sharing knowledge back and forth. Trust your instincts, but build on them and train them. Change your mind when knowledge changes. Push those of us who care for you to match your greatest effort with our own.

Let go of pain and anger you no longer need. Ride your anger when it strengthens you. Love yourself, love yourself, every chance you get. It's a brave fight you are fighting, and you well may win.

You are the architect of your own healing. And you don't have to die anymore.

REFERENCES

Barasch, M. I. *The Healing Path*. New York: Penguin, 1994.

Cousins, N. *Anatomy of an Illness*. New York: Doubleday, 1981.

Cousins, N. *Head First: The Biology of Hope and the Healing Power of the Human Spirit*. New York: Penguin, 1989.

Katoff, L. "Psychological study of long-term survivors of AIDS." *HIV/AIDS Clinical Insights,* 1994, *3*(1), 5–6.

Levine, J. "Androgyny, creativity and locus of control as predictors of depression in HIV positive women." Unpublished doctoral dissertation, California Institute of Integral Studies, San Francisco, 1993.

Moore, T. *Care of the Soul: A Guide for Cultivating Depth and Sacredness in Everyday Life.* New York: HarperCollins, 1992.

Storr, A. *Solitude.* New York: HarperCollins, 1994.

•

1993 CDC Criteria for a Diagnosis of AIDS

CD4+ (or T-Helper Cell) Count

CD4+ T cells less than 200 per microliter or
CD4+ percentage less than 14 percent

AIDS-Defining Clinical Conditions

- Candidiasis of bronchi, trachea, or lungs
- Esophageal candidiasis
- Invasive cervical cancer
- Disseminated (throughout the body) or extrapulmonary (outside of the lung) coccidiomycosis
- Extrapulmonary cryptococcosis
- Chronic intestinal cryptosporidiosis of more than one month's duration

Adapted from the Centers for Disease Control and Prevention, 1993 revised classification system for HIV infection and expanded surveillance case definition for AIDS among adolescents and adults. *Morbidity and Mortality Weekly Report,* 1992, *41*(No. RR-17), 2–15.

- Cytomegalovirus disease other than in liver, spleen, or nodes
- Cytomegalovirus retinitis with loss of vision
- HIV-related encephalopathy
- Chronic herpes simplex ulcers of more than one month's duration
- Herpes simplex bronchitis, pneumonitis, or esophagitis
- Disseminated or extrapulmonary histoplasmosis
- Chronic intestinal isosporiasis of more than one month's duration
- Kaposi's sarcoma
- Burkitt's lymphoma, immunoblastic lymphoma, or primary lymphoma of brain
- Disseminated or extrapulmonary mycobacterium avium complex or *M. kansasii* or other or unidentified mycobacterium species
- Mycobacterium tuberculosis, any site
- Pneumocystis carinii pneumonia
- Recurrent pneumonia
- Progressive multifocal leukoencephalopathy
- Recurrent salmonella septicemia
- Toxoplasmosis of brain
- Wasting syndrome due to HIV

APPENDIX II

•

Diet Diary and Nutritional Assessment Form

Your Diet Diary
•

Be sure to include everything you eat and drink, including random nibblings. Estimate amounts: one-half-cup carrots, twelve ounces soda or juice, and so on. Estimate water intake separately.

Day of Diary: 1   2   3   **Water**   **Calories**

Breakfast:

Morning Snacks:

Lunch:

Afternoon Snacks:

Dinner:

Evening Snacks:

Bedtime Snacks:

**Summary
Calories:**   Day 1   2   3   Average

Number of Servings: **Day 1**   **2**   **3**   **Average**

Solid Food

Meat, protein, eggs

Green or yellow vegetables

Fruits

Dairy products

Bread, grains, cereals

Potatoes, pasta, rice

High-sugar snacks

High-fat snacks

Other

Liquids (by cups or ounces)

Fruit juices

Vegetable juices

Clear soups and broths

Soda

Milk

Coffee, tea, diet soda

Water

Total

Your Nutritional Assessment
•

Part I: Who You Are, What You Eat, and What You Need

1. Who You Are

Name:

Age: Gender: M   F

If female, are you pregnant?

2. Your HIV Status

Year of diagnosis:

Estimated year of infection:

Stage of HIV:

Positive, no symptoms   x

Mild symptoms   x

AIDS, no symptoms   x

AIDS, mild symptoms   x

Active secondary infection (SI)   x

Active wasting   x

Stage of HIV by T4 cell (CD4) count, if known:

More than 500   x

More than 200   x

More than 100   x

More than 50   x

Less than 50   x

3. Your Weight Status

Height:

Ideal body weight (from Table II.1):

Usual weight (before infection or diagnosis):

Current weight:

As percentage of ideal body weight:

$$\frac{Current\ weight}{Ideal\ weight} \times 100 = \underline{\hspace{1cm}} percent$$

As percentage of usual weight:

$$\frac{Current\ weight}{Usual\ weight} \times 100 = \underline{\hspace{1cm}} percent$$

Prior episodes of rapid weight loss?   x

Associated with other infections?   x

Current weight loss?   x

How much?

Over how long?

4. What You're Eating

Average number of daily meals:

Average calories per day:

Average number of servings per day:

Protein (meat, eggs, tofu, etc.)

Vegetables

Fruits and juices

Dairy products

Complex carbohydrates (bread, grains, cereals, potatoes, pasta, rice)

High-sugar snacks

High-fat snacks

Vitamins and Minerals:

Combination multivitamin x

Combination trace-element supplement x

Specific Vitamins and Antioxidants:

Vitamin	Amount	Times a Day
1.		
2.		
3.		
4.		
5.		

(If more, continue on a separate page.)

Specific Trace Elements (zinc, selenium, etc.):

Element	Amount	Times a Day
1.		
2.		
3.		

(If more, continue on a separate page.)

Dietary Supplements:

Oral Supplements (medical foods) or

Enteral Supplements (taken into the stomach):

Supplement	Amount	Times a Day
1.		
2.		

(If more, continue on a separate page.)

Total Parenteral Nutrition, or TPN (taken into the vein)

5. How You Spend Your Energy

Type of Work (circle one):

Heavy   Moderate   Sedentary   None

Type of Exercise (circle one):

Heavy   Moderate   Mild   None

Frequency of Exercise (number of times a week):

Summary, Part I:

Average calories per day (from Section 4)   _____

Recommended calories per day (from Table II.2)   _____

Recommended change   _____

Average protein per day (from Table II.3)   _____

Recommended protein per day (from Table II.2)   _____

Recommended change   _____

Part II: Improving Your Nutrition

6. Current Medications

Over-the-Counter (nonprescription):

Name	Dose	Times a Day	Purpose
1.			
2.			
3.			
4.			
5.			

Prescription:

Name	Dose	Times a Day	Purpose
1.			
2.			
3.			
4.			
5.			
6.			
7.			

(If more, continue on a separate page.)

Alternative Treatments (herbs, others not listed above):

1.

2.

3.

4.

5.

(If more, continue on a separate page.)

Recreational Drugs, If Used (include alcohol and cigarettes):

Type of Drug	*Amount*	*Frequency of Use*
1.		
2.		
3.		
4.		
5.		

(If more, continue on a separate page.)

7. How You Get Your Food

Who does the shopping (circle one)?

Self   Others at home   Feeding program

Is cost a major factor in purchasing decisions?   x

Who prepares meals (circle one)?

Self   Others at home   Friends   Feeding program

How is your food prepared?

Facilities (circle all that apply):

Sink   Stove or hot plate   Oven

Microwave   Refrigerator   Freezer

None

Methods (circle all that apply):

Fresh, raw   Frying   Steaming

Broiling   Slow-cook   Ready to eat

Prevention:

Raw foods prewashed?   x

Rapid refrigeration or freezing:

Between preparation and eating?   x

After eating? x

Regular system of discarding refrigerated foods? x

Preparer washes hands before food preparation? x

8. Favorite Foods

Food Group	*Degree of Preference (1 = love, 3 = tolerate)*		
Meat, Eggs, Other Protein			
1.	1	2	3
2.	1	2	3
3.	1	2	3
4.	1	2	3
Vegetables			
1.	1	2	3
2.	1	2	3
3.	1	2	3
4.	1	2	3
Fruits and Juices			
1.	1	2	3
2.	1	2	3
3.	1	2	3
4.	1	2	3
Dairy Products			
1.	1	2	3
2.	1	2	3
3.	1	2	3
4.	1	2	3

Bread, Grains, Cereals

1.   1   2   3

2.   1   2   3

3.   1   2   3

4.   1   2   3

Potatoes, Pasta, Rice

1.   1   2   3

2.   1   2   3

3.   1   2   3

High-Sugar Snacks

1.   1   2   3

2.   1   2   3

3.   1   2   3

High-Fat Snacks

1.   1   2   3

2.   1   2   3

3.   1   2   3

4.   1   2   3

Comfort foods—foods that elicit good memories and make you feel loved, peaceful, or happy:

1.

2.

3.

4.

5.

6.

9. Special Problems:

Trouble eating or swallowing? (Circle all that apply):

Mouth infections or ulcers	Throat pain
Dry mouth	Dental pain
Choking or coughing	Pain with chewing
Insufficient teeth for chewing	

Appetite loss:

Triggers (circle all that apply):

Pain	Nausea
Diarrhea	Early satiety (fullness)
Apathy	Depression
Fatigue	Change in taste or smell
Confusion	

Tested for malabsorption?   x

Metabolic regulation disturbed (fevers, night sweats)?   x

10. Summary of Recommendations (See Text)

TABLE II.1
•
Estimating Ideal Body Weight

Men

height _____ # inches over 5 feet _____ × 6 = _____

add   106 pounds

total for men   _____

Women

height _____ # inches over 5 feet _____ × 5 = _____

add   100 pounds

total for women   _____

Adjustment for Frame (choose one):

small   × 0.9 =

medium   × 1 =

large   × 1.1 =

Ideal Body Weight   _____

To Determine Frame Size

height (inches)   _____ × 2.5 = A _____

wrist circumference (inches)

                        _____ × 2.5 = B _____

A divided by B =   _____

                                                                Frame size is

if less than 9.6 (men) or 9.9 (women)   large

if more than 10.4 (men) or 10.9 (women)   small

all others   medium

TABLE II.2
•
Daily Calories Needed, Men

___

Add:

weight _____ × 6.2 = _____

height _____

number of inches over 5 feet × 12.5 = _____

plus 816

subtotal _____

Subtract:

age _____ × 6.8 = (____)

subtotal _____

Multiply:

Activity Level (choose one):

bedridden × 1.2

minimal activity × 1.3

normal activity × 1.3–1.5

strenuous activity × 1.6 = _____

Special factors (choose one):

none × 1.0

attempting gain × 1.2

active illness/wasting × 1.6 = _____

Number of Calories Needed _____

Amount of Protein Needed (choose one):

maintenance: calories needed × 0.031 = _____ Grams

anabolism (repletion):

calories needed × 0.042 = _____ Grams

TABLE II.2 (continued)

•

Daily Calories Needed, Women

Add:

weight _____ × 4.4 = _____

height _____

number of inches over 5 feet × 4 = _____

plus 910

    subtotal _____

Subtract:

age _____ × 4.7 = (_____)

    subtotal _____

Multiply:

Activity Level (choose one):

    bedridden × 1.2

    minimal activity × 1.3

    normal activity × 1.3–1.5

    strenuous activity × 1.6 = _____

Special factors (choose one):

    none × 1.0

    attempting gain × 1.2

    active illness/wasting × 1.6 = _____

Number of Calories Needed _____

Amount of Protein Needed (choose one):

maintenance: calories needed × 0.031 = _____ Grams

anabolism (repletion):

    calories needed × 0.042 = _____ Grams

TABLE II.3
•
Protein Sources

	Serving Size	Grams
Protein		
meat and poultry (at 7 grams/ounce)	four ounces	28
fish (except shellfish or canned fish)	four ounces	28
shellfish or canned tuna or salmon	four ounces	14
egg	two	14
tofu	four ounces	7
frankfurter	one	7
luncheon meats	two ounces	14
Vegetables		
corn, peas, lima beans	one-half cup	3
cooked dried beans and lentils	one-third cup	3
green vegetables and salads:		
raw	one cup	2
cooked	one-half cup	2
tomato	one large	2
tomato or vegetable juice	one cup	4
Fruits and Juices	not applicable	0
Dairy Products		
cheese:		
cottage cheese, ricotta	one cup	14
grated Parmesan	two tablespoons	7
Swiss, American, blue,		
mozzarella, etc.	two ounces	14
milk	eight ounces	8
yogurt	eight ounces	8
pudding	one-half cup	3
ice cream	one-half cup	3
Complex Carbohydrates		
pasta	one cup	6
rice	one cup	9
potatoes	one cup	6
cooked cereals, grains	one-half cup	3
puffed cereals	one cup	2

TABLE II.3 (continued)
•
Protein Sources

	Serving Size	Grams
bagel, English muffin, bun	one	6
bread	one slice	3
cornbread	four ounces	6
popcorn	one cup	1
saltines, similar crackers	six	3

High-Sugar Snacks

	Serving Size	Grams
cake (angel, yellow, etc.)	three-inch square	6
vanilla wafers	six	3
cookies, small	two	3
frozen yogurt	one cup	9

High-Fat Snack

	Serving Size	Grams
peanut butter	two tablespoons	14

Combinations

	Serving Size	Grams
pizza	one fourth of 10″	13
casseroles, chili	one cup	20
macaroni and cheese	one cup	13
spaghetti and meatballs	one cup	13
soup:		
bean or chunky	one can	12
broth or cream (milk is extra)	one cup	3

APPENDIX III

•

List of Caloric Values

Meats (cooked, 3 oz.)

Corned beef—canned	210
Ground beef—broiled	
regular	245
lean	230
extra lean	215
Oven-cooked roast	
lean and fat	205–225
lean only	155–165
Pot roast—braised/sim-mered	
lean and fat	225–330
lean only	190–235
Steak—sirloin, broiled	
lean and fat	240
lean only	180
Veal cutlet— broiled/braised	185

Ground lamb—broiled	305
Leg of lamb—roasted	
lean and fat	235
lean only	160
Lamb shoulder chop— broiled	
lean and fat	285
lean only	175
Ham—canned, heated	160
Ham—cured, roasted	
lean and fat	205
lean only	135
Pork loin—roasted	
lean and fat	270
lean only	205
Pork loin chop—broiled	
lean and fat	290
lean only	215

Source: Calories & Weight: The USDA Pocket Guide.

Pork shoulder—braised

lean and fat	295
lean only	210

Poultry
Chicken—fried
Breast half, medium

meat only	160
flour coating	215
batter-dipped	365

Drumstick, medium

meat only	80
flour coating	120
batter-dipped	195

Thigh, medium

meat only	110
flour coating	160
batter-dipped	235

Chicken—roasted
Breast half, medium

meat only	140
meat and skin	190

Drumstick, medium

meat only	75
meat and skin	110

Turkey—roasted (3 oz.)

light meat only	135
light meat and skin	165
dark meat only	160
dark meat and skin	185

Eggs

Deviled—large (1)	125
Fried—large (1)	95
Hard or soft—large (1)	80
Omelet—plain, with milk and fat added, large (1)	105
Poached—large (1)	80

Scrambled—with milk
and fat added, large (1) 105

Seafood (3 oz.)

Clams	80
Crabmeat	85
Cod—breaded, fried	180
Fish—battered, fried	185
Fish sticks—frozen (3)	175
Flounder	115
Haddock	110
Ocean perch—breaded	190
Oysters—breaded, large (3)	155

Salmon

baked or broiled	145
canned, drained	125

Sardines—Atlantic, drained	175

Shrimp

canned	100
French-fried, large (5)	210

Tuna—light, drained

canned in oil	170
canned in water	110

Luncheon Meats (2 oz.)

Bacon—cooked, slices (3)	140

Bologna

beef or pork	180
chicken or turkey	115

Frankfurter—heated (1)

beef or pork	150
chicken or turkey	110
Ham—chopped	140

Ham

boiled, regular	90
boiled, lean	75

Luncheon Meats (2 oz.)

Pork sausages

patty (1)	100
links (2)	95
Salami	140

Vienna sausage—

canned (3)	135

Organ Meats

Beef liver—fried (3 oz.)	195

Chicken liver

cooked (1)	45
cooked (3 oz.)	195

Vegetables (1/2 cup)

Alfalfa sprouts—raw	5
Artichoke (1)	55
Asparagus—cooked	20

Beans

lima, cooked	110
snap, cooked	25

Bean sprouts

raw	15
cooked	30
Beets—cooked	25
Beet greens—cooked	20

Broccoli

flowerets, raw (3)	10
chopped, cooked	25
5-in. spear (3), cooked	30

Brussels sprouts,

cooked	30

Cabbage

plain raw	10
shredded, cooked	15
coleslaw	70

Carrots

shredded, raw	25
sliced, cooked	35

Cauliflower

raw (4)	10
cooked	20

Celery

raw (1)	5
diced, cooked	10
Chives (1 tbsp.)	trace
Collards—chopped	10

Corn

kernels	90
cream-style	90
on the cob, 5-in. ear (1)	80

Cucumbers—raw

(6–8 slices)	10
Eggplant—cubed, cooked	15

Lettuce

head (1 cup)	5
loose-leaf (1 cup)	5

Mushrooms

raw	10
cooked	20
Okra—sliced, cooked	30

Onions

raw (2 tbsp.)	5
cooked	30
Peas—green, cooked	65

Peppers

chopped, raw	20
cooked, medium (1)	20

Potatoes

au gratin	175
baked, medium (1)	220
boiled w/o skin, sliced	65
hash browns	155
mashed (homemade)	80–115
mashed (flakes)	110
puffs, oven-heated (10)	175

Potatoes

salad	130
scalloped	120
Pumpkin—canned	30
Radishes—medium (4)	5
Sauerkraut—heated	15

Spinach

raw, pieces (1 cup)	5
chopped, cooked	20

Squash

summer, raw	10
summer, cooked	20
winter, baked, cubed	40
winter, boiled, mashed	45

Sweet potatoes

baked, peeled, medium (1)	115
candied, 2.5 x 2 in. (1)	145
canned, pieces	90
canned, mashed	115

Tomatoes

raw, medium (1)	25
cooked	25
Tomato sauce	35

Turnips

raw	20
cooked	15
Turnip greens—cooked	15

Vegetable Juice (6 oz.)

Tomato juice	30
Vegetable juice cocktail	35

Fruits (¹/₂ cup)

Apples—raw (1)	80

Applesauce

sweetened	95
unsweetened	50

Apricots

raw (3)	50
canned in juice	60
canned in syrup	105
dried halves	105

Avocados

California, 4 oz.	140
Florida, 8 oz.	245
Bananas—raw (1)	105

Blueberries

raw	40
frozen, unsweetened	40
frozen, sweetened	95
Cantaloupe—raw, ¹/₄ melon	60

Cherries

sour	40
sweet	50

Cranberry sauce

(¹/₄ cup)	105
Dates—dried, pitted	115

Fruit cocktail

in juice	55
in heavy syrup	90

Grapefruit

raw (¹/₂)	40
canned, in juice	45
in light syrup	75
Grapes—raw	55

Honeydew melon—raw

6–7 inch, ¹/₈ melon	55
cubed	30
Kiwi fruit—raw (1)	45
Nectarine—raw (1)	65
Orange—raw (1)	60

Peaches

raw (1)	40
sliced	35

Fruits (½ cup)

Peaches—canned	
in juice	55
in light syrup	70
in heavy syrup	95
Peaches—dried	
halves	100
Peaches—frozen,	
sweetened	120
Pears	
raw (1)	100
canned, in juice	60
canned, in syrup	100
Pineapple	
raw	40
canned in juice	75
canned in syrup	100
Plantains—cooked	110
Plums	
raw (1)	35
canned in juice	75
canned in syrup	115
Prunes—dried (5)	85
Raisins (1/2 oz.)	40
Raspberries	
raw	30
frozen sweetened	130
Rhubarb—cooked	140
Strawberries	
raw	25
frozen sweetened	110
Tangerines—raw (1)	35
Watermelon—raw	25

Breads (one slice)

Bagel (whole)	165
Cracked wheat	65
French	70
Italian	70

Pita	
white	125
whole wheat	115
Pumpernickel	60
Raisin	70
Rye	65
White	
regular slice	65
thin slice	55
Whole wheat	60

Fruit Juice (6 oz.)

Apple juice/cider	85
Apricot nectar—	
canned	105
Cranberry juice—	
canned	110
Grape juice	
canned/bottle	115
concentrate	95
Grapefruit	
fresh	70
canned	
unsweetened	70
canned sweetened	85
concentrate	75
Lemon (1 tbsp.)	5
Lime (1 tbsp.)	5
Orange	
fresh/concentrate	85
canned	80
Pineapple—canned	105

Milk (1 cup)

Buttermilk	100
Lowfat—1 percent	105
Lowfat—2 percent	120
Skim	85
Whole	150

Cheese (1 oz.)

American	105
Blue—crumbled	
(¼ cup)	120
Cheddar	115
Cream cheese	100
Feta—crumbled	
(¼ cup)	90
Mozzarella	80
Parmesan—grated	
(1 tbsp.)	25
Provolone	100
Swiss	105

Rolls

Croissant	230
Dinner	85
Hot dog/hamburger	130
Hard	155
Submarine	145

Specialty Breads

Biscuits	
homemade	115
refrigerated	
dough	55
Banana bread	150
Coffee cake	100
Cornbread	160
Danish pastry	395
Doughnuts	
plain	165
glazed	245
English muffin	130
Muffin	
blueberry	165
corn	165
bran	125
Pancake	90

Toaster pastry	210
Waffle	
homemade	205
frozen	100

Crackers

Cheese (10)	50
Graham (2)	55
Matzoh (1)	120
Oyster (10)	45
Rye wafers (2)	50
Saltines (2)	25
Whole wheat (2)	30

Snacks

Ice cream (½ cup)	135
Frozen yogurt (½ cup)	105
Chocolate chip cookie (1)	50
Peanut butter cookie (1)	80

Cereals (1 oz.)

All-Bran	70
Bran flakes	90
Cheerios	110
Corn flakes	110
Grits	
regular/quick	110
instant	80
Corn Pops	105
Cream of Wheat	100
Frosted flakes	110
Frosted Mini-Wheats	100
Grape-Nut Flakes	100
Honey Smacks	105
Nature Valley Granola	130
Oatmeal	
regular	110
instant	105
Raisin bran	85

Cereals (1 oz.)

Rice Chex	110
Rice Krispies	110
Shredded Wheat	100
large biscuits	85
Special K	110
Total	100
Wheaties	100

Pastas

Macaroni	75
Noodles	100
Rice	
brown	115
instant	90
white	110
Spaghetti	75

APPENDIX IV

•

Vitamin Supplementation Sources

Jarrow Formulas
182411/2 South Robertson Blvd., Los Angeles, CA 90035
310–204–6936

Rainbow Light
207 McPherson Street, Santa Cruz, CA 95060
408–429–9089

Twin Lab
2120 Smithtown Avenue, Ronkonkoma, NY 11779
516–467–3140

APPENDIX V

•

Types of Studies to Evaluate Drug Effects

There are several ways to study a drug's actions. We can take an animal—a mouse or a monkey, for instance—and design a situation that is roughly comparable to the situation we want to study in humans. Mice, for example, can be infected with a mouse retrovirus, which acts on them the way HIV acts on us. Then we can expose these mice to a drug, see its effects, and infer from those effects its potential effect on people.

We call these *animal studies*.

This is a good way to start looking at a question, as mice are more expendable than people. Mice, however, are *not* people; so the inferences may not hold true. In addition, it's hard to evaluate these studies, because doses are hard to compare.

We can also take cells, from people or animals, and grow them in a dish in the lab. We can use cells already infected with HIV, or we can infect them in the petri dish, measuring viral production in that culture. Then we can add a drug and study its effect on those cells.

These are called *in vitro* studies—which translates roughly into "studies in the soup."

In vitro studies may give us more worthwhile information; if we use human cells, we are at least examining our own species, judging effects on our own cells. And we're still not putting people at risk. But this model ignores the tremendous complexity, and the whole universe of interrelated responses and compensations, within an intact, living organism. And again, doses are hard to compare to real-life situations.

We can study the natural history of people who have used a particular drug and people who have not—not designing the drug's actions and results, but simply reporting what has happened. These are called *retrospective* studies; they carry less weight in the scientific community because of a lack of control. We didn't plan the study in advance; we didn't find a way to exclude other variables, other influences, that may have contributed to the final outcome.

We can also observe people directly. We can divide them up into groups: people who use a drug, for example, and people who don't. We can then see what is different in their outcome.

These are called *observational* studies. The drawback here is that people have chosen the group they belong to. There may be other characteristics associated with those who made that choice that independently influence outcome.

We can take people who are all roughly the same. We can design the study in advance, randomly divide the group, give the drug to some and not to others, and compare the outcome.

These are called *prospective, randomized, controlled* studies—the untreated group, having the same characteristics as the treated group, acts as a *control,* or comparison point, for the subjects in the treated group.

We can then eliminate the effect of subjective bias in the participants by not telling the subjects or controls whether they're getting the real drug or just a *placebo*—an inert substance made to look like the real drug. We can eliminate bias in the doctors, too, if we also keep them in the dark about who is getting what, until the experiment is ended and the code is broken.

These are then called *prospective, randomized, double-blinded, placebo-controlled* studies. When performed with enough subjects for results to be significant—not subject to chance—they are the gold standard for clinical research.

These are the kinds of results a drug company must show to get a drug to market.

Most research, especially initial research, is not done in this way. It takes large numbers of subjects to obtain significant results. The studies are expensive. And we run the risk of hurting people if what we give them is not good for them. No one, for example, would take two hundred HIV-infected people and shoot half of them up with cocaine for three weeks to see if it wrecked their immune system. It wouldn't be ethical. But it's important to evaluate any research that you hear reported, giving the results the weight they deserve while recognizing opportunities for error due to study design.

Most studies looking at recreational drugs and their effects on HIV are either animal studies, in vitro studies, or retrospective observational studies. Studies on antioxidant vitamins, discussed in Chapter Four, are largely in vitro studies.

The Food and Drug Administration requires that any prescription drug, for use in HIV or any other illness, be evaluated with prospective, randomized, double-blinded, controlled studies prior to approval for use. These studies are generally done in phases. The nature of Phase I, Phase II, and Phase III studies is discussed in Chapter Sixteen.

APPENDIX VI

•

HIV Flow Sheet

HIV Flow Sheet

Name: Baseline weight:

Date tested positive: Measured height:

Measurements:

DATE					
Weight					
Body cell mass					

Routine Labs:

DATE					
Hematocrit					
White count					
Absolute neutrophil count					
Albumin					
Triglycerides					
LFTs up?					

Serial Labs:

DATE					
CD4					
CD8					
CD4%					
Viral load					

One-Time Labs: DATE   DATE

Hep B S Ag _____ _____   HSV Ab   _____ _____

Hep B S Ab _____ _____   CMV Ab   _____ _____

Hep Be Ag _____ _____   Toxo Ab   _____ _____

Hep C Ag _____ _____   G6PD   _____ _____

Hep A Ab _____ _____   Erythropoetin _____ _____

Annual Labs:

DATE _____ _____ _____

B12 _____ _____ _____

Folate _____ _____ _____

Magnesium _____ _____ _____

Testosterone _____ _____ _____

DHEA _____ _____ _____

PPD _____ _____ _____

Controls _____ _____ _____

Stool for O&P   1) _____   2) _____   3) _____

1) _____   2) _____   3) _____

1) _____   2) _____   3) _____

Rectal pap _____ _____ _____

Serial Labs:

DATE						
TIBC						
Prealbumin						
D-xylose						
Sudan stain						
Amylase						
LDH						
SGOT						
SGPT						
Alk phos						
Bilirubin						
GGTP						

APPENDIX VII

•

Recommended Schedules for Prophylaxis of Infection

At Initial Evaluation
•

Vaccinations

1. Pneumococcal vaccination if not done within preceding six years. Should be repeated every six years.
2. Consider influenza vaccine, if CD4 count over 300.
3. Hepatitis B vaccine series if hepatitis antibody–negative and any IV drug use or sexual activity. Also recommended for health care workers, or if sexual partner or household members are carriers of hepatitis B. Hepatitis A vaccine if antibody negative.
4. Consider diphtheria/tetanus booster every ten years. Alternatively, tetanus booster with injury if none for five years.
5. No live vaccines, even when otherwise indicated for travel.

Tuberculosis

1. Isoniazid (INH) prophylaxis for any patient with positive PPD. Dose is 300 milligrams a day for at least twelve months. Add vitamin B_6 to regimen. Discontinue if transaminase levels are three to five times normal values.
2. Consider other regimens if in an area where multidrug-resistant tuberculosis is present.
3. Prophylaxis also recommended for PPD-anergic patients if at high risk (homeless, IV drug users, migrant farm workers). Some recommend prophylaxis for high-risk groups, regardless of PPD status.
4. Anergy panel required with PPD. HIV-positive patients can be anergic even with high CD4 counts.

CD4 Nadir 200 or Less
•

Pneumocystis Carinii Pneumonia (PCP)

1. Initiate PCP prophylaxis with trimethoprim-sulfamethoxazole, one double-strength tablet per day. Also provides protection against toxoplasmosis.
2. If not tolerated, attempt desensitization protocol. If drug reaction is severe or does not resolve with desensitization to at least the equivalent of one double-strength tablet three times a week, attempt dapsone, 100 milligrams per day. Assess first for G6PD deficiency.
3. Atovaquone 750 milligrams twice a day if above not tolerated.
4. Aerosolized pentamidine a poor choice, as remainder of body, other than lungs, not protected. Prophylaxis failures with aerosolized pentamidine reported at 11 percent, and at 18.5 percent for those with prior PCP episode. If used, dose is 300 milligrams per month.
5. Some use intravenous pentamidine, at 300 milligrams per month, as a fallback strategy.

Prophylaxis may be initiated earlier if there is a previous PCP infection, chronic thrush, or unexplained fever greater than 100 degrees for more than two weeks. Some begin PCP prophylaxis at CD4 count of 250, as it has been reported that 18 percent of cases of PCP occur in those with CD4 counts above 200 within the previous six months.

CD4 Nadir 100 or Less
•

Mycobacterium Avium Complex (MAC)

Azithromycin, 1,200 milligrams once a week, or clarithromycyn, 500 milligrams a day; watch for drug interactions with protease inhibitors. Rifabutin not preferred with PIs. Some doctors start at CD4 nadirs of 75, some at 50. I start at 100.

Toxoplasmosis ("Toxo")

Trimethoprim-sulfamethoxazole for PCP prophylaxis is effective. If intolerant, and desensitization unsuccessful, dapsone 50 milligrams a day and pyrimethamine 50 milligrams a week are effective against toxo and PCP. Not frequent in the United States; incidence high in Europe.

Deep Fungal Infections

Prophylaxis following treatment for esophageal candidiasis is warranted. Some also prophylax against cryptococcus. Fluconazole, 200 milligrams a day, is recommended. Itraconazole and ketoconazole also used, but latter drug lowers testosterone levels. Resistant organisms reported with long-term use of fluconazole.

Cytomegalovirus (CMV)

Oral gancyclovir, 1,000 milligrams three times a day, appears to reduce chance of CMV.

APPENDIX VIII

•

HIV Intake Physical

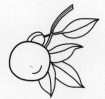

HIV Intake Physical

Date:

Patient Name:
Birthday: Age: Weight

T: P: BP: RR: **Meds**
UA: Antiretrovirals:
Current Problems: PMH   Date

                                       HIV (+)
                                       AIDS dx?
                                          by:
                                       Weight, baseline   Treatment:
                                       CD4 nadir
                                       Viral load max

Current C/O: **FH**

                                                                 Prophylaxis:
                                            SH

                                             | Cigs
                                             | Etoh
                                             | Other
                                             | Work
                                             | Sex   Symptoms:
                                             | Barrier protection
                                             | Support systems
                                             | IDU
                    HCM | Partner? (+/–)   Anabolics:
ROS   **HIV**   **Date**

Thrush   Pneumovax
Trouble   DT
  swallowing   Flu
PO   PPD and   **Other**
Vision   controls   Hep B status: Allergy
Libido   O & P
Erection   Nut. consult
Ejaculation   Toxo titers   Hep A status:
Diarrhea   CD4
Discharge   P24 antigen
Mood   B2 microglobulin
Memory   Pap   Nutritional   Alternative
Skin   Eye exam   Supplements   Treatments
HSV   GGPD
OHL   Erythropoetin
                    Chest X ray

Physical Exam

HEENT   Fundi [ ]   Thrush [ ]   Mental Status:

Neck   Extremities

Breasts   Neuro

Heart   Skin

Lungs   Genitals

Abdomen   Rectum

Back

ASSESS:

Staging: Treatment HIV:

[ ] Viral load   [ ] Antiretrovirals   Nutrition:

[ ] T-cell subsets   1)   [ ] BIA

                                2)   [ ] Exercise

Immunization: 3)   [ ] Vitamin supplements

[ ] Pneumovax   4)   [ ] Protein-calorie

[ ] Hepavax   5)   supplements

[ ] Fluvax   [ ] Immune-based therapies [ ] Appetite enhancers

[ ] DT   [ ] Acyclovir   [ ] Nutrition consult

                                [ ] Other

Evaluation: [ ] Anabolics

[ ] Chem panel, CBC   Prophylaxis:

[ ] B$_{12}$ [ ] PCP

[ ] Gonorrhea   [ ] MAC   [ ] Cytokine blockers

[ ] Toxo titers   [ ] CMV   [ ] Other

[ ] CMV titers   [ ] FUNGAL

[ ] Amylase   [ ] Other

[ ] Folate

[ ] Chlamydia   Social:

[ ] Erythropoetin level   Problems, new: Assessed Referred

[ ] GGTP   [ ] [ ] Barrier protection

[ ] Magnesium   [ ] [ ] Rx adherence

[ ] RPR   [ ] [ ] Support systems

[ ] G6PD   [ ] [ ] Volunteerism

[ ] Testosterone   [ ] [ ] Work satisfaction

    total   [ ] [ ] Shelter

    free   Treatment: [ ] [ ] Money and Rx costs

[ ] DHEA   [ ] [ ] Depression

[ ] Anal pap   [ ] [ ] Violence/abuse

[ ] Cervical pap   [ ] [ ] Recreational drug use

[ ] Chest X ray   [ ] [ ] Other

[ ] PPD/controls   Treatment,   Strong points

[ ] Eye exam   symptoms:

[ ] Other   Goals for change

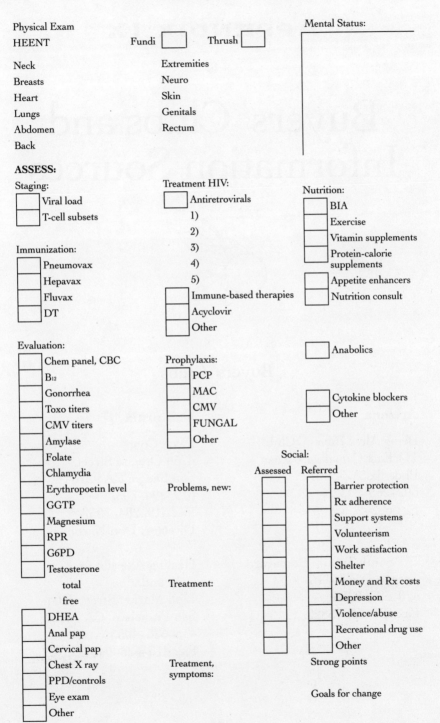

APPENDIX IX

•

Buyers' Clubs and Information Sources

Buyers' Clubs

Arizona

Being Alive Buyers' Club
111 East Camelback Road
Phoenix, AZ 85012
602–265–2437
Fax 602–265–9951

SAFE
151 South Tucson Boulevard
Tucson, AZ 85716
520–322–6226
Fax 520–622–5822

California

PWA Coop
4234 Oregon Street
San Diego, CA 92104
619–294–7057
Fax 619–294–7057
Director: Don Narbone

Healing Alternatives
    Foundation
1748 Market Street #204
San Francisco, CA 94102
415–626–4053
Fax 415–626–0451

CFIDS Buyers' Club
1187 Coast Village Road
 #1–280
Santa Barbara, CA 93108
800–366–6056
Founder: Rich Carson

National AIDS Nutrient
 Bank
P.O. Box 2187
Guerneville, CA 95446
707–869–1996
Fax 707–869–2562
Director: Michael Onstott

District of Columbia

Carl Vogel Foundation
1010 Vermont Avenue, NW,
 Suite 510
Washington, DC 20005–3405
202–638–0750
Fax 202–638–0749
Director: Ron Mealy

Florida

Wholesale Health
909 NE 18th Street
Fort Lauderdale, FL 33305
888–666–6743
954–764–1587
Fax 954–764–2393
Director: Mel Smith

Health Link
3213 North Ocean
 Boulevard, #6
Fort Lauderdale, FL 33308

800–456–4792
Fax 305–565–8289
Director: Marie Wansiki

AIDS Manasota
2080 Ringling Boulevard, #302
Sarasota, FL 34237
941–954–6011
Fax 941–951–1721
Director: Donna Fruiza

Georgia

AIDS Treatment Initiative
828 West Peachtree Street,
 Suite 210
Atlanta, GA 30308
404–874–4845
Fax 404–874–9320
Director: Jamey Rousey

Massachusetts

Boston Buyers' Club
29 Stanhope Street
Boston, MA 02116
800–435–5586
617–266–2233
Fax 617–450–9412
Director: Paul Schur

New York

PWA Health Group
150 West 26th Street #201
New York, NY 10001
212–255–0520
Fax 212–255–2080
http://www.aidsnyc.org/PWAHG
Director: Sally Cooper

DAAIR
31 East 30th Street, #2A
New York, NY 10016
212–725–6994
888–951–5433
Fax 212–689–6471
Director: Fred Bingham

Texas

Buyers' Club (Prince Street
    Market)
P.O. Box 131594
Houston, TX 77219
800–350–2392
713–520–5288
Director: Fred Walters

Newsletters and Information Sources
*Particularly recommended. See Figure 19.1 for Internet availability.

AIDS Action Baltimore
2105 North Charles Street
Baltimore, MD 21218
410–837–AIDS

**AIDS Treatment Data
Network***
259 West 30th Street
New York, NY 10011
212–260–8868

AIDS Treatment News*
P.O. Box 411256
San Francisco, CA 94141
415–255–0588

**AMFAR Experimental
Treatment Directory**
733 3rd Avenue,
    12th Floor
New York, NY 10017
212–682–7440

**BETA (Bulletin of
Experimental Treatments
for AIDS)***
San Francisco AIDS
    Foundation
P.O. Box 6182
San Francisco, CA 94101
415–863–AIDS

The Body Positive
2095 Broadway, Suite 306
New York, NY 10023
212–721–1346

GMHC's Treatment Issues
Department of Medical
    Information
129 West 20th Street
New York, NY 10011
212–807–6655

HEAL Quarterly
P.O. Box 1103
Old Chelsea Station
New York, NY 10113
212–873–0780

HIV AIDS Treatment Information Service
800–448–0440

HIV Alive
HIV Community Coalition
1255 23rd Street NW,
Room #4103
Washington, DC 20037
202–884–8857

League Against AIDS
2699 Biscayne
Boulevard, #4
Miami, FL 33137
305–576–6420

Linea de Información del SIDA
800–322–SIDA

National Information & Crisis Hotline
American Social Health
Association
P.O. Box 13827
Research Triangle Park,
NC 27709
800–342–AIDS

National Institutes of Health
Government clinical trials
information
800-TRIALS-A

PI Perspective and Facts Sheets*
Project Inform
347 Delores Street,
Suite 301
San Francisco, CA 94110
800–822–7422

Positively Aware
1258 West Belmont
Avenue
Chicago, IL 60657
312–472–6397

POZ Magazine
800–883–2163

PWA Advocacy Hotline
800–558–AIDS

PWA Coalition Hotline
50 West 17th Street
New York, NY 10011
212–532–0568
800–828–3280

PWAC Newsline
PWA Coalition
31 West 26th Street
New York, NY 10010
800–828–3280

Treatment Update
517 College Street,
Suite 324
Toronto, Ontario M6G 1A8
Canada
416–944–1916

Vancouver PWA Society Newsletter
1107 Seymour Street
Vancouver, BC V6B 5S8
Canada
604–681–2122

APPENDIX X

•

Partial List
of Feeding Programs

Atlanta

Project Open Hand
176 Ottley Drive
Atlanta, GA 30307
404–577–7341

Baltimore

Moveable Feast
3401 Old York Road
Baltimore, MD 21218
410–243–4604

Boston

Community Servings
125 Magazine Street
Roxbury, MA 02119
617–445–7777

Chicago

Open Hand Chicago
909 West Belmont Avenue,
   Suite 100
Chicago, IL 60657
773–665–1000

HIV Coalition (HIVCO)
Hand-to-Hand Food Program
1471 Business Center Drive,
   Suite 500
Mt. Prospect, IL 60056
847–391–9803

Denver

Project Angel Heart
Denver Center for Living
415 East 9th Avenue
Denver, CO 80218
303–830–0202

Eugene

HIV Alliance
1966 Garden Avenue
Eugene, OR 97403
541–342–5088

Los Angeles

Project Angel Food
7574 Sunset Boulevard
Los Angeles, CA 90046
213–845–1800

Miami

Food for Life Network
111 SW Third Street
Miami, FL 33130
305–375–0400

Minneapolis

Open Arms of Minnesota
5005 Bryant Avenue South
Minneapolis, MN
   55419–1211
612–331–3640

New Haven

Caring Cuisine AIDS Project
   New Haven
P.O. Box 636
New Haven, CT 06503
203–624 0947

New Orleans

Food for Friends
2533 Columbus Street
New Orleans, LA 70119
504–944–6028

New York City

God's Love We Deliver
166 Avenue of the Americas
New York, NY 10013
212–294–8100

Philadelphia

Metropolitan AIDS Neigh-
   borhood Nutrition Al-
   liance (MANNA)
P.O. Box 30181
Philadelphia, PA 19103
215–496–2662

Portland

Daily Bread Express
HIV Day Center
Ecumenical Ministries of
   Oregon
3835 SW Kelly Avenue
Portland, OR 97201
503–223–3444

St. Louis

Food Outreach, Inc.
4579 Laclede Avenue
Suite 309
St. Louis, MO 63108
314–367–4461

San Diego

Mama's Kitchen
1875 2nd Avenue
San Diego, CA 92101
619–233–6262

San Francisco

Project Open Hand
2720 17th Street
San Francisco, CA 94110
415–558–0600

Seattle

Chicken Soup Brigade
1002 East Seneca
Seattle, WA 98122
206–328–8979

Washington, DC

Food and Friends
58 L Street SE
Washington, DC 20003
202–488–8278

APPENDIX XI

•

Water Safety

Studies reported by the Environmental Protection Agency show that 65–97 percent of untreated water supplies throughout the country had cryptosporidium oocysts present. You have essentially three options for obtaining water that is likely to be free of cryptosporidium:

1. *Boiling water* for one minute at sea level or three minutes at altitudes over 6500 feet will eliminate the risk of cryptosporidium infection.

2. *Water filtration systems* are available that can remove oocysts. There are very specific and stringent standards that these filters must meet, and the Center for Disease Control (CDC) divides them into three types. The first is the microstraining filter, which removes particles 0.1–1 micron in size and must be labeled "absolute" 1 micron. The second type of unit is the reverse osmosis unit, which passes water through a tightly stretched membrane. Finally there are units that are NSF certified for "cyst reduction." While there are many such units available on

TABLE XI.1
•
Partial List of Approved Manufacturers.

Manufacturer	Price	Information
PUR	$50–80	Available at many major retailers and in faucet or countertop models. 1-800-PUR-LINE for more info.
Teledyne Instapure F5	$35	New, inexpensive faucet model with inexpensive replacement filters. Available at major retailers. Do not confuse with other Instapure products that are not safe for you. 1-800-525-2774.
Amway Corporation	$150–250	Both compact and countertop units available through local Amway distributors.
Multi-pure Drinking Water Systems	$170–250	*Consumer Digest* Best Buy. Several models available through local distributors.

the market, Robert Lehmann, author of *Cooking for Life,* recommends the PUR filter system (1–800–PUR-LINE) as the least expensive and a very good product. This is an on-the-tap filter system which meets the NSF standards and is available at many local retailers (K-mart, Target, etc.). A partial list of approved manufacturers is shown in Table XI.1. For a complete list of approved manufacturers or to check on a specific product, call the National Sanitation Foundation at 800–673–8010. Also please remember that the important question to ask when buying a water filter is whether it is "NSF certified for cyst reduction" and be sure to change the filter as required by the manufacturer.

3. *Bottled water* can be a safe alternative. However, it is very important to note that just because water is bottled does not mean that it is safe for you. Some brands of bottled water contain simply the unprocessed municipal water supply! Unfiltered spring waters like Evian and Volvic, which are bottled from deep source aquifer (nonsurface

water reserves) are unlikely to be contaminated with cryptosporidium, but do not meet the Center for Disease Control's standards for safety.

The following is a partial list of bottled waters processed to ensure safety from cryptosporidium: Deer Park, Great Bear, Naya, Poland Springs, Saratoga, Calistoga, Crystal Geyser, Vivanti, and Wissahickon.

To be considered free from cryptosporidium contamination, bottled waters should have been treated by one of the processes described above. If in doubt about whether your usual choice is safe for you, the best option is to speak to the manufacturer—they are usually friendly and helpful, but be sure that you get a very specific answer as to what processes they use, rather than general assurances about the quality of the water!

REFERENCES

Cenko, D. "Avoiding cryptosporidium: Safe food, safe water, safe sex." *BETA*, March 1996, 33–36.

GMHC Nutrition Counseling Department. "Cryptosporidia and the water supply." *Treatment Issues*, 1994, *8*(9), 15.

Lehmann, R. *Cooking for Life*. New York: Dell Publishing, 1997.

National Sanitation Foundation. *Drinking Water Treatment Units Certified by NSF International*, 1996.

•

Antiretrovirogram
Reverse Transcriptase Inhibitors

Nucleoside Analogues

AZT _____   D4T _____

3TC _____   DDI _____

DDC _____   Other _____

Non-Nucleoside Analogues

Nevirapine _____

Delaverdine _____

Efavirenz _____

Other _____

Drugs of Other Classes

Protease Inhibitors

Indinavir _____   Nelfinavir _____

Ritonavir _____   Saquinavir _____

Other _____   Other _____

All Other Antiretrovirals

Hydroxyurea _____

Other _____

Other _____

Legend:

Prior use, contraindicated due to severe adverse event: CROSS OUT.

Prior use, avoid if possible due to undesirable effects: BRACKET.

Prior use, progression: "⟶ PROGRESSION."

Prior use, reason for change not clear: "⟶ CHANGED."

Not used, contraindicated for this patient: BRACKET CONTRAINDICATION.

Not used, no contraindication: LEAVE BLANK.

GLOSSARY

●

Absolute neutrophil count. A measure of immune competence; neutrophil percent plus band percent, multiplied by total white cell count. Should be 1000 or more for safety.

Acyclovir. A medicine used to treat or suppress herpes infections. Sold under the trade name Zovirax.

AIDS. Acquired immunodeficiency syndrome. Preceded by HIV infection.

Albumin. A protein found and measured in the blood. Used to transport substances through the body. Levels used as indicator of nutritional status.

Allergy. A part of the immune response that causes our bodies to react to substances with inflammation, itching, rash, or other symptoms. Because of excessive activation of some parts of the immune system in people with HIV, allergic responses are more common.

Alpha interferon. A factor or cytokine used in the treatment of chronic active hepatitis B.

Anabolic hormones/anabolic steroids. Substances that favor anabolism, or the building or repletion of lean body mass or bone.

Anabolism. The process of building up or adding to lean body mass or bone.

Androderm. The brand name for a patch that delivers testosterone through the skin.

Androgenic. Causing the development of male sex characteristics, such as increased body hair or deeper voice. Androgenic substances tend also to be anabolic.

Anemia. A reduced amount of red blood cells in the blood.

Anorexia. Loss of appetite.

Anthropometry. A technique for estimating lean body mass by measurement of parts of the body.

Antibiotics. Medicines used to kill or suppress infecting organisms.

Antibodies. Substances made by the B-cell branch of the immune system to attack cells, organisms, or substances recognized as foreign.

Antidepressants. Medicines that address the chemical component of depression.

Antioxidants. Substances that alter molecules in the body in a way that reduces oxidative stress.

Antiretroviral. A drug used against retroviruses, such as HIV.

Antiretrovirogram. A review of antiretroviral drugs and your use of them. See Appendix XII.

Arachidonic acid. A fatty-acid component of cell membranes. The building block of many cytokines.

Atrophy. Ceasing to grow, or becoming smaller because growth is not supported.

Azithromycin (Zithromax). Antibiotic used for MAC prophylaxis.

AZT. Prior name for zidovudine, or ZDV, an antiretroviral drug used against the HIV virus. Trade name is Retrovir.

B cells. Cells of the immune system that are involved chiefly in the manufacture of antibodies.

Bacteria. A type of infecting organism.

Bactrim. Trade name for trimethoprim-sulfamethoxazole, a drug used against pneumocystis and other organisms. Another trade name is Septra.

Band. An immature neutrophil type of immune cell.

Beta-carotene. A natural source of Vitamin A, found in orange and yellow vegetables.

Bioavailability. How much of a drug you take into your body gets in to do its job.

Body cell mass. Similar though not identical to lean body mass. Includes intracellular contents, without including bone or fat.

Bone densitometry. A radiological study that assesses bone density.

Branched-chain DNA (bDNA) assay. A test for measuring HIV viral load.

CD4 cell. The T-helper cell, a part of the immune system that is attacked in HIV disease.

CD4 memory cells. Cells that already recognize a specific invader and no other, and whose offspring will do the same.

CD4 nadir. The lowest CD4 count, or T4 or T-helper cell count, you have ever had.

CD4 naive cells. Cells that are not yet specific for a given invader. They live longer, and can help to recognize and fight new infections by different organisms.

CD8 cell. The T-suppressor cell, a part of the immune system that is activated against HIV.

Candida. A type of fungal, or yeast, organism.

Candidiasis. Fungal infection.

Carpal Tunnel Syndrome. A tightening of the pathway through which nerves travel to the hand; can result in pain, abnormal sensation, or weakness. May be associated with the use of growth hormone.

Cellular immunity. The part of our immune response that is carried out by T cells.

Cervix. The lowest part of the uterus, or womb.

Chlamydia. A sexually transmitted disease.

Cidofavir (Vistide). An anti-CMV drug that may also have activity against PML.

Clarithromycin (Biaxin). Antibiotic used for MAC prophylaxis. Contraindicated with ritonavir; dose adjustment required with other protease inhibitors.

Condyloma accuminatum. Venereal warts, the result of sexual transmission of the human papilloma virus (HPV). May predispose to cancer at the site of infection.

Convergent therapy. A group of interventions aimed at fighting the same problem by different pathways. Used to describe antiretroviral combinations or comprehensive nutritional therapy.

Cortisol. A hormone made by the body. Levels rise in response to stress. May be implicated in loss of bone mineral density.

Cryptococcus. A fungal organism that can cause meningitis and sometimes other illness.

Cryptosporidium. An organism that can cause diarrhea.

Cytokines. Factors made by the immune system that have multiple effects on immune response and wasting.

Cytomegalovirus. An organism that can infect the retina. Can also cause diarrhea and other illness.

Dehydroepiandrosterone (DHEA). A hormone from which testosterone and estrogen are made. Deficiency may be implicated in depression or in wasting.

Diabetes mellitus. Elevated blood sugar as a result of insulin deficiency or insensitivity.

Didanosine (DDI). An antiretroviral drug. Trade name is Videx.

Dilantin. Trade name for phenytoin, a drug used to treat or protect against seizures.

DNA. The portion of the cell that carries all reproductive information. Necessary for replication.

Dual energy X ray absorptiometry (DEXA). A way to measure lean body mass.

D-xylose test. A test for malabsorption.

Dysplasia. An abnormal pattern of cell growth, which can precede transition to cancer.

Efavirenz (Sustiva, DMP 266). A NNRTI antiretroviral dosed once a day.

Electrolyte. One of many elements found throughout the body that help regulate essential reactions.

ELISA. Enzyme-linked immunosorbent assay. A screening test used to detect HIV. Sensitive, but not highly specific.

Esophagus. The tube that connects the mouth and stomach.

False negative. A test result that does not detect the presence of a substance when the substance is in fact present. More common if testing method used is specific but not sensitive.

False positive. A test result that suggests the presence of a substance when the substance is not in fact present. More common if testing method used is sensitive but not specific.

Fentanyl (Duragesic). A narcotic in patch form that can be absorbed through the skin; used to provide steady pain control.

Flushing. Increased blood flow to the face or upper body, resulting in increased skin color and a sensation of warmth.

Folate. A form of folic acid, necessary for many reactions in the body.

Foscarnet. A medicine used to treat CMV. Trade name is Foscavir.

Free radicals. Breakdown products of reactions in the body. Can do damage to surrounding cells. Neutralized by antioxidants.

Gancyclovir (DHPG). A medicine used to treat CMV. Trade name is Cytovene.

Gastritis. Inflammation or irritation of the stomach lining.

Glucose intolerance. A reduced ability of cells to take up sugar from the blood. May proceed to diabetes mellitus.

Glutathione. Part of the body's system of antioxidant protection.

Gonorrhea. A sexually transmitted disease.

Growth hormone. A genetically engineered version of human growth hormone. Administration leads to anabolism—increase and retention of lean body mass—in people who have wasted. Sold under the trade name Serostim.

Hepatitis. Inflammation of the liver. Infectious causes can be the hepatitis A, B, or C virus. Infection with either B or C may progress to a chronic state. A vaccine is available for hepatitis B. Hepatitis may result from other causes.

Herpes simplex. A viral infection that can result in cold sores, a painful or itching rash, or ulcers.

Herpes zoster. A reactivation of varicella, the chicken pox virus. Results in painful blisters in a defined area. Must be treated quickly to avoid lasting pain after resolution.

Highly Active Retroviral Therapy (HAART). Combination therapy with three or more antiretroviral agents, one of which is generally assumed to be a protease inhibitor.

Historical controls. A group of people or statistics chosen from the past and used as comparison for subjects under study.

HIV. Human immunodeficiency virus, the organism responsible for HIV disease and AIDS. Transmitted by contact with blood and body fluids from an infected person.

HIV-negative. Lacking the presence of antibodies to the HIV virus.

HIV-positive. Infected with the HIV virus, as evidenced by the presence of antibodies in the blood.

Homeostasis. The body's ability to maintain and regulate its own balanced environment, separate and distinct from the environment that surrounds it.

Host. An organism that is infected with another organism.

Human papilloma virus (HPV). The organism responsible for genital warts. Infection can cause cellular changes that predispose locally to cancer.

Humoral immunity. The part of our immune response that is regulated by antibodies made by B cells.

Immune system. A complex system with which the body protects itself against that which it recognizes as foreign.

Immunocompromised. No longer able to mount an adequate immune response against invading organisms or processes.

Immunosuppressed. Immunocompromised.

INH. Trade name for isoniazid, a drug used against tuberculosis.

Intravenous. Through the vein.

JC virus. The causative agent of PML.

KSHV. A herpes virus now known to predispose to Kaposi's sarcoma.

Lactase. An enzyme used to break down lactose. Often deficient in HIV-infected people.

Lactose. A sugar found in milk and milk products.

Lactose intolerance. A deficiency of lactase, resulting in abdominal discomfort after eating milk products.

Lamivudine. A new antiretroviral drug used against HIV, currently in trials.

Lean body mass. The part of our bodies that is neither water nor fat, and is inside the cells.

Leukotrienes. Part of the body's immune response.

Libido. Interest in or appetite for sex.

Long-term nonprogressors. People with HIV infection who have not gotten worse for many years despite no treatment. Many are now seen to be slow progressors, rather than nonprogressors.

Lumbar puncture. A spinal tap. The outer lining of the spinal canal is penetrated, and some of the fluid that is present to bathe the spinal cord is drawn off for examination.

Lymphocytes. Cells of the body's immune system. There are two basic types: B cells, which regulate antibody production, and T cells, which regulate cell-mediated immunity. These cells have multiple interactions.

Macrophages. Mature monocytes. They can release HIV virus when activated.

Malabsorption. An impaired ability to transport nutrients across the gut wall.

Marinol. Trade name for dronabinol, a drug used to counter wasting. Active ingredient is tetrahydrocannabinol (THC), the active compound in marijuana.

Matched controls. People followed in a study without intervention, or without the condition under study in experimental subjects, so serve as a comparison point for changes in those under study.

MDMA. An illegal recreational drug with psychedelic properties. Protease inhibitors, especially ritonavir, restrict elimination of this drug with potentially lethal consequences.

Megace. Trade name for megestrol acetate, a medicine used to slow or stop wasting.

Medium-chain triglycerides. A type of fat source that is easily absorbed.

Meningitis. Infection or inflammation of the lining of the brain.

Metabolic rate. The speed of metabolism.

Metabolism. The way in which the body uses nutrients to provide for the maintenance of its structure and function.

Methotrexate. A drug used chiefly in cancer chemotherapy.

Microsporidium. An organism that can cause refractory diarrhea.

Monoclonal antibodies. Antibodies made by genetic engineering, designed to target a specific infection.

Monocytes. Cells of the immune system that are infected by the HIV virus and used as factories for its production. When activated to become macrophages, they release new virus.

Monokines. Immune factors made and released by monocytes and macrophages.

Monotherapy. The outmoded practice of treating HIV with only one antiretroviral drug, thereby ensuring eventual resistance and progression.

Mycobacterium avium complex. Opportunistic organisms that are similar to the tuberculosis organism, but cause illness only in those who are immunosuppressed.

Myelopathy. Damage to the spinal cord.

Nandrolone Decanoate (Deca-Durabolin). A powerful anabolic hormone given intramuscularly to replete lean body mass. Also used to treat osteoporosis. It is highly androgenic.

Needle exchange programs. Programs that offer clean unused needles in exchange for used needles to injection drug users without charge. Goal is to halt the spread of HIV through dirty needles.

Nelfinavir (Viracept). A protease inhibitor.

Neoplasia. An abnormal pattern of cell growth signaling the transition to cancer.

Neopterin. A substance made by macrophages. Levels measured are used as an indirect marker of HIV activity.

Neuropathy. Damage to nerves.

Neurosyphilis. Infection of the nervous system with syphilis.

Neurotransmitters. Chemical compounds released by brain cells to communicate with other brain cells.

Nevirapine. A drug used in combination antiretroviral therapy for HIV. Not yet approved.

Nonoxynol-9. A spermicide developed for birth control that has some activity against the HIV virus.

Nonsteroidal anti-inflammatory drugs (NSAIDs). A group of drugs used to reduce fever, pain, and inflammation.

Nutrition. The process by which the body provides materials for its structural and functional needs.

Nutritional competence. The body's nutritional status; its ability to nourish itself and maintain its structure and function.

Omega-3 fatty acids. A form of fat found in fish oils.

Oocyst. The egg of a parasite, such as cryptosporidium or giardia.

1592. A new nucleoside analog said to have the power of a protease inhibitor.

Opportunistic infection. An infection that is normally obliterated or suppressed by an intact immune system, but that becomes a threat when the body can no longer defend against it because of immunosuppression.

Osteopenia. Reduced bone mineral density (thin bones).

Osteoporosis. Severely reduced bone mineral density, which can predispose to fractures.

Oxandrolone (Oxandrin). A powerful oral synthetic anabolic hormone with minimal androgenic properties.

P24 antigen. A part of the HIV virus that can be found and measured in the blood early in infection, before the development of HIV antibodies, and again at more advanced stages.

Pancreatitis. Inflammation of the pancreas, an organ that makes enzymes, to aid in digestion, and insulin, which permits cells to take up glucose, the basic source of energy for the body.

Pap smear. Short for Papanicolaou smear, a scraping of surface cells of the cervix or rectum to permit microscopic examination for changes that might progress to cancer.

Pathogens. Organisms that cause illness.

PCR RNA. A new test for viral load.

Pelvic inflammatory disease (PID). An infection that ascends from the cervix to the fallopian tubes and/or ovaries of the female reproductive system.

Pentamidine. A medicine used to treat pneumocystis carinii pneumonia.

Pentoxifylline. A cytokine blocker under study in wasting. Available by prescription. Sold under the trade name Trental.

Peripheral neuropathy. Damage to peripheral nerves.

Placebo. An inert substance given to some subjects in a placebo-controlled trial to provide a basis for comparison in testing the efficacy, safety, and side-effect profile of an active drug.

Placebo effect. The phenomenon of improving in response to a treatment or medication, independent of its physiologic value.

Prealbumin. A protein found in the blood. Used as a measure of current nutritional status.

Progressive multifocal leukoencephalopathy (PML). A disease caused by JC virus. Attacks white matter of brain.

Progressive resistance exercise. Weight lifting or similar exercise designed to build lean body mass.

Prophylax. To practice prophylaxis.

Prophylaxis. Treatment in the absence of a given infection, at a time when its presence becomes likely, in order to avoid or suppress clinical illness.

Prostaglandins. Substances made by the body that affect immune response and the function of many organ systems.

Prostate specific antigen (PSA). A test for amount of prostate growth. Used as a screening test for prostate cancer.

Psychoneuroimmunology. The study of the mechanisms by which what we feel influences our immune status and hence our health, and of the effects of this influence.

Pyrimethamine. A drug used against toxoplasmosis.

RDA (recommended dietary allowance). The minimum amount of a nutrient recommended per day for prevention of malnutrition in a healthy, unstressed person.

Replication. Reproduction, making copies of oneself.

Retinitis. Infection or inflammation of a part of the eye called the retina.

Retrovirus. A virus that, unlike most organisms, replicates itself starting with RNA. It inserts its RNA into the host's, and thus causes the host to reproduce it.

RNA. Part of the process of replication. In most organisms, RNA is made by associating with DNA, which carries the genetic information. Retroviruses start with RNA.

Saquinavir. A new antiretroviral drug currently being tested for its effectiveness against HIV.

Sensitive. Able to detect the presence of a substance. A test that is sensitive may not also be specific. Some positive test results, if a test is sensitive but not specific, may not be correct. The possibility of a false-positive result cannot be excluded.

Serotonin. A neurotransmitter that is reduced in depression. Medicines are available to enable us to use what serotonin remains more efficiently.

Sinusitis. Inflammation or infection of the sinuses. Requires early and aggressive treatment in HIV infection.

Somatostatin-A. A genetically engineered version of one of our body's own hormones. Helps to slow gut movement. Used to help treat refractory diarrhea. Sold under the trade name Sandostatin.

Specific. Able to exclude the presence of a substance. A test that is specific may not also be sensitive. In such a case some negative results may be false negatives.

Stavudine (D4T). An antiretroviral used against the HIV virus. Sold under the trade name Zerit.

Sublingual. Under the tongue.

Sudan blue stain. A test for the amount of fat in the stool. A high fat content suggests poor absorption.

Support group. A group of people with similar issues and concerns who meet together regularly to share their feelings, experiences, and strengths with one another.

Syphilis. A sexually transmitted disease. Left untreated, it can infect the brain and produce permanent damage.

T4 cell. The T-helper cell, a part of the immune system attacked by the HIV virus. Now called the CD4 cell.

T-cell subsets. A series of tests that measure the amounts of different types of T cells in the blood.

Testoderm. The brand name for a patch that delivers testosterone through the skin.

Testosterone. A male sex hormone.

Thalidomide. A powerful cytokine blocker currently under study.

TMP-SMX (trimethoprim-sulfamethoxazole). A drug used, in particular, against pneumocystis carinii pneumonia (PCP). Sold under the trade names Bactrim and Septra. Also protects against toxoplasmosis.

Theraband. A broad elastic band of varying strengths used for do-it-yourself progressive resistance exercise. Sold by the foot at some physical therapy offices.

TPN. Total parenteral nutrition, food delivered directly through a large vein in elemental form. Used when the gut cannot absorb nutrients, to halt or ameliorate wasting.

Trace elements. Substances needed in minute quantities for body functions. Must be obtained from the diet.

Triglyceride. A form of fat carried in the blood.

Trimethoprim-sulfamethoxazole (TMP-SMX). Bactrim or Septra. Increased in states of active infection.

Toxoplasmosis. A disease caused by an organism that can infect the brain of an immunocompromised host. Can be acquired through eating raw meat or changing litter boxes.

Urethra. The opening at the tip of the penis through which men urinate or ejaculate.

Viral burden. Viral load.

Viral load. The amount of virus present.

Viral load maximum. The highest viral load you have ever had.

Virucidal. Capable of killing virus.

Virus. An infecting organism that must take over the reproductive apparatus of the cells in the organism it infects, in order to reproduce itself.

Virustatic. Capable of suppressing, but not eliminating, viral infection.

Vitamins. Substances normally not made in the body that are essential for bodily reactions. Must be obtained from the diet, except for vitamin D, which the body can make if exposed to sunlight.

Western blot. A confirmatory test for the presence of antibodies to the HIV virus. More specific than the ELISA test. Used to confirm positive ELISA results.

Xerostomia. Dry mouth. Usually due to medications, but sometimes a result of reduced production due to changes in salivary glands induced by illness.

Zalcitabine (DDC). An antiretroviral drug used against the HIV virus. Trade name is Hivid.

Zidovudine (ZDV or AZT). An antiretroviral drug used against the HIV virus. Sold under the trade name Retrovir.

INDEX

●

THE AUTHOR

●

Mary Romeyn, M.D., is an internist on staff at Saint Francis Memorial Hospital in San Francisco with a private practice specializing in HIV and patient advocacy. She is Medical Director of the Andrew Ziegler Foundation and a member of the Scientific Advisory Committee of the San Francisco AIDS Foundation and HIV Care, Incorporated.